NURSING
EDUCATION
in the Clinical Setting

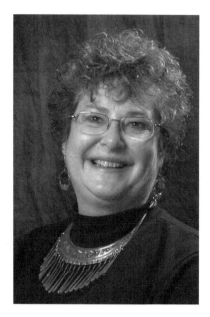

ABOUT THE AUTHOR

Roberta J. Emerson, RN, PhD

Roberta Emerson received her Bachelor of Science in Nursing (1969) and her Master of Science in Nursing (1971) from the University of Washington. In 1988, she received her PhD in Educational Leadership from Gonzaga University in Spokane, Washington. Her dissertation explored the design and testing of an instrument to quantifiably measure creativity in the application of the nursing process. She began her teaching career at Shoreline Community College in Seattle in 1971 and since that time has taught in associate, baccalaureate, and master's degree programs in Oklahoma, Louisiana, and Washington. She is currently an Associate Professor at the Intercollegiate College of Nursing/Washington State University College of Nursing in Spokane, Washington, where she has taught since 1981. She was awarded the College of Nursing's first Excellence in Teaching Award, and the next year was one of five faculty recognized for their quality teaching by Washington State University. Her primary teaching foci are medical-surgical nursing, and pathophysiology and pharmacology taught at both the undergraduate and graduate levels. Until recently she maintained a clinical practice in critical care, and is now a CCRN Alumnus.

NURSING EDUCATION

in the Clinical Setting

Roberta J. Emerson, RN, PhD

CCRN Alumnus
Associate Professor
Intercollegiate College of Nursing
Washington State University
Spokane, Washington

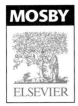

MOSBY

ELSEVIER

MOSBY
ELSEVIER

11830 Westline Industrial Drive
St. Louis, Missouri 63146

NURSING EDUCATION IN THE CLINICAL SETTING   ISBN-13: 978-0-323-03608-5
Copyright © 2007 by Mosby, Inc. an affiliate of Elsevier Inc.   ISBN-10: 0-323-03608-2

NOTICE

Nursing is an ever-changing field. Standard safety precautions must be followed, but as new research and clinical experience broaden our knowledge, changes in treatment and drug therapy may become necessary or appropriate. Readers are advised to check the most current product information provided by the manufacturer of each drug to be administered to verify the recommended dose, the method and duration of administration, and contraindications. It is the responsibility of the licensed prescriber, relying on experience and knowledge of the patient, to determine dosages and the best treatment for each individual patient. Neither the publisher nor the editor assumes any liability for any injury and/or damage to persons or property arising from this publication.

The Publisher

ISBN-13: 978-0-323-03608-5
ISBN-10: 0-323-03608-2

Acquisitions Editor: Kristin Geen
Project Manager: Tracey Schriefer
Designer: Teresa McBryan

Printed in the United States of America

Last digit is the print number: 9   8   7   6   5   4   3   2   1

To my students,
who have taught me so much.

Reviewers

Mike Aldridge, MSN, RN, CCRN, CNS
Instructor in Clinical Nursing
School of Nursing
University of Texas, Austin
Austin, Texas

Lynn Allchin, RN, PhD
Assistant Professor
School of Nursing
University of Connecticut
Storrs, Connecticut

Laura Bonanno, RN, BSN, CRNA, MS
Faculty, Nurse Anesthesia Program
School of Nursing
Louisiana State University
Baton Rouge, Louisiana

Julia Campbell, RN, MSN
Assistant Clinical Professor
College of Nursing
University of Missouri, St. Louis
St. Louis, Missouri

Eleanor Chester, MSN, MS, APRN, BC
Assistant Professor
College of Education, Nursing, and
Health Professions
University of Hartford
Hartford, Connecticut

**Catherine Clarey-Sanford, MSN, RN,
  LWOCN**
Assistant Professor
College of Nursing
Hope College
Holland, Michigan

Bronwynne C. Evans, PhD, RN, CNS
Associate Professor
Arizona State University College
of Nursing and Healthcare Leadership
Tempe, Arizona

Sally Fletcher, MSN, APRN, BC
Assistant Professor of Clinical Nursing
School of Nursing
University of Rochester
Rochester, New York

Anne Herzog, RN, MSN
Professor of Nursing
Cypress College
Cypress, California

Karen Karlowicz, EdD, RN
Assistant Professor of Nursing
School of Nursing
Old Dominion University
Norfolk, Virginia

**Joanne Laframboise-Otto, BSN,
  MSN, RN**
Assistant Professor
Nursing Program
Santa Fe Community College
Gainesville, Florida

**Natasha Leskovsek, RN, BSN, MBA,
  MPM, JD**
Nurse Attorney
Heller, Ehrman, White, & McAuliffe LLP
Washington, DC

Sofia Llahana, BSc Nursing, PGDip, MSc, DNSc, RGN, CNS
Clinical Nurse Specialist in Endocrinology
University College London Hospitals NHS Foundation Trust
London, England

Melanie Matthews, RN, MSN
Associate Professor
School of Nursing
Union University
Jackson, Tennessee

Cynthia Mitchell, MSN
Clinical Associate Professor
College of Nursing
University of Missouri, St. Louis
St. Louis, Missouri

Diana Openbrier, PhD, ARNP-BC
ARNP
Stephen's Family Practice
Jacksonville, Florida

Leona Pie, MPH, BSN, RN, BC
Associate Professor
Nursing Program
Capital Community College
Hartford, Connecticut

Kathleen Poindexter, RN, MSN, PhD
Associate Professor
College of Nursing
Michigan State University
Lansing, Michigan

Kathie Records, PhD, RN
Associate Professor
Washington State University
Intercollegiate College of Nursing
Spokane, Washington

Sarah Tvedt, RN, MS
Nursing Education Specialist
Mayo Clinic
Rochester, Minnesota

Helen Zsohar, PhD, RN
Associate Professor
College of Nursing
University of Utah
Salt Lake City, Utah

About this Book

The opportunity to be part of the experiential learning of nursing students is an opportunity to touch the future of the nursing profession unlike any other experience. You will find that working with students in the clinical setting and sharing a passion for the profession of nursing within this intimate relationship is profoundly rewarding. Over the years of teaching students in these environments, faculty impart more than knowledge and skills; they convey their own personal approaches to thinking about and practicing nursing. They pass these approaches on so tangibly that graduates have reported "hearing my instructor's voice" years after completing their education.

This book provides a practical approach to clinical nursing instruction for novice faculty in associate degree and baccalaureate programs, for graduate students interested in nursing education, and for more experienced faculty who are searching for new knowledge and approaches that will enhance their teaching. Practicable suggestions grounded in relevant educational theory are provided, and common questions and issues that arise when teaching nursing students in clinical settings are addressed. Incorporated within the text are illustrative scenarios, discussion questions, and exercises designed to facilitate thoughtful application of the content.

It is equally important to understand what is *not* addressed in this book. The focus of this text is the instruction of nursing students in clinical settings; a thorough discussion of all aspects of the faculty role is beyond its scope. For an in-depth exploration of the other facets of the academic role for nursing faculty, including classroom instruction, Billings and Halstead's *Teaching in Nursing: A Guide for Faculty* (2nd ed.) (2005) is highly recommended.

It was observed by Plato nearly 2500 years ago that the unexamined life is not worth living. The skill of critical reflection is widely used in nursing today, in clinical practice, education, and personal professional development. One of our central activities as educators is helping students become practitioners who regularly reflect on their care of patients to improve the quality of that care (Westburg & Hilliard, 2001). Successful development of reflective skills in our students is highly dependent on faculty role modeling. Reflection requires a keen awareness of experiences and being enthusiastic about learning from them (Westburg & Hilliard, 2001). Used by faculty to enhance their own growth, reflection facilitates learning from the act of teaching. As we help others learn from their experiences, so too do we learn. As we endeavor to prepare nurses who are not only competent but also thoughtful about their practice, we likewise need to develop a thoughtful awareness and openness to learning from our own experiences by attending to the thoughts and feelings associated with them. Reflection has the potential to revitalize teaching for even the most experienced faculty (Shellenbarger, Palmer, Labant, & Kuzneski, 2005). The heart of the technique is the identification and critical examination of the assumptions that undergird our actions by studying them from a variety of perspectives (Brookfield, 1995). Taking the time to periodically critically reflect while reading this book will significantly enhance both the quality and the quantity of learning. This is a good time to start a personal learning and teaching journal, using the activities suggested here and recording clinical experiences that leave behind heightened emotions. Journaling is an active learning approach for augmenting the reflective process (Blake, 2005). Jot down your thoughts related to the reflective exercises presented in this text. And for the clinical teaching stories, record the event and specifically what was significant about it. What are the thoughts and feelings experienced during and after it occurred? Critically reflective activities are embedded throughout this book. Additional exercises and questions for use with students are incorporated within the text and in the "Clinical Toolbox" (Chapter 20).

To further facilitate the transition to the role of academic clinical faculty, a "Clinical Toolbox" is provided at the conclusion of the text (Chapter 20). The Toolbox is filled with a variety of resources including sample approaches for teaching and evaluation, suggestions for preparing anecdotal notes, and references such as the *Student Nurses' Code of Conduct*.

When your students graduate and embark on their own professional practice journey, what will they hear when your voice comes to mind? What will they carry into their future practice that is a reflection of your teaching, your caring, your values and beliefs about nursing? Clinical nursing instruction is the door to the real world of nursing. What students experience as they step through it will impact the view they see and the future world they create. Clinical nursing faculty hold the key.

References

Billings, D.M., & Halstead, J.A. (Eds.) (2005). *Teaching in nursing: A guide for faculty* (2nd ed.). St. Louis, MO: Mosby.

Blake, T.K. (2005). Journaling: An active learning technique. *International Journal of Nursing Education Scholarship*, 2(1), Article 7. Retrieved August 15, 2005, from http://www.bepress.com/ijnes/vol2/iss1/art7

Brookfield, S.D. (1995). *Becoming a critically reflective teacher*. San Francisco, CA: John Wiley and Sons; Jossey-Bass.

Shellenbarger, T., Palmer, E.A., Labant, A.L., & Kuzneski, J.L. (2005). Use of faculty reflection to improve teaching. *Annual Review of Nursing Education*, 3:343-357.

Westburg, J., & Hilliard, J. (2001). *Fostering reflection and providing feedback: Helping others learn from experience*. New York, NY: Springer.

Contents

UNIT V   *Endings and Beginnings*

UNIT VI   *Clinical Educator Resources*

NURSING
EDUCATION
in the Clinical
Setting

UNIT I

Orienting New Faculty to the Teaching Role

Clinical Nursing Practitioner to Clinical Nursing Faculty: a Challenging Transition

- ▦ A CHALLENGING TRANSITION
- ▦ *REFLECTION EXERCISE 1: ASSUMPTIONS ABOUT ACADEMIA, TEACHING, AND LEARNING*
- ▦ APPOINTMENTS, ROLES AND EXPECTATIONS IN ACADEMIA
- ▦ ACADEMIC CLINICAL INSTRUCTION: SKILLS AND COMPETENCIES
- ▦ LEARNING CLINICAL TEACHING
- ▦ ADAPTATION ADVICE
  Learn About the System
  Establish a Support System
- ▦ *REFLECTION EXERCISE 2: EXAMINING THE POWER OF EXPERIENCE*
  Seek Balance in Self-Care
- ▦ SUMMARY

▦ A CHALLENGING TRANSITION

Welcome to academia: new geography, new culture, and new opportunities. Academia is very different terrain from the roles and functions of nursing practice. "Although experienced in clinical nursing, …[new faculty] are entering an unfamiliar culture with its own policies, procedures, practices, and role expectations—a culture they have only previously encountered as students" (Bellack, 2003, p. 383). Even for a recent graduate of a master's or doctoral program, having more current insights into the academic culture, the unknown far exceeds the known. Expectations and assumptions of academia at the outset, grounded primarily in personal experiences as a student, are often inaccurate. In fact, this frame of reference can be an impediment to the transition, distorting the view of this new landscape. The culture of academia has its own language, norms, and rules, both overt and covert. Assimilation there is as challenging as learning to fully function in a foreign country, and culture shock is a universal experience for novice faculty! This chapter provides suggestions designed to make the ride less bumpy, more satisfying and rewarding.

The transition from clinician to nurse educator has been called "a transformational journey" by one author in documenting her own experience (Neese, 2003). What this image communicates best is the evolutionary quality of the process. The learning of novice faculty, as for nursing students, is "…not an immutable structure consistent across time and situation…" (Neese, 2003, p. 261).

As is true in the development of clinical expertise, educational expertise is derived from experiential learning emanating from a knowledge base of theories and principles, as well as empirical evidence of the application of these theories to educational practice. Evidence-based teaching, nursing educational practices based upon the knowledge generated by nursing educational research, has been slow to evolve (Yonge et al., 2005). To be open to the new, it is necessary to describe preexisting assumptions, and then challenge them through critical reflection. Some "unlearning" needs to occur, both to create space for new learning and to avoid falling back into teaching as one was taught, an approach that may not incorporate the optimum. In an editorial for the *Journal of Continuing Education in Nursing*, Patricia Yoder-Wise (2002) suggested a new motto, appropriate to both education and practice: "Go unlearn something today! It will make more room for all that we have to learn" (p. 195). So, a good place to begin is to make an assumption list: what is assumed about academia, teaching, and learning in the clinical setting? Take a moment now to jot down some thoughts. The suggestions below provide a starting place.

REFLECTION EXERCISE 1

Assumptions About Academia, Teaching, and Learning

- Faculty in nursing education are ...
- Working in an academic setting, I expect my job satisfaction will be most related to ...
- From the perspective of a student, clinical courses are ...
- Faculty teaching clinical courses are ...
- The best clinical learning experiences are ...

Return to this list periodically to critically reexamine what you have written. What has changed? What has been affirmed; what has been unsubstantiated; what should be added?

APPOINTMENTS, ROLES, AND EXPECTATIONS IN ACADEMIA

This is a broad and general discussion of academic appointments, roles, and expectations, primarily focused on those that relate to clinical instruction. The topic is further explored in Chapter 19, but for more specific details, see Billings and Halstead's (2005) *Teaching in Nursing: A Guide for Faculty* (2nd ed.).

The term *appointment* is used to describe the process of being hired by an academic institution into a faculty position. The type of appointment depends on the mission and needs of the institution and the education and experience of the individual applicant. The basic requirement of accrediting bodies for teaching in nursing educational programs is a minimum of a master's degree in nursing, but appointment to certain positions often requires a doctoral degree. Due to the shortage of available qualified faculty, it is common in many nursing programs today for graduate nursing students to be appointed to teaching assistant (TA) positions, especially to teach clinical courses. In most cases, TAs are not considered faculty positions, and they are not held accountable for all of the role functions attributed to those appointments.

Faculty appointments may be full-time or part-time, and may be geared toward one of several tracks (temporary or term, tenure, clinical, or research scientist). Positions within a track are then typically delineated by rank, the titles of which may vary by track (e.g., Instructor, Assistant Professor, Associate Professor, Professor). The specific role(s) of each position can vary markedly. The classic role of faculty in an academic setting has three components: teaching, scholarship, and service. In nursing, the practice component is an additional, often required, element. Despite the demands of other role aspects, performance in the teaching role has been found to be the primary concern for novice faculty (Siler & Kleiner, 2001).

It is essential that specific responsibilities and expectations are clearly delineated for each prospective faculty member. Faculty hired to teach only clinical practicum courses are often given temporary rather than permanent appointments, with a specific term such as 1 to 3 years. Each new term of appointment should be preceded by the academic equivalent of a contract, typically a letter of appointment from the chief nurse executive (Dean or Chair) of the nursing program. This letter should delineate the specific role expectations and the salary offered. Faculty teaching clinical courses are often part-time employees, so the role expectations should include the percentage assigned to the appointment. A workload formula is typically applied to calculate the actual time allocation this percentage reflects. For instance, if a semester practicum of 4 credits is equal to a 50% workload, a faculty member should expect to spend 20 hours each week on work related to that course. Clinical courses are usually allocated 3 hours of time per credit, so a student in this course would spend 12 hours per week under the tutelage of the faculty (contact hours). The remaining 8 hours of the faculty workload would encompass the additional work for the course, for example, preparing and grading assignments, documenting performance, and preparing evaluations. Either the appointment letter or the faculty handbook should provide information related to the benefits available with the position. Benefits may include, in addition to health care insurance and a retirement program, such amenities as reduced tuition or an allocation of funds set aside for participation in continuing education programs.

Faculty salaries in public institutions and national mean salaries for the academic ranks are part of the public domain. It may be possible to negotiate salary, so doing some research and identifying assets brought to the position are well worth the time and effort. The following list in Box 1-1 identifies personal experiences and skills that might be useful in salary negotiations for the clinical practitioner entering academia.

The feelings associated with the first weeks in a new practice position, the uncertainties and insecurities, are actually quite similar to those of novice faculty. Awkwardness with a new role comes with the territory. But the statement once

> **BOX 1-1**
> **Factors to Consider When Negotiating Salary**
>
> **Education**
> - Highest degree achieved in nursing
> - Degrees held in other fields
>
> **Certifications**
> - National certifications (e.g., CCRN, CNS, ARNP)
> - Specific skills certifications (e.g., ACLS, NRP)
>
> **Teaching experience**
> - Other schools of nursing
> - In practice teaching experience (e.g., preceptor experience, in-service classes, patient groups)
>
> **Clinical practice experience**
> - Years of practice in specific areas, including role descriptions (e.g., 5 years as staff and charge nurse in ICU)
> - Leadership, management, and research experiences in specific roles (e.g., manager of surgical services, data collector for clinical drug testing)
>
> **Scholarship**—experience in writing and publishing
>
> ---
>
> *CCRN,* Critical Care Registered Nurse; *CNS,* clinical nurse specialist; *ARNP,* Advanced Registered Nurse Practitioner; *ACLS,* advanced cardiac life support; *NRP,* Neonatal Resuscitation Program; *ICU,* intensive care unit.

made by Francis Bacon about knowledge being power remains a valuable adage. Learning as much as possible about the role of faculty in the clinical setting and how best to carry out that role will result not only in personal rewards but also in the generation of new nurses who will be optimally equipped to address the health care needs of the future.

ACADEMIC CLINICAL INSTRUCTION: SKILLS AND COMPETENCIES

The heart and soul of nursing education is the clinical practicum, where nursing knowledge is shaped into professional practice. Consider the goals of the clinical learning experience, regardless of the specific learning context. Within that framework, many of the abilities needed for clinical practice are likewise needed for clinical instruction (Table 1-1).

Incorporating previous practice experiences into the teaching role can be very beneficial to new faculty; it can enhance teaching in a small group setting and can help highlight what information is most important in the practical sense (Diekelmann, 2004), especially in the area of clinical instruction. One of the most meaningful learning opportunities for students is being instructed by way of faculty storytelling. Whether it's a classic clinical case being presented for critical analysis, an example of excellent practice, or a story that illustrates one's own mistakes—one shared with humor and self-awareness—all such stories

TABLE 1-1

Clinical Learning Goals and Acquired Clinical Practice Abilities Relevant to Teaching

CLINICAL LEARNING GOALS	ACQUIRED CLINICAL PRACTICE ABILITIES
Professional nurse role development	Professional nurse practical experience
Theoretical knowledge application	Strong theoretical knowledge base
Communication skills development	Strong communication skill foundation and experience
Skill in performing caring therapeutic nursing interventions	Practice experience in providing caring therapeutic nursing interventions
Ability to evaluate ethical aspects of clinical practice	Experience with ethical decision making in practice situations
Collaborative and leadership skills development	Interdisciplinary and leadership experience

make nursing practice more real for students; the practice of nursing becomes more tangible when experiences are related with openness and honesty.

Novice faculty also will find a difference in how some of their clinical practice abilities play out in the teaching role. For instance, the organizational skills required to provide care to a group of patients or function as a charge nurse are quite different from those needed to provide clinical supervision to students. Working with beginning nursing students is not the same as precepting new nurses in practice or serving as a resource to other nurses. Novice faculty working with students in the clinical setting tend to focus on the patient, as they did in their own practice (Scanlan, 2001). As a clinical instructor, it is important to broaden the perspective, taking into consideration the learning of the student as well. In action, as a nursing faculty member in the clinical setting, the role is more one of "query and quest" than of "know and show."

And finally, new knowledge has to be obtained and new skills have to be developed before one can successfully fulfill the role of clinical nursing faculty. Experience as a professional nurse includes little exposure to the legal issues and their ramifications as associated with academia. An understanding of the theoretical foundations of the clinical nursing practicum, models of clinical nursing education, and the characteristics of today's students provide the foundation for the methods of instruction and the evaluation of student learning.

LEARNING CLINICAL TEACHING

The focus of nursing education at the master's level traditionally has been primarily on preparing advance practice nurses. Graduate preparation for nursing education has been inconsistent and insufficient for decades. Consider that those who teach our children from kindergarten through high school are required to have formal preparation in education itself, including classroom observation and student teaching! The need for formal academic preparation in nursing education has gained notice of late, but the movement is still in its infancy. Novice clinical teachers without this preparation are hampered by significant educational knowledge deficits. They lack the knowledge required to design clinical learning experiences—a lack evident in both clinical instruction methods and the evaluation of student functioning in that setting (Oermann, 2004). To become scholarly teachers who (1) choose relevant information from the literature to direct their teaching, (2) contribute their own experiences to the literature, (3) evaluate student outcomes most effectively, (4) purposely seek evaluation of their own teaching, and (5) participate intelligently in curriculum design and revision, graduate preparation in nursing education is the ideal (Allen & Field, 2005). However, with or without such preparation, learning to teach in the clinical context remains profoundly experiential, a form of on-the-job training.

Far more effort has been put into identifying effective clinical teaching behaviors than in examining how clinical instruction is learned, but the results of one particular study serve as useful guideposts on this transformational journey. Interviewing both novice and expert clinical teachers, Scanlan (2001) identified five processes by which clinical teaching is learned: (1) trial and error; (2) cognitive processes (reflection, problem solving, hypothesizing); (3) participating in workshops/conferences; (4) reading the literature; and (5) "intangible processes" such as intuition.

Experience, past and present, is a powerful teacher, and when learning clinical teaching, novice faculty draw extensively from these sources (Scanlan, 2001). Learning by trial and error, testing an approach, and keeping or rejecting it based on results is a difficult and stressful way of learning anything, from riding a bicycle to learning clinical instruction. Progress is a constant struggle, for both faculty and students if this is the only method novice faculty have to rely on. Fortunately, other sources of experiential learning are available. Personal experiences as a student provide positive role models to emulate and negative behaviors to reject. These can be extremely potent influences. Typically, prior clinical faculty whose personalities and approaches most conformed to how the now novice faculty learned were those selected as the most positive role models. But sometimes, with the wisdom gleaned from the passage of time, novice faculty were able to recognize that some of the behaviors they found most negative at the time they were clinical students had the most impact on their learning and eventual practice.

Another experiential resource identified by Scanlan's research (2001) was that of observing nursing student-faculty interactions that occurred while they were working in practice. These scenarios provided novices with insight, but unless the subtleties of the context were understood, the novices were subject to making errors in interpretation. For example, a staff nurse might overhear a faculty member providing constructive feedback to a student after the performance of a skill. The nurse might interpret what she hears as an instance of the instructor being *too* positive and ignoring student errors the nurse had seen with her own eyes. However, it could be that what the nurse did not hear was the student's earlier self-assessment, which may have been overly critical. The faculty member may have been trying to assuage the student's self-esteem at that particular moment and had not yet provided suggestions for improvement that would be forthcoming.

Next, the experience gained from teaching itself, exemplar experiences and having met explicit challenges such as dealing with specific student problems, added to the confidence of novice faculty. However, when novice faculty faced difficult situations that challenged their assumptions about an individual student or teaching itself, they were often left confused and unsure. So, logically, novice faculty reported turning to those they perceived as expert faculty. Learning from other clinical faculty, listening to their stories, and using them as sounding boards to validate assessments and approaches, were reported as being useful strategies. But novices, warns Scanlan (2001), may select their faculty role models simply because they have the same views, thereby rejecting other potentially valuable resources. And perhaps even more significant, beginning faculty accepted the input from more experienced clinical teachers almost without question, while at the same time feeling vulnerable to both these colleagues and students who might challenge them.

The expert clinical faculty in Scanlan's study (2001) depicted the couched and elusive means of learning clinical teaching as instinctive or intuitive in nature. Although very familiar with the intuitive aspects of expert nursing practice, the novice faculty in her study simply did not feel sufficiently competent in their new role to rely on its educational equivalent as a basis for operation. Benner (2001), in delineating the performance characteristics of the expert clinician, indicates these individuals have "…an intuitive grasp of each situation…" and that they work "…from a deep understanding of the total situation…" (p. 32). Benner explains that expert nurses no longer rely upon analytic principles (i.e., rules, guidelines, maxims) to connect their understanding of the situation to an appropriate action. Expert nurses use analytic problem-solving methods only when faced with experientially new situations or when their initial comprehension of the problem proves to be incorrect. That this is a capacity developed with time by some faculty is easily extrapolated. But, as in clinical practice, this level of functioning is not automatically attained by all faculty who teach in the clinical setting. Experience, as Benner (2001) noted, does not necessarily denote the practitioner's length of time in a position. Instead, it refers to "…a very active process of refining and changing preconceived theories, notions, and ideas when confronted with actual situations" (p. 178). This, indeed, is learning from experience.

The additional sources of learning about clinical teaching reported in Scanlan's study (2001) were those of attending conferences and reading literature pertaining to teaching. These continuing education/development type of processes were described as deriving their value by way of stimulating the participants' reflection and causing them to think differently about teaching. The worth of reflection continues to be affirmed.

As part of the process of reflecting upon teaching, faculty can benefit greatly from examining the role of prior experience in forming their beliefs about and approaches to clinical instruction. This is the foundation for the "teach as you were taught" method. This approach is not inherently wrong unless it is the single process of learning the craft faculty use and its origins remain unexamined. Brookfield (1995) tells us "...The influences that shape teachers' lives and that move teachers' actions are rarely found in research studies... " Instead, they are located "...in a complex web of formative memories and experiences...." And he says that "...the images, models, and conceptions of teaching [are] derived from our own experiences as learners" (p. 49). In her study, Scanlan (2001) reported that expert clinical faculty found reflection to be directly associated with learning to teach. The following reflection exercise, part of creating what Brookfield (1998) calls "an autobiography of learning", is open-ended. Set aside some time to record initial thoughts about it now. Then later, return to your log to spend some more time critically examining what was written earlier to see what additional insights can be revealed. Write down those thoughts as well. Remember, this is a journey.

REFLECTION EXERCISE 2

Examining the Power of Experience

Think back to your experiences as a student and to the clinical instructors from whom you learned the most.

◆ What behaviors of these teachers were most helpful to you in learning to perform technical skills?

◆ What behaviors of each of these teachers were most helpful to you in understanding and applying theoretical knowledge in the clinical setting?

Now, consider why these behaviors were helpful to you.

◆ How did they make you feel?

◆ Do you think these behaviors would be helpful to *any* student in *any* clinical setting? Why or why not?

◆ Would you apply any of them in your own clinical teaching?

Think back, if you can, to a clinical experience you had as a student in which your interaction with the teacher evoked strongly negative feelings. Briefly write a description of the situation.

Now, step back from the experience to look at your clinical instructor's behaviors.

◆ Do you feel the instructor contributed to your negative feelings? If so, how?

◆ What do you think the instructor might have done to help you in this situation?

Consider any observations you can recall of academic clinical faculty interactions with students that occurred while you were in practice.

◆ What impressions did these observations leave behind?

◆ What conclusions can you draw from reviewing these experiences?

▨ ADAPTATION ADVICE

Learn About the System

A smooth transition into the academic world and the role of clinical teaching faculty partially depends on learning as much as possible about the specific academic environment, as early as possible (Bellack, 2003; Diekelmann, 2004). The quality of formal academic orientation varies tremendously. It may be that part-time faculty (common circumstance for those teaching clinical courses) will receive very little orientation. The following suggestions for learning about the academic institution stand alone, with or without a concomitant orientation program.

One good way to begin learning about the system is to ask for a copy of the most recent report prepared for the nursing program's accreditation. This resource typically provides the curriculum vita (academic resumes) of all faculty, which can be useful for getting to know them, their backgrounds, and areas of expertise. It will also supply the school's organizational structure, with the lines of communication (who reports to whom). Identify by name the person to whom you will report, usually a coordinator for the course or a collection of courses. The school's strategic plan will be incorporated into the self-study. This can be very helpful, especially for new faculty with background in the business aspects of clinical practice, or it can initially appear too general and esoteric to be personally operational. The curriculum for each program is a part of the report. Initially, what is most important is information about prerequisite and subsequent courses related to your assigned clinical course. In general, you need to know what knowledge and skills students should be expected to have when they begin the course you are to be teaching.

Before moving to course-specific information, gather some general information related to school and faculty policies. A faculty handbook should be made available and provided to new faculty at the time they are hired. Do not try to read it like a textbook; look at the topic areas addressed and flag them so you can return to them as needed, and that will happen often! A copy of the student handbook should also become a part of this new library you are building. You need to know specifically what information is provided to students and what policies are documented. Be sure to pick these up annually, or whenever they are revised. Further discussion regarding academic policies is found in Unit 2: Legal and Ethical Issues in Clinical Nursing Education.

Next, gather materials and information specific to the assigned course. What is available varies, but typically a general syllabus, evaluation forms, and information for the students that is related to expectations and focus of the course (usually presented as course objectives) will be provided. Because typically a clinical course includes multiple sections, learning what other faculty have developed for their student groups can be very helpful. If it is acceptable, avoid reinventing the wheel; use as much of what others have tried and tested as you can, especially for the first semester. After that, your own unique "touches" can be added. A certain degree of standardization is essential when multiple faculty members are teaching a given course, particularly in terms of assignments and evaluation materials, but differences between clinical sites and faculty methods are to be expected. More detail related to course specifics is located in Unit 3: Setting the Stage.

Establish a Support System

Moving from a familiar context where boundaries have become clear, resources known, and where competency has been established, recognized, and rewarded, into the foreign landscape of academia can leave the novice disoriented and lost. The professional autonomy traditionally associated with academia carries with it a degree of role ambiguity that can produce considerable frustration and dissatisfaction. What has been found to most enhance job satisfaction in academia are faculty morale, their esprit, and the presence of positive social and emotional relations among faculty (Gormley, 2003). Clearly, establishing a support system within this new environment is of great benefit to novice faculty (Bellack, 2003; Diekelmann, 2004).

Major supports are available to academic faculty that can make the work of teaching easier, faster, and better. Clinicians who are novice faculty are used to working around others, so it comes as something of a shock that other faculty often are not around the school on a daily basis, and when they are present, they are incredibly busy (Siler & Kleiner, 2001; Diekelmann, 2004). Part-time faculty have obligations elsewhere, and full-time faculty may have committee, scholarship, and practice commitments, may be involved in community activities, or they may work extensively from home. This makes it difficult for novice faculty to find others to whom they can address their questions, and sometimes they hesitant to interrupt colleagues once they are located. It is imperative to identify approachable faculty early, and begin to develop collegial, perhaps even mentoring, relationships (Bellack, 2003). Novice faculty can be very enthusiastic about developing their new role as rapidly as possible, often becoming overwhelmed and overworked within a short time. The role of a mentor in guiding role development is extremely important. It is particularly crucial to have help in setting limits and realistic expectations, in understanding how to cope with problem situations, and in maintaining a sense of perspective. The novice faculty who learns how to work within the organization and whom to consult for advice and guidance can then begin to develop a network for learning and career development.

Consider asking some open-ended questions of others, such as: "What are six words that best describe the culture here?" "What are the expectations for attending other classes, for office hours, committee involvement, social interactions with students, and with other faculty and/or staff?" "Who do you consider to be the best clinical faculty?" "Who's the best person to ask about...?" If at all possible, expand your exploration of collegial support beyond the borders of the nursing school to the larger institution. At a minimum, this will give a broader perspective of academic life (Bellack, 2003). Attend social interactions such as lunchtime discussion groups, or journal clubs. Consider, too, a mutual support group composed of other novice faculty. Being part of such a group is a reminder that others are going through much the same adjustment period, and their encouragement and points of view can be extremely valuable.

Find the resources provided by the school for new faculty, and for students. If it is possible to obtain an orientation to the library and its services (literature searches, referencing services), do so. Get to know the library staff, how to obtain materials by inter-library loan, what materials are kept on reserve and what is in general circulation, and what can be accessed online. Ask and find answers to some of the following questions, and be open to generating more:

- Is there a teaching-learning center for faculty?
- Are development seminars or a formal mentoring program available?
- Where is the learning laboratory/resource center/skills lab? What does it contain? How is it operated?
- Is a technology resource center available for faculty? How is technical computer assistance obtained?
- How are audio-visual and computer learning materials obtained?
- Is a writing center available to help faculty and/or students?
- What support is available for students with learning or other disabilities?
- What support is available for those for whom English is a second language (ESL)?
- Is a tutoring program available for students?

Support personnel, in the secretarial services, business office, even custodial services, are also colleagues, with valuable roles within the academic environment. Establishing good working relationships with these academic equivalents of ancillary personnel can make it infinitely easier to obtain post-it notes, fill out the appropriate forms, and get an office rearranged! These are the individuals who know about the routine operational particulars and who can save hours of your time. Learn their names and their responsibilities; remember that their cooperation can make your work easier and more pleasant. Most importantly, respect their roles within the organization and treat them with friendly respect and not as servants (Bellack, 2003).

Seek Balance in Self-Care

Novice faculty enter academia as more than just experienced clinicians. Being a friend, a family member, and a community member are also a part of each person's role repertoire. It is imperative that "Physical activity, family and social networks, community involvement and cultural interests [be continued in order to] provide respite and renewal..." (Bellack, 2003, p. 384). This is a message routinely directed to students, but it is true for faculty too. We need to practice what we preach. Join a book club or a walking group, attend the symphony or theatre, take a yoga class, or schedule a favorite activity into the plan for the week. The stresses associated with new and different role demands, new colleagues, or possibly a move to a new city, make the need for balance that much more important. The major stress periods occur at the beginning and end of each term, so self-care interventions need to be in place early on and continued with the ebb and flow of academic demands. Clinical teacher is only one of your roles; don't allow it to overshadow the others.

SUMMARY

The transition from practice to academia is not a smooth and facile passage. Starting the journey by examining underlying assumptions about academia, teaching, and learning provides the cornerstone of a reflective process that will enable novice faculty to continuously learn about teaching, both intellectually and emotionally. Academic appointments, roles, and expectations have been reviewed as a foundation for discussing the skills and competencies of clinical instruction and how they are learned. Advice for adjusting to this role change was offered in terms of learning the academic system, establishing a support system, and balancing life in academia with life outside it. Despite the best possible orientation, the finest mentors and resources, and the answers to all conceivable questions, the anxiety associated with being a neophyte is destined to occur. Recording those feelings and thoughts along the way allows novice clinical faculty to gain knowledge about both learning and teaching through the potent portal of autobiography and facilitates transitioning from practitioner to educator.

References

Allen, M.N., & Field, P.A. (2005). Scholarly teaching and scholarship of teaching: Noting the difference. *International Journal of Nursing Education Scholarship, 2*(1), Article 12. Retrieved August 15, 2005, from The Berkeley Electronic Press website: http://www.bepress.com/ijnes/vol2/iss1/art12.

Bellack, J.P. (2003). Advice for new (and seasoned) faculty. *Journal of Nursing Education, 42*(9), 383-384.

Benner, P. (2001). *From novice to expert: Excellence and power in clinical nursing practice.* Upper Saddle River, NJ: Prentice Hall Health.

Billings, D.M., & Halstead, J.A. (Eds.) (2005). *Teaching in nursing: A guide for faculty* (2nd ed.). Philadelphia Saunders.

Brookfield, S.D. (1995). *Becoming a critically reflective teacher.* San Francisco, CA: Wiley and Sons, Jossey-Bass.

Diekelmann, N. (2004). Experienced practitioners as new faculty: New pedagogies and new possibilities. *Journal of Nursing Education, 43*(3), 101-103.

Gormley, D.K. (2003). Factors affecting job satisfaction in nurse faculty: A meta-analysis. *Journal of Nursing Education, 42*(4), 174-178.

Neese, R. (2003). A transformational journey from clinician to educator. *Journal of Continuing Education in Nursing, 34*(6), 258-262.

Oermann, M.H. (2004). Reflection on undergraduate nursing education: A look to the future. *International Journal of Nursing Education Scholarship, 1*(1), Article 5. Retrieved August 15, 2005, from The Berkeley Electronic Press website: http://www.bepress.com/ijnes/vol1/iss1/art5/

Scanlan, J.M. (2001). Learning clinical teaching: Is it magic? *Nursing and Health Care Perspectives, 22*(5), 240-246.

Siler, B.B., & Kleiner, C. (2001). Novice faculty: Encountering expectations in academia. *Journal of Nursing Education, 40*(9), 397-403.

Yoder-Wise, P.S. (2002). Learning and unlearning. *Journal of Continuing Education in Nursing, 33*(5), 195.

Yonge, O.J., Anderson, M., Profetto-McGrath, J., Olson, J.K., Sillen, D.L., & Boman, J., et al. (2005). An inventory of nursing education research, *International Journal of Nursing Education Scholarship, 2*(1), Article 11. Retrieved August 15, 2005 from http://www.bepress.com/ijnes/vol2/iss1/art11

CHAPTER 2

Theoretical Foundations of the Clinical Nursing Practicum

As in clinical practice, educational practice should be not only theory-based but also evidence-based. And again, as in clinical practice, much of the educational practicum is all too often carried out "the way we've always done it," without adequate consideration being given to what works and why, or why something else might work better. Educational research has been poorly funded and often underappreciated in the rarified air of academia. Anecdotal evidence is an unstable foundation for practice but often provides the fodder for research. Part of the problem is that of semantics. Philosophies, theories, and frameworks intermingle. Domains of knowledge are added to the mix. Abstraction becomes obfuscation. And then there are all those pedagogies! The neophyte faculty, without adequate educational background, cannot avoid feeling confused about what direction to take. This chapter provides clarification and gives structure to this terminology tangle as it apples to clinical nursing education.

▓ LEARNING THEORIES

Learning comes from experience, from reading a book, watching a movie, and simply living life. It is the process through which knowledge, in the broadest sense, is acquired and given meaning. The result of learning is growth—a change in thinking, feeling, or acting. Through the years, how learning occurs has been studied through the lenses of many disciplines—physiology, psychology, and sociology especially. Analysis of these findings has resulted in the evolution of theories that endeavor to explain how people learn. Theories are developed from the analysis of facts in relation to one another and then are used to explain phenomena. Knowledge obtained from such research has contributed to the theoretical underpinnings for entire conceptual structures—frameworks—for education. Learning theories are conventionally divided into two categories, behavioral and cognitive, although the cognitive theories are typically further separated into multiple groups.

Behavioral Learning Theories

Behaviorism has had more influence on education than any other single move-ment, and aspects of its principles continue to be applied appropriately and successfully today whereas others are roundly rejected. Pavlov, Thorndike, and B.F. Skinner were psychologists in the late 19th and early 20th centuries who developed the foundational principles of behaviorism (Braungart & Braungart, 2003; Vandeveer & Norton, 2005), originally derived from observations of learning in animals. There were many behavioral theorists, and behaviorists presented a variety of principles, but they all shared an elemental commonality. The fundamental premises of behaviorism are that all behavior is learned, and that learning is most influenced through manipulation of the environment (setting and conditions) in which it occurs and the rewards provided to encourage it (Braungart & Braungart, 2003; Vandeveer & Norton, 2005).

Educators embraced behaviorism. Seminal works were produced that guided education from kindergarten through college. By way of a tiny book that became the educators' handbook, Tyler (1949) carried behaviorism into the classroom, structuring learning experiences in a way that would help educa-tors achieve carefully delineated results (outcomes, goals) through the develop-ment of objectives. "The most useful form for stating objectives is to express them in terms which identify both the *kind of behavior* to be developed in the student and the *content or area of life* in which this behavior is to operate" (pp. 46-47; Thus were born behavioral objectives. Bloom, Engelhart, Furst, Hill, and Krathwohl (1956) endeavored to create a classification scheme of educational objectives addressing the cognitive domain, "...the recall or recognition of knowledge and the development of intellectual abilities and skills" through the use of observable action verbs (p. 7). In dedicating the book to Tyler, and emphasizing the role of observable behaviors in determining whether learning has occurred, Bloom added his name to the prestigious list of behaviorist educa-tors. As Bloom lead the efforts in the cognitive realm of knowledge, his colleague Krathwohl (Krathwohl, Bloom, & Masia, 1956) spearheaded work in the affective realm, but still with a decidedly behaviorist inclination. Here were objectives emphasizing "...a feeling tone, an emotion, or a degree of acceptance or rejection... attitudes, appreciations, values, and emotional sets or biases" (p. 7). Attainment of the objectives continued to be through highly structured, precisely delineated, and visible behaviors. In 1962, Mager raised behavioral objectives to a near art form. Objectives were reduced to their separate components: behavior ("...any visible activity displayed by a learner"), terminal behavior (behavior demonstrated by the learner "...at the time your influence over him ends"), and criterion ("...a standard or test by which terminal behavior is evaluated") (p. 2). Educators and students alike learned to construct behavioral objectives to guide teaching and identify measurable outcomes as the basis for evaluating learning.

Many aspects of behaviorist learning theories are well known and continue to be used in clinical educational settings, especially in the acquisition of technical skills (Box 2-1). In most cases, especially at the beginning of clinical nursing education, it is faculty who determine what is important to know, experience, and demonstrate. Although students' involvement in their own learning has increased, faculty retain the primary control and authority, even today. Knowledge grows as a house is built, one aspect or brick upon another. So prior knowledge forms a reference point for both the assimilation of new knowledge and the application transfer of knowledge from one learning experience to another. Knowing what prior knowledge is available can allow the teacher to intentionally assist the student in connecting new knowledge to old and thereby enhance overall understanding. Students learn to auscultate lung sounds after they have learned the anatomy of the lungs. Principles used to establish a sterile field to change a dressing transfer to the operating room. Technical skills are classically learned as procedures, following a relatively rigid, lockstep approach. Agency procedure manuals reinforce this programmed, sequential pattern. The behavioral objectives, carefully crafted to identify the desired learning outcomes, prescribe not only the learning experiences students will be exposed to but also

---

BOX 2-1

Behavioral Learning Theories: Sample Applications in Clinical Nursing Education

- Teacher-determined and -directed learning experiences
- Teaching in a sequential pattern, simple to complex
- Technical skill acquisition
- Use of behavioral objectives to identify learning outcomes and guide evaluation
- Development of teaching plans by students
- Use of nursing process and nursing care plans
- Application of positive reinforcement

the basis for student evaluation. The sequential, step-by-separate step format of the nursing process, and the resulting nursing care plans are a direct outgrowth of behaviorism. Any activity students are involved in that follows this procedural template, such as the development of teaching plans, reflects behavioral learning theories. Positive reinforcement, both written and verbal, is a powerful extrinsic learning reward, and rewarding the attainment of desired outcomes is key to behaviorism. The expectation of praise has thoroughly permeated not only education but also society as a whole.

Cognitive Learning Theories

The emphasis of cognitive theorists is not external to the learner, as in behaviorism, but rather emphasizes what occurs within the learner. To the cognitive theorists, the mental steps involved in acquiring, processing, and structuring information are the key foci to learning (Braungart & Braungart, 2003). There is a profound shift from passive to active learning and from teacher to learner. It is a logical progression then that the concept of an externally delivered reward for learning attainment is not a feature of these theories. Indeed, internal motivation, the learners' desire to learn is seen as the impetus to learning; their own goals are the origin of an inner uncertainty and strain that become the stimulus to learn (Braungart & Braungart, 2003). Just as behavioral learning theory has a common core, so too the mental aspects of learning are at the center of cognitive learning theories.

With this emphasis on the internal mental processes of learning, cognitive theorists advanced their field by attending to the various component processes from a host of perspectives (Braungart & Braungart, 2003; Vandeveer & Norton, 2005). These branches of the cognitive theory tree have been subdivided, rearranged, and labeled differently by assorted authors, contributing to an overall sense of disorder. Gestalt psychologists identified pattern recognition and reorganization as the source of the sudden insight of the same name. Information processing theorists provided a new understanding of short-term memory, the movement of information into long-term memory, and the different components of long-term memory (Braungart & Braungart, 2003; Vandeveer and Norton, 2005). Here too is the theoretical source of the many models for individual learning preferences and learning styles (auditory, visual, kinesthetic).

The changes in the mental processes facilitating learning that occur from infancy to adulthood are the basis of the work of a large group of cognitive developmental theorists (Braungart & Braungart, 2003; Vandeveer & Norton, 2005). This branch of cognitive theory introduced concepts such as learning readiness, which evolved to provide the foundation for Perry's research into ethical development (1970), Kohlberg's work in moral development (1984), and the identification of learning differences between children and adults (Knowles, 1980). Other researchers introduced concepts of social and cultural context into the learning and developmental mix (Braungart & Braungart, 2003). Being occasionally separated from the cognitive theorists because some of their early work incorporated aspects of behaviorism, these social cognitive theorists addressed learning through observation and defined learning into the context of interpersonal relationships. Collaboration and role modeling are central to these theories, but the centrality of the learner and the cognitive mental processes remain the core (Braungart & Braungart, 2003). Information processing theories and cognitive developmental theories informed what has come to be known as the *theory of multiple intelligences* (Gardner, 1983). This theory posits that each person begins life with an individual constellation of different ways of learning, each associated with a particular facet of awareness (e.g., musical-rhythmic, bodily-kinesthetic, logical-mathematical).

The diverse cognitive learning theories provide valuable guidance in clinical nursing instruction (Box 2-2). Insightful awareness gleaned from prior learning experiences, "…an intuitive grasp of each situation…," is foundational to the expert nurse in Benner's model of skill acquisition (Benner, 2001, p. 32). Simple, clear, and concise directions and explanations are more conducive to student learning. Too many extraneous stimuli interfere with learning, so trying to guide a student through the interpretation of lab results by the nurses' station or in a busy hallway may not be effective. Individual filters of culture, past experience, meaning, needs and goals, and the form of the stimuli (e.g., written, verbal, mathematics) all markedly influence to what the learner attends. So, a particular teaching approach that is effective with one student may not work with the next. And, logically, learning for adults (college students) differs in many ways from that of children. Knowing that information remains in short-term memory only briefly, then to be lost or moved into long-term memory reinforces the need to use techniques that facilitate that shift. Students are encouraged to group like concepts, mentally rehearse skills, and compare and contrast. This latter approach is very useful in the clinical setting, where a student might be asked to compare the manifestations of pneumonia to those of emphysema, or the presentation of a premature infant

---

BOX 2-2

Cognitive Learning Theories: Sample Applications in Clinical Nursing Education

- Recognition of student as individual
- Mental rehearsal
- Compare/contrast activities
- Questioning
- Journaling; reflection
- Concept mapping
- Role-play
- Emphasis on role modeling
- Student as active participant in learning
- Emphasis on teacher-student relationship

contrasted with one that is full term. Reviewing prior knowledge as a basis for assimilating new knowledge through the use of questioning and forming analogies can help a student see the relationship of preexisting to new knowledge.

Learning activities such as journaling and reflection, concept mapping, role-playing, discussion and debate all have their origins in cognitive learning theories. The importance of quality clinical role models for students is derived from social cognitive theories, as is our awareness of the significance of the social context in which learning occurs. Perhaps most important of all, students actively participate in the learning process, and indeed assume some responsibility and control of it. They identify their learning needs and goals, seek out learning experiences, explore resources, ask questions, and work collaboratively with faculty and peers. Learning is expedited when there is a trusting relationship between the teacher and the student. In addition to providing new perspectives on learning, cognitive learning theorists broke down many of the barriers between student and teacher.

■ EDUCATIONAL PHILOSOPHIES AND FRAMEWORKS

Educational philosophies and frameworks move beyond exploring simply how people learn to examine the environments and methodologies most conducive to learning (Vandeveer & Norton, 2005). It is often very easy to see the footprints of learning theories within these configurations of ideas. Changes in society have been a major influence on educational frameworks: how people perceive and relate to one another, how they view their world, and what they value. These form the essence of a philosophy. The system of concepts and thoughts that forms a philosophy provides an overall vision of what is fundamentally important. Philosophies can then be translated into structures that reflect back onto society, such as organizational and social policies, art, science, and educational frameworks. Educational frameworks are the conceptual structures that guide the sum of all aspects of teaching and learning, known as *pedagogies*. A certain amount of variation is found in how philosophies, educational frameworks, and the pedagogies are presented, both in their derivations and in the relationships between them. Table 2-1 illustrates the relationship of philosophies, educational frameworks, and the pedagogies they inform that are used in this text.

Current Educational Philosophies

With the evolution of society, humanity's perceptions of what is important, that is, what is valued, also have evolved. "Philosophy is the art of reason; reason is an attempt to put what is perceived about life's phenomena together...and make sense of it" (Bevis, 1989, p. 42). The identification of what is valued by society guides the construction of a system of beliefs. The assumptions upon which a philosophy is based eventually become embedded in the educational approaches used by faculty, the roles of teacher and student, and the character of their relationship to one another.

Philosophies, Related Educational Frameworks, and Pedagogies

PHILOSOPHY	EDUCATIONAL FRAMEWORK	PEDAGOGY
Realism	Behaviorism	Traditional (conventional; outcome-based; evidence-based)
Existentialism	Humanism	[Subtly affected traditional]
	Caring	Caring
	Adult education	Andragogy
	Postmodern	Interpretive:
		Critical
		Feminist
		Postmodern
		Phenomenologic
		Narrative

Although other philosophies have impacted nursing practice and education historically, current nursing education is primarily based on two very different philosophical perspectives: realism and existentialism. Interestingly, these perspectives can be seen as diametrically opposed, and yet both remain simultaneously viable within education today.

Realism, the philosophic theory that reality exists in the physical world and that truth is an observable fact, is the foundation of behaviorism (Csokasy, 2002, 2005). The organization of the world, as it was known in his time, is credited to Aristotle. He divided knowledge into social, physical, and life sciences (Csokasy, 2002). Behaviorism is seen both as an educational framework and as a learning theory. The tangible, observable outcomes of learning emphasized by behaviorism are consistent with realism's conviction that reality is solely a visible construct.

Directly or indirectly, changes in nursing education that began to appear in the 1960s reflected the philosophical position known as *existentialism*. From this perspective, the greatest value is placed on freedom of choice, and the individual is the basis of reality. A meaningful individual goal is locating personal meaning in existence (Csokasy, 2005). Existentialism remains the dominant philosophical standpoint of current 21st century society.

Current Educational Frameworks

"When philosophical concepts move into the realm of theory, philosophical thought is translated into hypotheses that can be tested. Thus, the conceptual construct is no longer philosophy; it is theory" (Bevis, 1989, p. 34). Applied to nursing, an educational framework "…is the conceptualization and articulation of concepts, facts, propositions, postulates, theories, phenomena, and variables relevant to a specific nursing educational system" (Bevis, 1989, p. 26). In Table 2-1, the educational frameworks that evolved from the philosophies are illustrated.

The educational framework of behaviorism emerged from the philosophical point of view of realism and the behavioral learning theories (Csokasy, 2005). This educational framework, and the pedagogy it informed, remains the dominant approach to nursing education today, in both classroom and clinical settings. The value of educational efficiency, characterized by rote memorization to produce rote recall, is at the heart of the behaviorist educational framework. Learning is highly structured, procedural, and hierarchical, with theory courses and clinical experiences built upon one another (Vandeveer & Norton, 2005). The incongruence of this framework and the traditional pedagogy it inspired, in light of the philosophical evolution of society, has become the source of increasing discomfort among nurse educators and is the driving force behind the recent pedagogic revolution.

Existentialism spawned several educational frameworks. From the position of existentialism, the role of education is to facilitate the overriding goal of identifying one's personal meaning for existence. Personal growth was at the heart of education (Csokasy, 2005). This emphasis on the individual and freedom of choice triggered the rise of humanism, a movement within society seen by some to be of sufficient impact to generate its own educational framework (Csokasy, 2005; Vandeveer & Norton, 2005). Freedom of choice carried an implicit obligation to take responsibility for one's own life, which included taking a more active role in the educational process. The active learning premise, as well as other components of cognitive learning theories, is found in all of the educational frameworks that developed from existentialism, but humanism was the first. Other disciplines contributed to humanism's educational framework, especially Maslow's hierarchy of needs (1954) and Rogers' valuing of the role of self-esteem and self-concept in learning (1961). Both of these theorists emphasized the individual and the potential of personal growth (Vandeveer & Norton, 2005). Nursing education embraced the tenets of humanism but remains true to much of the behaviorism model. Behaviorism was buffered by humanism. The holistic model became integral to nursing's unification of all parts of the individual. In nursing education, humanism sparked the development of integrated curricula and awareness that students were people with many other facets to their lives than school (Bevis, 1989). Relationships between teachers and students became more intimate, personal; this was especially true in the naturally smaller groups in clinical settings. Mastery of facts occurred within an environment designed to encourage exploration, independence, accountability, inventiveness, and even passion.

This existential-humanistic approach to individual freedom became the basis of a unique approach specific to nursing education: the caring curriculum (Bevis & Watson, 1989). The educational framework that was the starting point for what has come to be known as the *curriculum revolution* is perceived by some as distinctly separate from humanism, and by others as an outgrowth of it. This caring framework approaches nursing education through the integration of premises of existentialism, humanism, feminism, caring, and phenomenology (Bevis & Watson, 1989; Benner & Wrubel, 1989). As articulated by its architects,

Em Bevis and Jean Watson, "This framework accommodates an evolving professional consciousness and allows for methods that attend to the moral ideals and values that are relational, subjective inner experiences, while honoring intuition, persona, spiritual, cognitive, and physical senses alike…a transformative paradigm that is philosophically and morally consistent with phenomena and practices of human caring in both educational and clinical worlds" (Bevis & Watson, 1989, pp. 53-54). The application of the theory pedagogically, how it plays out in educational practice, is perhaps easier to understand.

Using the belief system of existentialism as a springboard, Knowles (1980) articulated the basis for an educational framework addressing teaching of adults (andragogy) as being differentiated from the education of children (pedagogy). The role of prior experience, active participation in learning, and individual determinations of meaning as presented in the cognitive learning theories are key to this framework. The freedom to choose what is personally relevant, drawn from existentialism, supports a pragmatic approach for the adult learner. Additional assumptions of adult learning theory include (1) adult learners work best in learning environments that provide opportunities for social interaction; (2) adult learners assume increased responsibility for their own learning; and (3) learning must be relevant for adult learners (Knowles, 1980; Forrest, 2004; Vandeveer & Norton, 2005). These concepts have been readily incorporated into the teaching of adults, but the use of the term *pedagogy* remains the dominate terminology at all educational levels.

The final educational framework derived from existential philosophy is that of postmodernism (Csokasy, 2005). This framework has been the generative force for a torrent of creative, sometimes esoteric, pedagogies believed by many to hold the future for nursing education. Postmodernism itself has no consistent single description. Generally, as both an educational framework and a cultural phenomenon affecting many other disciplines, it refers to what has come after the modern philosophies and conventional perceptions and to the products of nursing education, music, architecture, and so forth. Those conventions are being challenged; diversity, novelty, and change are being encouraged (Csokasy, 2005). Postmodernism, the most recent of the modern philosophies, marks the end of existentialism's influence; so the postmodern educational framework encompasses all that has gone beyond the past educational ones and has engendered a mélange of new pedagogies by so doing.

PEDAGOGIES—OLD, NEWER, AND NEWEST

Pedagogies evolve from, and are a reflection of, philosophies, educational frameworks, learning theories, and theories derived from other fields. Pedagogy is more than simply the art and science of teaching. It encompasses what we teach, how we teach it, why we do it that way, and how it is learned. It is "…a way of thinking about and comportment within education" (Ironside, 2001, p. 73). Table 2-1 outlines the pedagogies discussed here and the philosophies and educational frameworks from which they emanate. Although the origin of the word lies in the education of children, and an effort was made to differentiate the education of adults (andragogy), the term *pedagogy* receives its perspective from the contextual setting in which it is used. The unique aspects of educating adults, derived from adult learning theory, are routinely incorporated into the pedagogies used in higher and continuing education.

The instructional strategies and learning activities used in the clinical setting are based on assumptions embedded within the various educational schools of thought. How learning occurs, whether it is a passive or active process, what motivates the learner, how knowledge transfer occurs, and the relative impact of internal and external environments on learning vary from subtly to profoundly among the pedagogies. The roles played by the teacher and the learner—the amount of control, interdependence and independence—are enacted quite differently. These in turn inform the character of the relationship between student and teacher within each pedagogical approach. A final word: there is no perfect pedagogy appropriate to all aspects of nursing education. The pedagogies are not meant to be either exclusive or all-inclusive. The pedagogy appropriate for ethical discourse is not applicable when a student needs to learn how to perform a catheterization. Bits and pieces of different pedagogies may be mixed and blended. For instance, aspects of humanism are likely to ebb into the pedagogy derived from behaviorism.

Traditional Pedagogy

The pedagogical application of behaviorism is known by a number of names: traditional, conventional, outcomes-based, and evidence-based. This is the oldest of the approaches to nursing education and it remains the dominant one today. Classically, traditional pedagogy uses approaches to teaching and learning that are derived from behavioral learning theories. When it comes to clinical nursing practica with a heavy focus on skill acquisition, the traditional pedagogy is not only appropriate but also probably superior to any other (Bevis, 1993; Romyn, 2001). This is due to both the behavioral theory that supports procedural learning and the fact that the outcomes of skill acquisition "...can be assessed and judgments can be made as to whether the objectives of a particular learning experience were attained" (Romyn, 2001, pp. 5-6). In its purest application, traditional pedagogy places the student in a passive, receptive role; the teacher knows all, establishes the desired goals, designs and controls the learning environment, and determines when the desired outcome has been satisfactorily attained. Through the use of rewards and reinforcement, the preferred learning occurs; it is then strengthened and transferred through practice (Braungart & Braungart, 2003).

But other things happen in clinical courses besides skill acquisition. The beliefs, attitudes, and values of the profession are taken on; collegial interdisciplinary affiliations are established; ethical and social issues are explored, and so much more. Additionally, the student-teacher relationship and student role in learning are not conducive to preparing nurses to be life-long learners. Clearly, pure traditional pedagogy is not appropriate for all situations. Enter then the gentle touch of humanism and the respectful perspective of andragogy.

Traditional Pedagogy Moderated by Humanism and Andragogy

Retaining the stepwise, procedural aspects of the traditional model and accepting the tenets of these educational frameworks has had a profound impact on traditional pedagogy.

Humanism shifted the student role into an active mode and shifted learning into the internal environment of the student. Teachers became facilitators who valued each learner as unique and worthy (Braungart & Braungart, 2003; Vandeveer & Norton, 2005). In clinical courses, the interaction that occurs within small groups of students is especially supportive of learner self-growth.

Knowles (1980) named the "art and science of helping adults learn" (p. 43) andragogy and intended it to be an entire pedagogical perspective for adult learners. Instead, what has occurred is the absorption of the assumptions of the adult educational framework into not just the traditional pedagogy, but also into all the subsequent pedagogies used within higher education and beyond. Already assuaged by the effects of humanism, the facets of andragogy subsumed into traditional pedagogy offered teachers and students a new constellation of approaches to learning "...in an environment that encourages, builds, and maintains relationships" (Forrest, 2004, p. 76). Faculty treat students with respect, communicating a valuing of their feelings, ideas, and past experiences. With students collaborating with faculty to assess their learning needs, determine their goals and learning activities, and participate in their own evaluation, students both accept responsibility for and make a commitment to learning. The degree to which this is actualized in clinical instruction varies greatly, both from course to course and among faculty teaching different sections of the same course. All students who are chronologically adults do not necessarily conform developmentally to all aspects of andragogy. And, all principles of andragogy are not appropriate when the content is completely unfamiliar to students (Braungart & Braungart, 2005). In a clinical course for beginning nursing students, or at the beginning of a course in clinical setting that requires a significant amount of new knowledge (e.g., operating room, labor and delivery, pediatrics), more traditional pedagogical approaches characterized by increased teacher control and direction are very appropriate.

Caring Pedagogy

The educational framework of caring presented earlier formed the basis for a pedagogy unique to nursing. At its center is a reconceptualization of the relationship between the student and the teacher as highly interactive, connected, and infused with trust—by its very nature, a caring relationship (Evans, 2004; Bankert & Kozel, 2005; Vandeveer & Norton, 2005). This new partnership between and among teachers and learners has been identified as one embodiment of excellence in nursing education (Ironside, 2005). "The commitment to care about students is central to concepts of good teaching" (Scotto, 2003, p. 289). Instructional approaches in the clinical setting that enlighten the student in regard to alternative ways of thinking and intervening, clinical questioning, and seminar or clinical conference activities such as debates and role-playing from the position of the patient or family members are examples of caring pedagogy. Caring pedagogies assist nursing students to learn how to care for their patients. As faculty model caring behaviors in their interactions with students, patients, even mannequins in the Learning Resource Center, caring is nurtured in nursing students (Tarnow & Butcher, 2005). Additionally, the use of reflective journaling and real cases of patient experiences "...allows examination of the real-life complexities encountered in nursing practice" (Vandeveer & Norton, 2005, p. 274). Evans (2004) has identified the components of the caring curriculum and how faculty may operationalize them within the context of both the relationship they establish and the teaching methods they employ. The caring component is seen in a relationship in which both participants "...exhibit reverence for humanity, mutual respect,...self-respect, and self-care" (p. 221). Learning experiences that encourage dialogue, thereby increasing awareness of divergent ways of knowing and the role of context, and personal as well as professional growth are representative of caring pedagogy. Every teaching moment is an opportunity for faculty to model caring (Evans, 2004). Scotto (2003) defined caring as the offering of self, and it is exemplified through "...offering the intellectual, psychological, spiritual, and physical aspects one possesses as a human being to attain a goal" (p. 290). The principle that knowledge is constructed that was introduced in the caring pedagogy is carried forward into the newest, interpretive pedagogies. From this standpoint, what is known is context-dependent and therefore changeable and relative. Moral-ethical principles are embedded in this pedagogy because they are central to nursing practice. As important as it is for students "...to cultivate a strong knowledge base and reasoning skills and to develop psychomotor skills to efficiently meet patients' needs...[it is] equally important for nurses to develop awareness of themselves regarding their own psychologic and spiritual foundations so they may respond appropriately to others. Caring demands a great deal of self-awareness and self-development" (Scotto, 2003, p. 291). Tenets of feminism support efforts to diminish power inequities between student and teacher, and those of phenomenology facilitate making discernible what is concealed in the caring practice of nursing (Benner & Wrubel, 1989).

Interpretive Pedagogies

A group of new pedagogies (critical, feminist, postmodern, and phenomeno-logic) are also called *interpretive pedagogies* because a central issue of all of them is the interpretation of the context for learning (Ironside, 2001). All these pedagogies "...challenge...teacher-centered assumptions of outcomes-based nursing education and support the development of student-centered learning experiences" (Diekelmann & Lampe, 2004, p. 245). Faculty truly become colearners within these pedagogies; the security of objectives, even in clinical courses, is abandoned, and the focus shifts to what the students are thinking while learning along with them (Diekelmann & Scheckel, 2004). Multiperspective thinking, supportive of all aspects of diversity and alternative points of view, is also common to all of the interpretive pedagogies (Diekelmann, 2003). These pedagogies arose partially in response to the recognition by nurse educators that the behavioral approach of traditional pedagogy, while of value in preparing technically competent nurses, cannot adequately equip them to function as agents of social change in the essential transformation of the health care system (Romyn, 2001). Traditional pedagogy engenders highly structured learning experiences that are guided by objectives and evaluated based on outcomes. These new pedagogies "...shift to critiquing, examining, exploring, and deconstructing" student experiences to determine learning and meaning" (Diekelmann, 2001).

Critical pedagogy is grounded in principles of social activism and "...is the liberation of thought through analysis of power and relationships within social structure" (Vandeveer & Norton, 2005, p. 262). Rather than emphasizing the individual, critical pedagogy seeks the attainment of a collective good for the community, and emphasizes decentering authority and engendering empowerment. Application of critical pedagogy in any setting is through rational discussion and reflective journaling and is directed toward attaining an increased understanding of those who exist on the margins of society (Ironside, 2001; Diekelmann, 2003; Vandeveer & Norton, 2005). The role of the teacher in these applications is assumed to be that of a neutral mediator. This is contradictory to a pedagogy that negates neutrality, assuming everyone is affected by their unique external and internal environment; this is one of the limitations and criticisms of critical pedagogy (Ironside, 2001). In clinical nursing instruction, this pedagogy can be included in focused discussion in seminars and clinical conferences and contemplative analyses of practice incidents through the use of journaling. The purpose of these strategies is to assist students in recognizing existing injustices and inequities of power and hopefully to encourage them to explore the underlying issues and suggest potential actions for change (Vandeveer & Norton, 2005).

Feminist pedagogy is at minimum associated with, and at most subsumed by, critical pedagogy but engenders a unique spin on oppression by casting it as an issue of gender (Ironside, 2001; Vandeveer & Norton, 2005). In clinical education, the teacher with this perspective identifies gender bias and its resulting oppression in all social structures, especially education and the profession of nursing (Vandeveer & Norton, 2005). All aspects of existential educational frameworks come into play in feminist pedagogy: autonomy, independence, self-determinism, collaboration, and mutual trust. With its emphasis on identifying situations of male privilege and gender bias, students exposed to feminist pedagogy are more prepared to initiate social change; however, they may be ill-prepared for the existing patriarchal systems, and the diversity within the gender goes underrecognized (Ironside, 2001).

Postmodern pedagogy evolved from the concept of multiple realities and is a method of extracting and examining knowledge, deconstructing it in order to better understand it (Vandeveer & Norton, 2005). This is truly the most esoteric and abstract of the interpretive pedagogies. Knowledge is not seen as universal or transcendental but as being in a state of continuous, contextual flux, so relative that all bases for decision making are eliminated (Ironside, 2001). In settings where both vagueness and doubt are feasible and specific use of knowledge is not necessary, this approach may be applied, but definitive application is likely more theoretical and academic than sensible (Ironside, 2001; Vandeveer & Norton, 2005). Postmodern pedagogy has primarily been applied in nursing academia as a method of revealing the fundamental assumptions of current educational practices (Ironside, 2001). It could conceivably be used in any situation where the teacher desires to promote diverse understandings; however, the documentation providing evidence of actual advancement in the direction of applying the theory is negligible (Vandeveer & Norton, 2005). With underlying premises of ambiguity and the fluidity of knowledge, such guidance for the use of postmodern pedagogy in clinical nursing instruction will not likely evolve.

Phenomenologic pedagogy does apply to clinical education. It encompasses techniques by which lived human experiences are examined for common meanings through storied discourse (Ironside, 2001; Vandeveer & Norton, 2005). The commonalities are then integrated into the subject matter at hand. Phenomenologic pedagogy is highly contextual, speaking to the moment, place, and people currently at hand. A specific application of this pedagogy in nursing education, narrative pedagogy, is used by faculty, students, and clinicians through the communal sharing of their experiential stories with the intent of engendering increased understanding (Diekelman, 2001; Diekelmann & Lampe, 2004; Diekelmann & Scheckel, 2004; Ironside, 2001). All the elements of other pedagogies that support collegiality and trust in the teacher-student relationship, the contextual nature of knowledge and learning, and respect for diversity and individual growth are embedded in this pedagogy.

In the clinical practicum, principles of phenomenologic pedagogy have several valuable applications. Narrative pedagogy can be used by faculty to explore commonalities between student and teacher within the clinical context. Students are surprised to discover that faculty worry about many of the same things that they do, before, during, and even after a day in a clinical setting (Diekelmann & Scheckel, 2004). Faculty are reminded of the commonalities of anxiety when they are confronted with new tasks or are exposed to clinical queries and experience the fears of failure or inadequacy associated with a desire for perfection. The thoughts and feelings associated with attending major life experiences with patients—birth and death, terminal diagnoses and successful procedures—provide common ground for those who teach, those who learn, and those who practice. This pedagogy "…shifts the focus from a technical skills orientation to one that is concerned with the whole human being" (Vandeveer & Norton, 2005, p. 267).

Faculty can model eliciting aspects of patient experiences with the skillful use of open-ended, probative questions posed to patients at the bedside and to patient guests attending seminars or clinical conferences (Vandeveer & Norton, 2005). Students learn to listen to what is said and interpret the emotional undertones provided by nonverbal language when this approach is used. The ubiquitous interpersonal process recording (IPR) can be refocused to extract personal meaning as well as examine therapeutic communication skills. Reflective journaling allows students to identify and clarify their thoughts and feelings individually, which can then be shared in community discourse during seminars or clinical conferences. All of these learning experiences "...have the potential for promoting a more in-depth understanding and enhancing the caring aspects of students' clinical practice" (Vandeveer & Norton, 2005, p. 269).

DOMAINS OF LEARNING IN THE CLINICAL LEARNING CONTEXT

Following the convention of the American Psychological Association in 1948, a group of educational psychologists, lead by Dr. Benjamin Bloom, began a project to develop a classification system of levels of intellectual behavior within the three overlapping realms of learning: knowledge (cognitive), attitudes (affective), and skills (psychomotor). Classification systems were to be hierarchical, moving from the simple to the complex, building on and subsuming prior learning at each level (Bloom et al., 1956). These individuals were college examiners, what today would be called *accreditation site visitors*. The original intent was the creation of a theoretical framework that would enhance the consistency of communication among examiners, promote the development of ideas regarding testing, and facilitate test construction (Bloom et al., 1956). That such an endeavor was even initiated is an indicator of the pervasive influence of behaviorism! This was the first attempt to classify learning behaviors and provide concrete measures for identifying levels of learning.

Two systems were created, one for the knowledge or cognitive domain (Bloom et al., 1956), and one for the emotional/attitudinal or affective domain (Krathwohl et al., 1956). The publication of these classification systems, termed *taxonomies*, contributed to the development of systems for using instructional objectives (Mager, 1962) and reinforced the behavioral approach to curricular design (Tyler, 1949).

The group did not address the psychomotor domain, reflecting the learning of manipulative skills, although they recognized it as a distinct sphere of learning. They believed that it was insufficiently used in secondary education, so did not warrant the efforts involved in generating a taxonomy (Bloom et al., 1956). As time passed, and motor skills were seen as more important to many occupations, mechanical tasks, and even sports, others have explored learning in this domain, but in most cases this has resulted in applications of learning theories rather than generation of actual taxonomies leveling the intellectual behaviors associated with skill development (Adams, 1987).

In no other courses in nursing curricula do all three domains of knowledge come into play as they do in the courses taught in clinical settings. Students learn new cognitive skills and transfer and apply knowledge from their other courses. The affective domain, associated with emotions, attitudes, and values, is key in the development of caring professional nurses. And of course, the acceptable mastery of psychomotor skills is a major focus of clinical nursing education. Here too, the overlap of the domains is obvious. Students must demonstrate the knowledge of the principles guiding skill performance in order to carry out a skill safely and efficiently, and they must do so while interacting with the client with respect and sensitivity.

The conceptualization of these three interrelated domains of learning continues to be common parlance in education. Despite an abundance of criticism, the use of behavioral objectives is likewise universal. They continue to provide guidance for students and faculty in everything from the requirements of specific individual assignments (e.g., demonstrate an understanding of sterile technique when changing dressings) to those of entire courses or program levels (e.g., apply concepts of primary, secondary and tertiary prevention to the nursing care of adults experiencing acute and chronic illness). They direct the selection of learning settings and experiences and the subsequent evaluation of learning attainment. Objectives, or outcome indicators, are also used by the agencies responsible for accrediting overall programs of study in colleges and universities (e.g., provides compassionate, ethical care to individuals of diverse cultures, values, beliefs, and lifestyles).

Cognitive Domain

Six major classes of cognitive learning are identified. Presented in order of ascending complexity they are (1) knowledge, (2) comprehension, (3) application, (4) analysis, (5) synthesis, and (6) evaluation. Each class is further broken down into varying numbers of components. For example, the knowledge class may be divided into knowledge of specifics, then of ways and means to deal with those specifics, and finally, the knowledge of the universals and abstractions associated with a given field of study. Specific learning behaviors are associated with each level, as are verbs descriptive of those behaviors, which are to be used when writing objectives (Bloom et al., 1956). Depending on whether the learning is new or constructed based on prior learning, and the desired endpoint level of cognitive learning, faculty design the appropriate objectives. The verbs used also provide guidance for how the learning will be evaluated. For example, knowledge is the lowest cognitive level, so having a student state the normal range for serum sodium is reflective of this level. When the student explains the role of sodium in the body, comprehension is demonstrated. Interpreting the specific patient's hypernatremia as it relates to his Cushing's syndrome moves the cognitive learning to the level of application. Now, asking the students to compare the pathophysiology behind hypernatremia in a patient with Cushing's syndrome to that of another patient with diabetes insipidus shifts up a level, to analysis. Moving to synthesis, the student's plan of care can be explored in terms of interventions for the cause and manifestations of the patient's hypernatremia. And finally, the student would be directed to evaluate the results of their interventions with this patient, the quality of their critical thinking skills, and the extent of their overall grasp of the concept of sodium imbalance. Without encouraging rigid application of all the behaviors and action verbs, the six levels, or classes, of cognitive learning, with their ascending complexity, are very important in clinical instruction. The questions asked and the assignments provided cannot remain at the level of knowledge and comprehension if students are going to learn to base their practice on a full constellation of cognitive learning. This is a common problem for novice faculty in the clinical setting. Rote memory has its place, but only as a starting point for further cognitive learning.

Affective Domain

The affective domain relates to what may be perceived as the intangibles of learning—behaviors connoting values, emotion, appreciation, and attitudes. The group of educational psychologists charged with designing a taxonomy for this domain found their greatest challenge was in establishing a continuum of affective learning, the basis for the development of levels of learning within the domain (Krathwohl et al., 1956). Ultimately, their analysis resulted in five categories that they defined as receiving/attending, responding, valuing, organization, and characterization by a value or value complex. The category of *receiving/attending* is associated with behaviors indicative of the development of awareness. *Responding* equates to reacting to a situation, and doing so with satisfaction in that reaction. *Valuing* behaviors are those associated with choosing values and expressing a commitment and conviction to them. At the level of *organizing*, the internalized value is organized into a system of priorities. And, at the final affective domain level *(characterization),* the individual performs actions consistent with the internalized values, and develops a life philosophy consistent with those values (Krathwohl et al., 1956; Reilly, 1978).

Although the taxonomy for the affective domain published by Kathwohl, et al. (1956) can certainly be used as a basis for writing behavioral objectives, creating learning experiences, and evaluating learning, other approaches may be used as well. Depending on the content to be addressed, alternative frameworks related to values clarification, moral inquiry/ethical decision making, and professional codes of ethics may be more utilitarian for nursing education. Leveling in terms of hierarchical expectations for performance may evolve from the framework used.

In clinical nursing courses, learning experiences relating to the affective learning domain are plentiful and may be structured or spontaneous

---

BOX 2-3

Clinical Course Objective: Affective Domain With Behavioral Exemplars

Implements the professional nurse role with responsibility and accountability by:
- Applying legal, cultural, ethical, and professional standards of practice.
- Using resources efficiently.
- Collaborating effectively with other members of the health care team, peers, and faculty.
- Using effective, appropriate communication techniques with patients, colleagues, and faculty.
- Demonstrating respectful behavior in all interactions.

and unstructured. These might include the development of therapeutic communication skills such as listening and clarifying, attending to what patients are communicating verbally and nonverbally, responding to the multiple aspects of diversity between patients and families, and incorporating the values associated with the profession of nursing. Box 2-3 illustrates a clinical course objective from the affective domain and behavioral exemplars for use as indicators of attainment.

Psychomotor Domain

The psychomotor domain pertains to the learning of technical skills. As previously discussed, the educational psychologists who created taxonomies for the cognitive and affective domains did not endeavor to do so with the psychomotor domain. Rather than focus on levels of psychomotor learning, in discussions related to this domain attention is directed more typically toward the application of learning theories than toward the learning of skills. Behavioral and cognitive learning theories both provide relevant principles that serve to guide skill acquisition. Box 2-4 provides a list of activities and conditions known to facilitate learning, retention, and transfer of psychomotor skills.

BOX 2-4
Techniques and Conditions for Learning, Retaining, and Transferring Psychomotor Skills

Learning of psychomotor skills is enhanced by:
- Quality of teacher-student relationship
- Positive self-concept ("I think I can")
- Identifying similarities to prior learning
- Understanding the meaning/value/use of the skill
- Relaxation techniques for reducing performance anxiety
- Mental rehearsal, especially imagery
- Reduction of distracting stimuli
- Clear, straightforward directions
- Pacing (slow enough)
- Sequential progression (steps)
- Modeling (teacher) followed by imitation (learner)
- Guided (prompted) learning early in learning process
- Quality feedback, both to reinforce and correct
- Frequent feedback
- Return demonstration
- Reflection and self-critique

Retention of psychomotor skills is enhanced by:
- Regular practice
- Adequacy of feedback during learning

Transfer of psychomotor skill learning is enhanced by:
- Positive self-concept
- Problem-solving strategies

■ REVISED, TWO-DIMENSIONAL TAXONOMY

In 2001, Anderson et al. published a revision of Bloom's taxonomy of educational objectives. Objectives continue to remain central to the educational process. The reason for revising Bloom's handbook in regard to the cognitive domain was primarily to incorporate the knowledge about learning that has evolved over the intervening years. To more accurately reflect newfound respect for the complexity of learning, the new taxonomy has two dimensions, which are depicted in Figure 2-1. Objectives are designed for each facet of the knowledge dimension, at each category of the cognitive process dimension.

The knowledge dimension, shown vertically in the figure, is composed of four categories progressing along a continuum of concrete *(factual)* to abstract *(metacognitive)* (Anderson et al., 2001). The categories of *conceptual* and *procedural* are seen as overlapping in terms of abstractness; some procedural knowledge is more concrete than the most abstract conceptual knowledge. Factual knowledge encompasses the knowledge, terminology and specific elements fundamental to the discipline (e.g., medical terminology, stages of pregnancy, primary/secondary/tertiary prevention). Conceptual knowledge addresses the interrelationships between the elements, organizing systems and theories (e.g., nursing process, relationship of pathology to manifestations). Procedural knowledge includes the knowledge behind skills, algorithms, and techniques, and the determination of when they should be used. This separates the knowledge basis of skills from the actual performance of the skill (e.g., Leopold's maneuvers, sterile technique, community assessment, suicide assessment). The final

The Knowledge Dimension	The Cognitive Process Dimension					
	Remember -recognizing -recalling	**Understand** -interpreting -exemplifying -classifying -summarizing -inferring -comparing -explaining	**Apply** -executing -implementing	**Analyze** -differentiating -organizing -attributing	**Evaluate** -checking -critiquing	**Create** -generating -planning -producing
Factual Knowledge						
Conceptual Knowledge						
Procedural Knowledge						
Meta-cognitive Knowledge						

FIGURE 2-1 ■ Components of the revised taxonomy of educational objectives. (Adapted from Anderson L.W. et al. (2001). *A taxonomy for learning, teaching, and assessing: A revision of Bloom's taxonomy of educational objectives.* New York: Addison Wesley Longman.)

category of *metacognitive* knowledge includes the subtle influence of the affective domain, as it reflects self-knowledge, thinking about one's thinking. It also contains the knowledge required for strategic planning and the contextual, conditional, and heuristic features of the discipline (e.g., reflective practice).

The cognitive process dimension, shown horizontally in the figure, is composed of six categories (remember, understand, apply, analyze, evaluate, and create) on a continuum of progressive cognitive complexity (Anderson et al., 2001). This dimension is a clear evolution of the previous levels of Bloom's cognitive domain. It provides a conceptual basis for progressive development within the various aspects of the knowledge dimension. Inherent to this development are the educational goals of promotion of retention and transfer; "...retention focuses on the past, whereas transfer emphasizes the future" (p. 63). Transfer of learning is the litmus test for meaningful learning, and all of the categories beyond that of remembering are increasingly associated with the transfer of learning. Each of the process categories is further subdivided with hierarchical action verbs, in the same fashion as Bloom's taxonomy, to be used to guide objective construction, selection of learning experiences, and ultimately, the evaluation of learning.

This redesigned taxonomy addresses some of the problems encountered with the original work and applies advances in both teaching and learning. It can improve teachers' understanding of objectives in determining what is important for nursing students to learn in the clinical setting, given all the contextual constraints of today's health care system. And then, it can provide direction in selecting learning experiences, making the most of serendipitous learning opportunities, and affording meaningful feedback to students. Unfortunately, little has been published in the nursing education literature discussing and demonstrating the application of the revised taxonomy. Clearly, expert teachers should provide guidance for novice faculty by endeavoring to fill this gap.

▪ DEVELOPING CLINICAL EXPERTISE: NURTURING THE NOVICE

Patricia Benner, in her exploration of experiential learning and skill acquisition in clinical nursing practice (2001), endeavored to articulate how practical knowledge develops and evolves over time. When she alluded to practical knowledge, Benner was referring to the practical wisdom of clinical judgment. Textbook knowledge "...is not the same as recognizing when and how these characteristics manifest themselves in particular patients, with a range of variation. This clinical discernment must be learned in practice" (Forward, p. x). Benner elucidated a sequential development with discrete levels of practice and clinical judgment. Her model provides guidance to faculty in clinical practice settings.

An evolutionary process of learning occurs in nursing practice. Beginning with clinical learning as students, "Expertise develops when the clinician tests and refines propositions, hypotheses, and principle-based expectations in actual practice situations" (Benner, 2001, p. 3). In Benner's model, the first stage of development is that of novice. Nursing students are novices at the beginning of their education, but also return to this baseline level with each new clinical area, because of their lack of experience with contextual issues. The student, who reached the level of marginally acceptable performance (advanced beginner) taking vital signs in the nursing home, regresses to the novice stage when moved to an acute care setting. As neophytes, novices bring an armamentarium of limited, inflexible, and context-free rule-governed behaviors to their clinical practice. For novice practitioners, Benner suggested teachers provide guidelines and structure, because these students can typically take in little of the situations in which they find themselves. What Benner calls aspect recognition is the primary focus of the novice (Benner, 2001). Learning to discriminate between serous and serosanguinous drainage on a dressing, or distinguishing wheezes from normal bronchovesicular breath sounds are examples of aspect recognition. At the end of their formal education, graduates have reached Benner's level of advanced beginner and are capable of identifying aspects of clinical situations, but only if they have had prior experiences with similar situations (Benner, 2001).

Operating from the perspective of caring theory, Benner (2001) asserts that "Understanding caring as a practice, rather than as pure sentiment or attitudes apart from the practice, reveals the knowledge and skill that excellent caring requires" (Forward, p. *x*). Teacher-student relationships and learning environments that are supportive are most likely to foster the development of practical knowledge. To prepare nurses who are equipped to enter nursing practice and further develop their clinical judgment, the teacher in the clinical setting must nurture the novice.

SUMMARY

In light of the existing and predicted challenges facing those in nursing education, outcomes-focused, traditional pedagogy is still necessary but no longer sufficient (Diekelman, 2005). Teaching and learning occur within a unique, often intensely personal, relationship between teacher and student. This is especially true in the clinical learning environment, where theory literally comes alive. Faculty charged with providing instruction in the clinical setting need to have a theoretical foundation for their teaching. An understanding of the behavioral and cognitive learning theories, educational philosophies and frameworks, the variety of pedagogies currently explicated and their applicability for clinical instruction, the domains of knowledge, and Benner's (2001) research implications for working with novices is foundational to effective clinical instruction.

REFLECTION EXERCISE 3

Reflecting on Theoretical Foundations

Take a moment to consider the following questions. Record your responses in your log.

◆ What are the assumptions embedded in traditional pedagogy?

◆ How are these assumptions challenged by the newer and newest pedagogies?

◆ As an adult learner, what are your thoughts and feelings about the role of experience in learning? How might you use this insight in your own teaching?

References

Adams, J.A. (1987). Historical review and appraisal of research on the learning, retention, and transfer of human motor skills. *Psychological Bulletin, 101*, 41-74.

Anderson, L.W., Krathwohl, D.R., Airasian, P.W., Cruikshank, K.A., Mayer, R.E., Pintrich, P.R., et al. (Eds.). (2001). *A taxonomy for learning, teaching, and assessing: A revision of Bloom's taxonomy of educational objectives.* New York: Addison Wesley Longman.

Bankert, E.G., & Kozel, V.V. (2005). Transforming pedagogy in nursing education: A caring learning environment for adult students. *Nursing Education Perspectives, 26*(4), 227-229.

Benner, P. (2001). *From novice to expert: Excellence and power in clinical nursing practice, commemorative edition.* Upper Saddle River, NJ: Prentice Hall Health.

Benner, P., & Wrubel, J. (1989). *The primacy of caring: Stress and coping in health and illness.* Menlo Park, PA: Addison-Wesley.

Bevis, E.O. (1988). New directions for a new age. In *Curriculum revolution: Mandate for change* (pp. 27-52). New York: National League for Nursing.

Bevis, E.O. (1989). *Curriculum building in nursing: A process* (3rd ed.). New York: National League for Nursing.

Bevis, E.O. (1993). All in all, it was a pretty good funeral. *Journal of Nursing Education, 32*(3), 101-105.

Bevis, E.O., & Watson, J. (1989). *Toward a caring curriculum: A new pedagogy for nursing.* New York: National League for Nursing.

Bloom, B.S., Engelhart, M.D., Furst, E.J., Hill, W.H., & Krathwohl, D.R. (1956). *Taxonomy of educational objectives: The classification of educational goals. Handbook I: Cognitive domain.* New York: David McKay Company.

Braungart, M.M. & Braungart, R.G. (2003). Applying learning theories to healthcare practice. In S.B. Bastable (Ed.). *Nurse as educator: Principles of teaching and learning* (pp. 43-71). Mississauga, ON, Canada: Jones and Bartlett.

Csokasy, J. (2002). A congruent curriculum: Philosophical integrity from philosophy to outcomes. *Journal of Nursing Education, 41*(1), 32-33.

Csokasy, J. (2005). Philosophical foundations of the curriculum. In D.M. Billings & J.A. Halstead (Eds.), *Teaching in nursing: A guide for faculty* (2nd ed.) (pp. 125-143). Philadelphia: Saunders.

Diekelmann, N. (2001). Narrative pedagogy: Heideggerian hermeneutical analyses of lived experiences of students, teachers, and clinicians. *Advances in Nursing Science, 23*(3), 53-71.

Diekelmann, N. (2003). Thinking-in-action journals: From self-evaluation to multiperspectival thinking. *Journal of Nursing Education, 42*(11), 482-484.

Diekelmann, N., & Lampe, S. (2004). Student-centered pedagogies: Co-creating compelling experiences using the new pedagogies. *Journal of Nursing Education, 43*(6), 245-247.

Diekelmann, N., & Scheckel, M. (2004). Leaving the safe harbor of competency-based and outcomes education: Re-thinking practice education. *Journal of Nursing Education, 43*(9), 385-387.

Diekelmann, N.L. (2005). Creating an inclusive science for nursing education. *Nursing Education Perspectives, 26*(2), 64-65.

Evans, B.C. (2004). Application of the caring curriculum to education of Hispanic/Latino and American Indian nursing students. *Journal of Nursing Education, 43*(5), 219-228.

Forrest, S. (2004). Learning and teaching: The reciprocal link. *Journal of Continuing Education in Nursing, 35*(2), 74-79.

Gardner, H. (1983). *Frames of mind: the theory of multiple intelligences.* New York: Basic Books.

Ironside, P.M. (2001). Creating a research base for nursing education: An interpretive review of conventional, critical, feminist, postmodern, and phenomenologic pedagogies. *Advances in Nursing Science, 23*(3), 72-87.

Ironside, P.M. (2005). Working together, creating excellence: The experiences of nursing teachers, students, and clinicians. *Nursing Education Perspectives, 26*(2), 78-85.

Knowles, M.S. (1980). *The modern practice of adult education: from andragogy to pedagogy* (2nd ed.). Chicago: Follett.

Kohlberg, I. (1984). *The psychology of mental development: The nature and validity of moral stages.* San Francisco: Harper and Row.

Krathwohl, D.R., Bloom, B.S., & Masia, B.B. (1956). *Taxonomy of educational objectives: The classification of educational goals. Handbook I: Affective domain.* New York: David McKay Company.

Mager, R.F. (1962). *Preparing instructional objectives.* Belmont, CA: Fearon/Lear Siegler.

Maslow, A. (1954). *Motivation and personality.* New York: Harper and Row.

Perry, W.C. (1970). *Forms of intellectual and ethical development in the college years: A scheme.* New York: Rinehart and Winston.

Reilly, D.E. (1978). *Teaching and evaluating the affective domain in nursing programs.* Thorofare, N.J.: Charles B. Slack.

Rogers, C. (1961). *On becoming a person.* Boston: Houghton Mifflin.

Romyn, D.M. (2001). Disavowal of the behaviorist paradigm in nursing education: What makes it so difficult to unseat? *Advances in Nursing Science, 23*(3), 1-10.

Scotto, C.J. (2003). A new view of caring. *Journal of Nursing Education, 42*(7), 289-291.

Tarnow, K.G., & Butcher, H.K. (2005). Teaching the art of professional nursing in the learning laboratory. *Annual Review of Nursing Education, 3*; 375-392.

Tyler, R.W. (1949). *Basic principles of curriculum and instruction.* Chicago: University of Chicago Press.

Vandeveer, M., & Norton, B. (2005). From teaching to learning: Theoretical foundations. In D.M. Billings & J.A. Halstead (Eds.), *Teaching in nursing: A guide for faculty* (2nd ed.) (pp. 231-281). Philadelphia: Saunders.

CHAPTER 3

Philosophy and Models of Clinical Nursing Education

Clinical nursing courses must involve students in comprehensive, spirited learning experiences that reflect the realities of nursing practice. To accomplish this, a variety of clinical learning settings appropriate to the specific goals of each course are carefully selected. The quantity of direct student supervision provided by academic faculty varies with the specific clinical setting, the objectives of the course, and the experience level of the students enrolled. This is what is meant by the term *models of clinical instruction;* who is involved in the supervision, teaching, and evaluation of students in the clinical setting? Table 3-1 provides a brief description and listing of common clinical nursing education models currently in use.

The purpose of academic faculty in the clinical setting was well articulated by Bevis in 1988, and regardless of the model selected, this vision should hold true. First, there is safety—safety for those with whom students work and safety for students. Assuring this is primarily a supervisory activity rather than one of teaching. Clinical faculty must assure that students have an adequate understanding of their nursing care activities in order to carry them out safely. And they must also assure that students are personally safe in their environment and in carrying out their care. Bevis saw this aspect of clinical supervision as important, but less so than the overall purpose of truly teaching, that is, creating the learning environment, organizing the learning experiences, and facilitating discussions with students. This is what is most conducive to the application of theory to the art and science of nursing practice. To fulfill this purpose, the teacher's primary role in the clinical setting is to "…raise questions that require reading, observation, analysis, and reflection upon patient care" (p. 46).

TABLE 3-1

Models of Clinical Nursing Education

MODEL NAME	MODEL DESCRIPTION
Traditional model	Faculty directly supervise and teach one group of students.
Faculty-directed independent experiences model	Students function without direct supervision according to specifically delineated instructions.
Collaborative models	
Clinical teaching associate (CTA) model	Staff nurses supervise and teach students with faculty direction. Learning experiences, assignments, and evaluation may be shared.
Clinical teaching partner (CTP) model	Teaching, supervision, and evaluation are shared between faculty and agency clinical nurse specialist (CNS).
Clinical educator/paired model	Student/staff pairing. Faculty are responsible for theory integration and evaluation.
Preceptor model	Long-term student/staff nurse preceptor team. Preceptor teaches and supervises according to individualized learning goals with variable faculty oversight.

Expanding this philosophy, actualizing it in educational practice, means that the role of faculty in the clinical setting should be:

> ...to nurture the learner; to nurture the ethical ideal, to nurture the caring role, to nurture the creative drive, to nurture curiosity and the search for satisfying ideas, to nurture assertiveness and the spirit of inquiry together with the desire to seek dialogue about care, and to be available for that dialogue. The teacher's role is to interact with the students as persons of worth, dignity, intelligence, and high scholarly standards (p. 46).

Whatever model of clinical instruction is used, clinical nursing faculty need to assure, to the best of their ability, that this occurs. What this means is that even using a model of clinical education in which some or all of the student supervision is delegated to others, ultimately, it is the faculty's responsibility to guide and facilitate the student's overall learning experience, to teach themselves or assure it is well done by others. Academic clinical faculty cannot abrogate this responsibility to others who may have technical skill competency but lack the theoretical knowledge and skill to facilitate optimal student learning.

Additional factors impact the models of clinical nursing education used in nursing curricula and in any single clinical course today. Increased student enrollments, competition for clinical placements among other nursing and allied health education programs, higher acuity plus rapid patient turnover generating increased demands on staff nurses in acute care agencies, as well as burgeoning numbers and varieties of community-based health care services are only a few of the current forces that influence clinical nursing education. In addition, the faculty role demands for scholarship are escalating. Knowledge grows exponentially, driving nurse educators' concerns regarding "covering content" sufficiently to adequately prepare students to function in today's high pressure health care system, let alone what is envisioned for the future. Guidance for faculty teaching clinical nursing courses in this mercurial health care and educational milieu is found in their clarity of purpose.

TRADITIONAL MODEL

The oldest and most common model of clinical nursing education is the traditional one. In this model, academic clinical faculty provide direct supervision and teaching for a group of students in a given setting (Stokes & Kost, 2005). The number of students in the clinical group may be governed by state legislation, but 8 to 10 students is typical. Agency personnel may provide some assistance, but clinical faculty retain primary responsibility for supervision, instruction, and evaluation. This model is used most often for beginning students, in in-patient transitional care settings (assisted living centers, rehabilitation centers, nursing homes), and in clinical settings where the patient acuity is high, such as in acute care institutions.

This model theoretically provides the teacher with maximal control over both learning and evaluation. Faculty present both skills and concepts exactly as desired. They guide the students' thinking and acting, assuring accuracy and thoroughness. There is the sense that students are learning what they need to know, at the level they need to know it. When the time comes for evaluation, because they have provided direct supervision and instruction, faculty theoretically have the necessary information to provide the best possible feedback to students.

Reality, however, may not mirror theory when the traditional model is used. In acute care settings, students often must be placed in several different areas of the facility because no single unit can accommodate all of the students in a clinical section. With this arrangement, even allowing no time for faculty breaks or traveling from one unit to another, each student in a 10-student group would receive an average of only about 45 minutes of one-on-one interaction with the teacher in an 8-hour clinical day! Faculty endeavor to accommodate for this problem in a variety of creative ways. Skill performance in the clinical setting may be limited to a certain number or type of skills each day or to a specific grouping of students (e.g., only students assigned to 1 or 2 specified units may give medications on a given day). Faculty may determine a specific level of performance as being adequate for independence with a given skill (e.g., administering oral medications, or performing dressing changes). Under some circumstances, faculty may rely on agency staff nurses to provide some skill supervision (e.g., double-checking insulin doses or approving the selection of an IV fluid before administration). Typically, faculty find it necessary to use written work as the primary source of evaluating students' understanding and application of theory. Another approach may be altering student/patient assignment patterns, so that student-faculty interactions occur in small groups. For instance, two students may be assigned to one patient—each charged with responsibility for different aspects of care. A common method of reducing the number of students requiring direct supervision is the use of another model for some students, usually faculty-directed independent experiences. If more clinical time must be used to meet the supervisory goal of ensuring safety, logically there is less time available to fulfill the other aspects of clinical nursing education.

FACULTY-DIRECTED INDEPENDENT EXPERIENCES MODEL

The faculty-directed independent experiences model of clinical instruction is used in community-based settings and to decrease the number of students requiring direct faculty supervision in acute or transitional care settings. Community-based settings are located within a large geographic area, and faculty may be miles away from their students, although remaining accessible via pagers or cell phones and making periodic site visits to observe and interact with students. Schools, physicians' offices, clinics, out-patient and ambulatory care centers, daycare centers, shelters and centers for the abused and/or homeless, private residences, and industrial businesses all can be sites for clinical learning experiences.

Although these settings are most often assigned to students further into their nursing education, beginning students may benefit from carefully designed learning experiences that do not involve direct faculty observation and supervision. Faculty-directed independent learning experiences are part of a variety of clinical nursing courses and may use many different teaching strategies. Students in a maternity-nursing course may follow an expectant mother throughout antepartum and on into the postpartum stage, performing assessments and patient teaching along the way. In acute care settings, students may have off-service experiences in areas such as IV therapy, interventional radiology, and out-patient dialysis centers. In order for this model to successfully facilitate student learning, faculty must have excellent relations with the site, provide clear direction to the students, and build into the experience the means to assure student accountability and enable evaluation of learning.

When an understanding of the purpose of the particular learning experience is lacking, students often flounder and become bored. Time spent in a daycare center can be interpreted as nothing more than babysitting if students are not given adequate direction in terms of their learning activities. In the Clinical Toolbox (Chapter 20, p. 349) is a sample assignment for a faculty-directed independent experience in a community-based surgical center. Checking to be sure the student arrived is as simple as making a telephone call; methods of evaluating the student's learning might include a paper, presentation, group discussion, or reflective journaling.

COLLABORATIVE MODELS

Nursing education is very expensive, primarily because of the costs associated with clinical instruction where the student-faculty ratio is so high. From an academic perspective, collaborative models address this fiscal issue while endeavoring to provide excellent role models of expert nursing practice. Agency nursing staff and clinical faculty in all of these models share the instructional role. However, there is considerable variation in the degree to which each participant is involved in supervising, teaching, and evaluating the students. Although preceptor models could conceptually be included here, they are usually seen as separate from the collaborative models due to both the number of students and collaborators involved and the role assumed by academic faculty. With both collaborative and preceptor models, the staff nurses must be knowledgeable about the nursing program and its curriculum in general, the given clinical course in particular, and also the theoretical foundations of clinical nursing education, teaching-learning strategies, and methods of evaluation. In reality, this foundational knowledge is often lacking. Using these models without adequate preparation of the collaborators diminishes the value of clinical nursing pedagogies.

Clinical Teaching Associate Model

In the clinical teaching associate (CTA) model, staff nurses work with clinical faculty by taking on certain functions with a predetermined number of students (Stokes & Kost, 2005). Applications of this model reported in the literature are found in the acute care setting, with the intent of providing close student supervision while freeing up faculty time to fulfill other role obligations (Phillips & Kaempfer, 1987; De Voogd & Salbenblatt, 1989; Baird, Bopp, Kruckenberg Schofer, Langenberg, & Matheis-Kraft, 1994; Hunsberger et al., 2000). A faculty member collaborates with CTAs for a section of students, again limited to 8 to 10. CTAs supervise several students apiece on their own nursing units, with each student caring for 1 or 2 patients. In the classical CTA model, staff nurses are responsible for supervision and teaching, functioning as resources and role models for students whereas the faculty member supervises the CTAs and may not be on site (Phillips & Kaempfer, 1987; De Voogd & Salbenblatt, 1989; Baird et al., 1994). Faculty also may supervise and teach, and student evaluation may be shared or retained as a faculty function. Decisions related to learning experiences and assignments are shared to varying degrees (Stokes & Kost, 2005).

In Australia, some hospitals and community-based health care agencies have created Dedicated Education Units (DEUs) in which all nursing staff function as CTAs. The service settings provide pay upgrades for the nurses involved, in recognition of their additional responsibilities. The academic institution provides faculty supervision of the nurses and the educational programs ("Partnership Approach to Nursing Education," 1999).

In a recent modification of the model, staff nurses assumed the teaching role for a small number of students (usually 3 to 4) on their own unit in a more equal relationship with faculty, and both were involved in clinical supervision (Hunsberger et al., 2000). These co-teachers took on complimentary roles during student orientation, with staff addressing agency-specific aspects of policies, procedures, equipment, and documentation, whereas faculty provided information related to school and course policies. After orientation, the staff member worked with the students the first day of a typical 2-day/week clinical course, which had an increased focus on time management and technical aspects of care. Faculty were then freed to attend to other aspects of their academic role for the day, returning at the end of the day for a postconference with the students and CTAs. The second day, the clinical nursing faculty member would provide supervision and focus a greater emphasis on the theoretical aspects of care. Preparing evaluations and meeting with students to discuss their progress was also a shared activity between CTAs and faculty (Hunsberger et al., 2000).

Some of the benefits of the CTA model cited include the staff nurses' satisfaction with the opportunity to learn more about clinical instruction and grow professionally (Hunsberger et al., 2000). Students reported that they felt they benefited from two different perspectives, and that they were more accepted in the agency because of the staff nurses' relationships. Faculty were able to remain clinically involved, with reduced student contact hours and increased time for other faculty responsibilities (Hunsberger et al., 2000). Other evaluations of this model also have been positive from the perspective of students, faculty, CTAs, and nurse managers (Baird et al., 1994).

There are also some obvious concerns with the CTA model. First is the matter of the breadth and depth of the CTAs' knowledge of theory and approaches to clinical nursing education. If CTAs are actually teaching and not simply supervising skill performance, the academic institution should provide preparation and ongoing education in these areas. The additional time required to deal with student-related paperwork was far more than many CTAs anticipated, and in some cases, they may not be reimbursed for these time expenditures. Also, the demands involved in the supervision and teaching of students, on top of being accountable for the patients was felt to be arduous by some of the CTAs (De Voogd & Salbenblatt, 1989). The clinical agencies must "buy into the model" and support its application, philosophically and practically. From an academic faculty perspective, the increase in time available for other role responsibilities could be offset by the need to supervise CTAs and reduced impact on the students' education (DeVoogd & Salbenblatt, 1989). However, with the increasing emphasis on academic and service collaboration and the escalating costs of nursing education, the clinical teaching associate model holds great promise if these concerns are addressed.

Clinical Teaching Partner Model

The clinical teaching partner model (CTP) is another collaborative effort between health care agencies and academic nursing programs. In this model, originally described by Shah and Pennypacker (1992), a hospital-based clinical nurse specialist (CNS) and an academic faculty member share in the management of a group of students in the clinical setting. The faculty member may have a joint appointment, evenly shared and financed by the health care organization and the academic institution, but this was not the case in the model presented by Shah and Pennypacker. The CNS typically holds an adjunct faculty appointment with the academic institution. A wide variety of health care professionals from the service and educational arenas may be appointed to adjunct faculty positions. Academic institutions that use adjunct faculty in any capacity have policies and procedures for their appointment and role. Adjunct faculty may present selected content based on their area of expertise, teach an entire clinical or theory course, act as preceptors, or be used as part of a clinical teaching partnership. Remuneration of adjunct faculty likewise varies, primarily based on the specific role they are fulfilling for the academic institution. In the CTP model Shah and Pennypacker (1992) described, the CNS was employed on a per diem basis as needed by the academic setting while continuing to work for the hospital.

Together, the faculty and CNS determine how to divide the work and time requirements of the clinical course (Shah & Pennypacker, 1992). Typically, a 2-day/week clinical course would be divided between the two. Evaluation is a shared responsibility. The CNS is fully oriented by the college or university and provides orientation to faculty and students regarding policies and procedures of the health care agency. The CNS is evaluated annually according to academic guidelines. As with the CTA model, faculty are freed from the full-time commitment to the course, so are able to pursue their scholarly efforts. Disadvantages of this model are the same as with the CTA model, but may be partially defused due to the CNS' advanced degree and exhaustive academic orientation. It cannot be assumed, however, that the CNS has the educational knowledge base necessary for teaching. Many of the advantages are the same, with the addition that the CNS is a Master's prepared nurse with an academic appointment, enhancing the potential for collaborative projects, research, and publications (Shah & Pennypacker, 1992). In this model, the faculty member deals with only one collaborator in the clinical setting, potentially providing more consistency and better communication. The advantages of this, however, may be diminished by the fact that in the CTA model there is a lower ratio of staff nurses to students, potentially allowing for closer supervision and better teaching of students than does the clinical partner model.

Clinical Educator/Paired Model

One final collaborative model has been reported in the literature. Like the CTA model, this approach uses staff nurses, but differs markedly in the ratio of student to educator. Student/clinical educator pairs are created. Faculty may use this model on a 1- to 2-day basis with a selected number of students, thus freeing up time that can be used to work with other, nonpaired students (Stokes & Kost, 2005). On the other hand, one faculty member may work with 8 to 10 pairs for a full academic term (Roche, 2002). Some might see this model as a derivation of the preceptor models, but they are typically used with senior students; here there is more faculty involvement and less student independence. The faculty responsibility is "...to integrate theory and clinical practice, cultivate deliberate reflection on practice patterns and decision making, and evaluate the students' progress in meeting defined goals" (Roche, 2002, p. 366).

Advantages and disadvantages of the clinical educator model are consistent with those of other collaborative models. Significantly higher scores in clinical decision-making skill were obtained by students in the clinical educator model as compared with those in the traditional model of clinical education (Roche, 2002). This model is particularly appropriate for specialized student experiences, such as critical care and emergency departments. Like faculty-directed independent experiences, this approach can be used periodically for some students to enrich their overall learning experiences, while increasing faculty time for supervision and teaching of other students using the traditional model.

PRECEPTOR MODELS

In preparing beginning practitioners, preceptors are characteristically used toward the end of the program, often as a clinical capstone experience. Students have the opportunity to explore a specific area of nursing practice, while being socialized into the role of practicing nurse. Students identify their goals and faculty assign a preceptor for a one-to-one relationship for a given period of time, usually several weeks (Stokes & Kost, 2005). A preceptorship can be developed anywhere an interested expert nurse practices. In addition to acute and critical care in adult and pediatric settings and in-patient maternity units, students may choose to explore nursing practice in a wide variety of community-based agencies, rural and even international experiences (Mallette, Loury, Engelke, & Andrews, 2005).

Depending on the application, a variable amount of faculty oversight is provided, but significantly less than in the collaboration models. Like the collaborative models, preceptor programs release faculty to attend to other role demands while students receive the benefits of working in a close relationship with expert practitioners. Again, however, teaching may be delegated to those without adequate preparation. It has been documented that preceptors tend to ask students lower-level questions than do faculty (Myrick, 2002). This observation leads naturally to recommendations for appropriate preparation (Alspach, 2000; Trevitt, Grealish, & Reaby, 2001) and suggests that faculty need to "precept the preceptor" regarding teaching and learning approaches (Myrick, 2002).

Preceptorships provide an opportunity for students to "put it all together." Encouraging students to think about and care for the whole patient is important to both faculty and preceptors. Eventually students become more holistic in their views, although initially they focus on performing as many technical skills as possible. Student nurses learn how to think like a nurse in this intimate interpersonal relationship, and they learn the centrality of caring to nursing practice (Nehls, Rather, & Guyette, 1997).

The tenet that the preceptor model should be limited to students who are at the end of their formal educational experience has been challenged increasingly (Nehls, Rather, & Guyette, 1997; Beeman, 2001). The individual attention afforded to a student over a prolonged time and the opportunity for the preceptor to truly get to know the student and spent time in dialogue regarding the application of theory to caring practices could be profoundly beneficial to beginning students (Nehls, Rather, & Guyette, 1997). These students are able to share their perceptions of their learning needs and of their actual experiences as they are addressing them; they hear expert nurses articulate their clinical decision-making process; and they obtain a more accurate understanding of nursing practice earlier in their educational experience than they would otherwise (Beeman, 2001).

SUMMARY

An assortment of models of clinical nursing education are currently being applied in an array of settings for students at various points in their educational process. The forces impacting nursing education, especially the shortage of qualified faculty and the cost of clinical education, generate impetus for the search for creative alternative methods. It is imperative that academic faculty assure students they will receive more than just supervision for the sake of safety concerns, regardless of the model chosen or created. Students, as novice learners, need to "learn how to learn—how to think critically—how to gain insights and find meanings—how to see patterns and how to capitalize on their paradigm experiences" (Bevis, 1988, p. 46). Faculty must assure that those to whom clinical education is delegated are capable of creating the environment, activities, and dialogue that will produce this outcome, or they must retain that responsibility themselves.

REFLECTION EXERCISE 4

Becoming a Nurse

Take a moment to think back to your own experiences as a student in the clinical setting.

◆ What clinical education models were part of your experience?

◆ If you experienced a nontraditional model, what feelings do you remember experiencing associated with faculty being at a distance? What role did the faculty play in the overall learning experience?

Now think beyond the supervision of skill performance.

◆ What do you remember now about learning what it is to be a nurse? Who contributed to that process? How did they accomplish that?

◆ Write a brief narrative of a particularly meaningful experience.

References

Alspach, J.G. (2000). *Preceptor handbook: From staff nurse to preceptor* (2nd ed.). Aliso Viejo, CA: American Association of Critical Care Nurses.

Baird, S.C., Bopp, A., Kruckenberg Schofer, K.K., Langenberg, A.S., & Matheis-Kraft, C. (1994). An innovative model for clinical teaching. *Nurse Educator, 19*(3), 23-25.

Beeman, R.Y. (2001). New partnerships between education and practice: Precepting junior nursing students in the acute care setting. *Journal of Nursing Education, 40*(3), 132-134.

Bevis, E.O. (1988). New directions for a new age. In *Curriculum revolution: Mandate for change.* (pp. 27-52). New York: National League for Nursing.

De Voogd, R., & Salbenblatt, C. (1989). The clinical teaching associate model: Advantages and disadvantages in practice. *Journal of Nursing Education, 28*(6), 276-277.

Hunsberger, M., Baumann, A., Lappan, J., Carter, N., Bowman, A., & Goddard, P. (2000). The synergism of expertise in clinical teaching: An integrative model for nursing education. *Journal of Nursing Education, 39*(6), 278-282.

Mallette, S., Loury, S., Engelke, M.K., & Andrews, A. (2005). The integrative clinical preceptor model: A new method for teaching undergraduate community health nursing. *Nurse Educator, 30*(1), 21-26.

Myrick, F. (2002). Preceptorship and critical thinking in nursing education. *Journal of Nursing Education, 41*(4), 154-164.

Nehls, N., Rather, M., & Guyette, M. (1997). The preceptor model of clinical instruction: The lived experiences of students, preceptors, and faculty-of-record. *Journal of Nursing Education, 36*(5), 220-227.

Partnership approach to nursing education. (1999). *Australian Nursing Journal, 7*(3), 31.

Phillips, S.J., & Kaempfer, S.H. (1987). Clinical teaching associate model: Implementation in a community hospital. *Journal of Professional Nursing, 3*(3), 165-175.

Roche, J.P. (2002). A pilot study of teaching clinical decision making with the clinical educator model. *Journal of Nursing Education, 41*(8), 365-367.

Shah, H.S., & Pennypacker, D.R. (1992). The clinical teaching partnership. *Nurse Educator, 17*(2), 10-12.

Stokes, L. & Kost, G. (2005). Teaching in the clinical setting. In D.M. Billings and J.A. Halstead (Eds.). *Teaching in nursing: A guide for faculty* (2nd ed.) (pp. 325-346). Philadelphia: Saunders.

Trevitt, C., Grealish, L., & Reaby, L. (2001). Students in transit: Using a self-directed preceptorship package to smooth the journey. *Journal of Nursing Education, 40*(6), 225-228.

CHAPTER 4

Today's Student, Tomorrow's Nurse: Characteristics and Clinical Educational Implications

An e-mail circulates through colleges and universities describing the incoming freshman class nearly every fall. Typically it focuses on historical and experiential reference points that these new students lack; implications for instruction are left to the reader. Life experiences define each generation; so, more than technologic advances or age, each generation reflects the societal changes that have impacted it (Darling, 2002). Each generation encompasses about a 20-year period. Some variation exists in terms of the year ranges used as generational cut-off points. The most common ones are applied here. For the most part, current nursing faculty were born between 1946 and 1960, what is known as the Baby Boom generation. The generation born between 1961 and 1981, following the Baby Boomers, is referred to as Generation X. Today, there are still plenty of students, and some faculty as well, who are representative of this generation. But the literature tells us that the newest generation, born after 1981, is markedly different from its predecessors in terms of attitudes and behaviors (Skiba, 2003). Additionally, this generation is predicted to diametrically reverse many of the trends initiated by the Baby Boom generation. Lest that observation be seen as overly negative, it is also predicted that this may be a true powerhouse generation, a generation of greatness with technologic adeptness and strong leadership potential (Howe & Strauss, 2000). Faculty have found it a challenge to make the necessary changes in their teaching approaches to adequately respond to the Gen-X student (and some have never accomplished it!). But the next generation will require revolutionary changes in teaching. This new generation

49

of students, who are just beginning to appear in higher education institutions, goes by a variety of names: generation Y, millennials, echo boomers, digital generation, net generation, generation next, and nexters (Clausing, Kurtz, Prendeville, & Walt, 2003; Skiba, 2003; Howe & Strauss, 2000). For clinical nursing faculty to be most effective, they must understand what today's students perceive nursing to be and why they made it their career choice. This knowledge, along with the characteristics of these two most current generations, has significant educational implications in the clinical setting.

WHAT IS NURSING?

A close relationship exists between how students see nursing and why they choose it as a career. The most current literature addressing student perceptions of nursing is drawn from Generation Xers, because this generation of students are just now appearing in programs of nursing.

Cook, Gilmer, and Bess (2003) found that beginning students' definitions of nursing could be broken down into categories consistent with nursing as a verb, as a noun, and in terms of a transaction. These categories with representational examples are found in Box 4-1.

These findings are similar to those of other studies conducted internationally, with some notable differences. In the United States, caring and nursing were not necessarily considered to be one and the same. Caring was definitely part of nursing, but these students defined nursing in broader terms. In a study of nursing students conducted in Norway, the concept of care provided the connection between nursing as a subject and nursing as a function (Granum, 2004). Although the students in the study by Cook et al. (2003) seemed to have quite an understanding of the characteristics that augment nursing's individuality as compared with other professions, they did not select traits typically used to describe professional identity (e.g., independence, leadership, critical thinking qualities, commitment to the profession). Caution must accompany

---

BOX 4-1
Beginning Students' Definitions of Nursing

Nursing as a verb	Nursing as a noun	Nursing as a transaction
Caring	Holistic system	Promotion of health
Nurturing	Connecting system	Treatment of illness
Teaching	Delivery system	Prevention of illness
Implementing	Discipline	Promotion of self-care
Assessing/analyzing		
Advocating		
Managing		

From Cook, Gilmer, and Bess, 2003.

any interpretation of these findings; however, the implications related to clinical nursing education are significant. The authors recommend that beginning nursing students need exposure to theories and application practice in areas such as "…ethics, patient-provider communication, finance and health policy, law, cultural competence, and interdisciplinary issues" (p. 317). Much of this can be accomplished in clinical courses and can provide the fodder for analysis and discussion resulting in perceptions of nursing that more accurately reflect its professional identity.

■ WHY CHOOSE NURSING?

What drives the selection of nursing as a career option is important to educators in recruiting students, and in fashioning their educational experiences. The choice is based on preconceptions, right and wrong, and the individual's attitudes and values. As students proceed through their education, the current realities and future projections engender an evolution of thought about what nursing is.

Again, the recent literature provides insight primarily about Generation Xers' selection of a career in nursing, because the Net Generation students are still new to the scene. In a qualitative study of beginning nursing students who had not yet been exposed to any clinical experience, Beck (2000) identified eight themes governing the selection of a career in nursing. The 27 students had a mean age at the time of the study of 24 ± 6.48, so they were likely born between 1970 and 1982—definitely Gen-Xers with a few early Net-Gens. These themes, in order of decreased frequency, are summarized in Box 4-2.

Beck's findings (2000) are not significantly different from those of previous research. However, health care and nursing have undergone major changes recently. Opportunities for direct patient care have decreased; nursing now involves more management skills because the nurse more often directs and supervises patient care delivered by others. Early clinical courses in nursing may

---

BOX 4-2

Reasons for Choosing Nursing as a Career

- Extreme desire and genuine love of helping others.
- Because it is a profession characterized by mutual benefits (nurse and patient).
- Previous caring experiences confirmed the inclination.
- Exposure to role models in the health care field.
- Actual observation of practicing nurses.
- Dissatisfaction with original career selection.
- Intentionally chose nursing because medical education was not seen as a viable option.
- Attraction to sciences and interest in the human body.

From Beck, 2000.

reinforce an increasingly obsolete perception of nursing; beginning courses need to provide a more realistic picture of nursing practice. Clinical courses must include experiences that positively illustrate the depth and breadth of nursing practice. The dissonance between preconceptions and reality may drive our students to seek other career options. If we fail to help our current students "…experience satisfaction and pleasure in working through others and in working in environments where constraints may be placed on them that will prevent them from always doing what ideally they would like to do with their patients" (p. 322), we face a grim future of disillusioned practitioners.

▨ GENERATIONAL CHARACTERISTICS

The influences of social forces and life experiences on each generation are profound. The Baby Boomers can be used as a baseline because comparisons are often made between this generation and the two that follow it.

Current Workforce: Baby Boomers

The end of World War II and the subsequent positive economic environment brought a period of calm optimism to the United States. Baby boomers experienced their childhood at a slower pace, so they are comfortable with delayed gratification (Darling, 2002). But they do want positive feedback, because they want to do well. Plenty of documentation, with less frequent feedback is expected (Billings, 2004). Technology common to society in general, and education and health care specifically, is often overwhelming to this generation; it was not part of their early educational experiences and came late, if at all, to their private lives. As students, they often require additional assistance in learning how to use computers, and become easily flustered with learning activities that require them to access web-based resources. The traditional model of pedagogy is comfortable and familiar to Boomers. They expect the teacher to be in charge, to determine what is important to be learned and then to teach it to them (Darling, 2002). The more structure, the better for these students, and challenging the instructor is the exception, not the rule. At the same time, these students expect to assume responsibility for their own learning (Billings, 2004). Finally, this generation is characterized by the expectation of a permanent career with the same institution (Darling, 2002). Organizational loyalty and commitment are the norm, with the expectation of financial remuneration and recognition for work well done (Billings, 2004). Baby Boomers comprise the entrenched work force. They are the dominant generation in nursing practice today.

Emerging Workforce: Generation X

Men and women born between roughly 1961 and 1981 comprise Generation X and are known as the "emerging work force." In their mid-twenties to mid-forties, many members of Generation X are still in the educational system and will progressively take over the practice arena. Box 4-3 provides a summary of the characteristics of this group.

BOX 4-3
Characteristics of Generation X (1961-1981)

- Independent; self-starting learners
- Technologically literate and dependent
- Excel at multitasking
- Adapt well to change
- Want flexibility, autonomy, and options in learning and life
- Lack interpersonal skills
- Impatient with process; outcome oriented
- Expect immediate gratification
- Desire to be trusted and respected for work performed
- Desire fun and balance of work and personal life
- Want to be lead, not managed
- Value money and material goods
- Daring, and expect to be challenged

Gen-Xers are significantly different from the Baby Boomers in a number of ways. Having grown up as the latchkey kids of working parents or single-parent households, Gen-Xers have developed a high level of independence (Darling, 2002). When their parents returned home, they became the center of attention; consequently, they developed high self-esteem, seen by some as arrogance (Wieck, 2003). They are creative problem-solvers, yet lack basic math skills and may have lower than expected reading capabilities (Darling, 2002; Wieck, 2003).

Growing up in a media-rich environment, most Gen-Xers see computers as a necessity and accessing information via the Internet as an expectation (Darling, 2002). Those who are less than literate with computers can find themselves left in the dust, both at work and at school. Members of Generation X expect a learning environment that is entertaining and stimulating and provides them with immediate feedback on demand (Darling, 2002; Wieck, 2003). Gen-Xers are able to consume and process information rapidly, and multitasking is so familiar it is nearly innate. They want their educational experiences to be flexible and to have a variety of options from which to choose (Wieck, Prydun, & Walsh, 2002; Billings, 2004; Darling, 2002). Relevance is essential to learning for Gen-Xers, who may demand that the value of learning experiences be made clear to them before they will participate (Darling, 2002).

Two observations of this emerging workforce have particular impact on education: Gen-Xers seem to be impatient with process, and they lack interpersonal skills (Wieck, Prydun, & Walsh, 2002). Both of these qualities can be attributed to their intensive exposure to television and less so, to computers. Gen-Xers prefer to be goal-directed and outcome-oriented, and become impatient with meandering meetings or classes. In school or the workplace, Gen-Xers want to be participative in determining goals and the means to attain them.

They have no inclination to defer to authority figures, on the job or at school (Wieck, 2003). The problems this can pose in both nursing education and practice are obvious. Some Gen-X nursing students may resist performing what they see as menial skills, beneath the "kind of nurse" they plan to be.

Having seen their Baby Boomer parents sacrifice home-time for work-time, and then lose the jobs they had worked for many years, Gen-Xers plan to be mobile, not staying long in any position and certainly not working their way up a job ladder. They are determined to have both their family and diversionary time, creating balance in their lives they did not see in their own childhood (Wieck, 2003). Money and the material wealth it can bring are important to Gen-Xers too, so they seek positions that will pay well without the expectation of long hours (Wieck, Prydun, & Walsh, 2002; Wieck, 2003).

The members of Generation X bring challenges and a new energy to nursing education and practice. They are adventurous and entrepreneurial, and with their skills in technology they seem to be ideal workers for the new millennium. At the same time, the differences in their attitudes and values generate friction with those of the entrenched Baby Boom workers and faculty.

Newest Generation: Net-Gen

In many important ways, individuals born after 1981 are remarkably different from both of the preceding generations. There is a tendency to focus on technology, especially the Internet, as the source of this difference, but that would be overly simplistic. Each generation is defined by its past, present, and future. This new generation reflects a sharp break from Gen-Xers and a direct reversal of the trends Baby Boomers established in their youth (Howe & Strauss, 2000). The Net Generation embodies some of the most positive attributes of their predecessors. They have the capacity to become the next great generation for America (Howe & Strauss, 2000). It has been said that this generation will comprise the ideal workforce. They bring to the table the can-do attitude of the World War II era, the work ethic of the Baby Boomers, and the technical know-how of Generation X (Zemke, Raines, & Filipczak, 2000). A partial listing of the characteristics of this generation is provided in Box 4-4.

Tapscott (2000) dubbed this generation the Net Generation because they are the first generation to grow up in an entirely digital technologic environment. Computers and digital cameras are ubiquitous; cell phones have instantaneous messaging and immediate photo transmission capabilities. All of these technologies are being connected increasingly to the Internet, producing a worldwide network of communication and resource access. This generation is "bathed in bits" and totally unintimidated by the technology. Tapscott predicts that it is through their use of digital media that Net-Geners will develop a culture that will superimpose over the rest of society. Young people growing up as part of the Net Generation use digital media in every aspect of their lives—to learn, work, and play.

As significant as technology is to the development of this generation, other social influences also have contributed to the evolution of this new generation. This is the most ethnically and racially diverse generation in American history

---

BOX 4-4
Characteristics of the Net Generation (1981-2002)

- Technologically addicted
- Social inclusion and globalization
- Embrace diversity
- Curious and creative
- Possess a strong work ethic
- Collaborative team players
- Highly mobile
- Highly intelligent
- Optimistic
- Self-sufficient and assertive
- Respect and admire their parents
- Rule followers
- Anticipate multiple career changes

(Howe & Strauss, 2000). This inherent diversity, combined with their ability to communicate electronically with friends and colleagues around the world virtually instantaneously, means that the preoccupation of prior generations with differences between people and groups is dissolving for the Net Generation (Tapscott, 2000).

This is the era of the wanted and protected child. Net-Geners were raised in an environment in which they were made to feel special, where trust and confidence blossomed, where pressures to excel were rewarded and resulted in high achievement (Howe & Strauss, 2000). Net-Geners lack the competitive orientation of preceding generations, preferring to collaborate and support those they work or study with (Clausing et al., 2003). From the perspective of Net-Geners, reward for their efforts lies in the personal meaning of the work and in the opportunity to learn something new. But their expectation is that feedback will be immediate and available on demand (Billings, 2004).

Linear processing of information is incongruent with computers and hence the assimilation of information. Instead, the Net-Gen learner appears to be collecting information randomly, collating it into patterns, and reflecting on the resulting formulation before coming to a conclusion (Murray, 2004; Clausing et al., 2003). The result is more rapid and meaningful learning, a sort of intellectualized gestalt.

A significant difference in this generation is their attitude toward adults and aging (Tapscott, 2000; Clausing et al., 2003). Net-Geners admire and respect their parents and other adults and insist they are more mature than might be expected (Howe & Strauss, 2000). The preoccupation with youth that is common to Baby Boomers, and even to some degree with GenXers, is far from the case among Net-Geners. They face the future with optimism, and multiple changes of not just workplace but career hold no trepidation for them. Carrying their patience, trust, and action orientation into the community, this generation will "…set high standards, get organized, team up, and do civic deeds" (Howe & Strauss, 2000, p. 66).

The individuals comprising the Net Generation, as they mature and make their mark on the world, will function as an orchestrated collective. They will derive power and vigor from connection and conformity, and honor from responsibility (Howe & Strauss, 2000). They bring new skills and a new mindset to nursing education and hold great promise for the profession of nursing.

IMPLICATIONS OF GENERATIONAL DIFFERENCES FOR NURSING CLINICAL EDUCATION

In a classroom packed with students, opportunities to individualize teaching approaches are limited. Fortunately, this is not true of teaching in the clinical setting. The ability of faculty to personalize their approach to students in this learning environment surely contributes to the quality of teacher-student relationships and to the overall value of the learning experience. Part of this individualization lies in accounting for generational differences among students and their expectations of a career in nursing.

The incorporation of generational differences into clinical instructional methods should begin with a personal assessment by each faculty member. The first two parts of the reflection exercise that follows this discussion may be useful as a starting point. Obviously, technology is a huge part of nursing, education, and the world in which all living generations exist. As a faculty working with students of both Generation X and the Net Generation, technologic competence is an important issue. Acknowledge deficits and discomforts and seek assistance from the resources available in the academic and clinical settings. If computer charting is used in the facilities where your students will be, learn the system yourself in advance and get to know the personnel that will be most helpful later in the event assistance is needed. If the clinical course uses an online format such as Blackboard, gain some competency with it before classes begin, and again, identify someone who can serve as a resource. If possible, consider developing a personal website. If it is available, sit in on a class offered to students at the beginning of the program that addresses accessing and evaluating Internet resources. Soon such courses will be obsolete! There will likely be library materials that may be useful. Build the goal of enhancing personal computer competency into a long-term development plan (see Unit VI). Most likely, students will have a range of computer competencies. Net-Geners will be supportive and inclined to help their colleagues and faculty alike.

Specific activities for getting to know the students in a clinical group will be explored later, in Unit III, but a part of this time should include some discussion of how each student learns best, what their perceptions and expectations are about nursing in general and this course specifically. Generational differences will likely emerge as a common theme. Assess computer and technologic expertise, comfort with group and individual work, and communication skills. Ask the students to identify their commitments outside of school, and what they do for fun and to reduce their stress. Encourage balance from the beginning.

For the course itself, spell out the expectations clearly on paper and review them with the group at the beginning of the course. Have some general plan for providing feedback to the students, and then discuss their individual expectations for frequency and format. Talk with the students about what is "set in stone" and what is flexible within the confines of the setting and course, providing options for experiences and assignments whenever possible. Encourage the use of electronic media: calculators and portable reference materials such as drug guides. Clarify with the students the appropriate use or curtailment of cellular phones in the clinical setting. Try to break up sitting time with active time; even the college standard of 50-minute periods may prove difficult for some students to endure. And inject fun and humor appropriately. A former colleague began every clinical conference, seminar, and class with a joke, encouraging students to provide them whenever possible.

SUMMARY

Special people are drawn to nursing, for different reasons and with different expectations and goals. To a certain degree, these differences are generationally derived. To provide the best possible clinical learning experience to each individual student, an understanding of these differences is essential. The Nursing Education Advisory Council of the National League for Nursing recently developed a series of standards, "Hallmarks of Excellence in Nursing Education" ("Anonymous," 2004). Part of one of these hallmarks is "Students are excited about learning, exhibit a spirit of inquiry and a sense of wonderment..." (p. 98). Clinical faculty are in a unique position to ignite that excitement, foster the inquiry, and promote wonderment and awe for nursing in our practitioners of the future. The better we know our students, the better we can accomplish those goals.

REFLECTION EXERCISE 5

Nursing and Generational Differences

◆ Think back to what contributed to your selection of a nursing career. What were your expectations of nursing practice? What have you found to be personally rewarding? Disappointing? What are your feelings about the future of nursing and your place in it?

◆ What are your own preferences for learning? How are they similar or different from those associated with your generation?

◆ Consider the themes identified in Beck's (2000) study. Given the current health care environment, what clinical learning experiences could help students address them?

◆ As a clinical faculty, how might you become aware of and accommodate generational differences among your students while avoiding stereotyping?

◆ How might generational differences affect how students might interact during clinical conferences or other group situations? What might you do to facilitate group interaction?

References

Anonymous. (2004). Hallmarks of excellence in nursing education. *Nursing Education Perspectives, 25*(2), 98-101.

Beck, C.T. (2000). The experience of choosing nursing as a career. *Journal of Nursing Education, 39*(7), 320-322.

Billings, D. (2004). Teaching learners from varied generations. *Journal of Continuing Education in Nursing, 35*(3), 104-105.

Clausing, S.L., Kurtz, D.L., Prendeville, J., & Walt, J.L. (2003). Generational diversity—the Nexters. *AORN, 78*(3), 373-379.

Cook, T.H., Gilmer, M.J., & Bess, C.J. (2003). Beginning students' definitions of nursing: An inductive framework of professional identify. *Journal of Nursing Education, 42*(7), 311-317.

Darling, L. (2002). Learning: Generation does matter! *Element K Newsletter.* Retrieved October 26, 2004, from http://www.elementk.com/training_advice/htm/05-02-learninggen.asp

Granum, V. (2004). Nursing students' perceptions of nursing as a subject and a function. *Journal of Nursing Education, 43*(7), 297-304.

Howe, N. & Strauss, S. (2000). *Millennials rising: The next great generation.* New York: Vintage Books.

Murray, J.P. (2004). Nursing: The next generation. *Nursing Education Perspectives, 25*(3), 106.

Skiba, D.J. (2003). The net generation: Implications for nursing education and practice. In NLN Living Book (Chapter 1). Retrieved October 26, 2004, from http://www.electronicvision.com/nln/chapter01/chapter_01.htm.

Tapscott, D. (2000). The rise of the net generation: Growing up digital. Retrieved October 27, 2000, from http://www.growingupdigital.com/

Wieck, K.L. (2003). Faculty for the millennium: Changes needed to attract the emerging workforce into nursing. *Journal of Nursing Education, 42*(4), 151-157.

Wieck, K.L., Prydun, M., & Walsh, T. (2002). What the emerging workforce wants in its leaders. *Journal of Nursing Scholarship, 34*(3), 283-288.

Zemke, R., Raines, C., & Filipczak, B. (2000). *Generations at work: Managing the clash of veterans, Boomers, Xers, and Nexters in your workplace.* New York: Amacom.

Legal and Ethical Issues in Clinical Nursing Education

CHAPTER 5

Rights and Responsibilities: The Clinical Setting

■ ESTABLISHING CLINICAL CONTRACTS
■ AGENCY POLICIES AND PROCEDURES
■ REGULATORY LAWS
  Confidentiality and the Health Insurance Portability and
    Accountability Act
  Student Safety and the Occupational Safety and Health Administration
■ ACCREDITATION
  Joint Commission on the Accreditation of Healthcare Organizations
■ SUMMARY
■ *REFLECTION EXERCISE 6: CLINICAL AGENCY POLICIES
  AND PROCEDURES*

When discussing legal and ethical issues related to nursing education, the focus is typically on the educational program, its faculty, and the student. In teaching clinical courses, however, it is also important to have some understanding of legal and ethical issues pertinent to the sites at which students are placed. Faculty need this information so they can conform to the agencies' requirements and also assist the students in gaining an appreciation of these topics from the agencies' perspective.

It is true that faculty teaching clinical courses are responsible for the selection of sites for student placement that will best meet the course objectives and also for negotiating contracts between the nursing program and these settings (Stokes & Kost, 2005). However, such an expectation of novice faculty is rare. Instead, novice faculty are more likely to be assigned to clinical settings that have already been established. In either instance, faculty are expected to be aware of the rights and responsibilities of the agency, both in relation to the nursing program and its students as specified in the contract, and more generally as stipulated in the agency's policies and procedures. The affiliation contract also addresses those obligations to be reciprocated by the nursing program to the clinical setting and its personnel. Regardless of the setting, agencies expect nursing students to be aware of applicable standards developed by the Occupational Safety and Health Act. One of the most important concerns of health care agencies is student and faculty compliance with the requirements of the Health Insurance Portability and Accountability Act (HIPAA). At health care sites, students are often involved in accreditation team visits, usually made by the Joint Commission on the Accreditation of Healthcare Organizations (JCAHO).

61

Students need to understand the concept of accreditation in general and to understand specifically their role if they are approached by a surveyor. An understanding of the rights and responsibilities of the clinical settings used in the course is essential for a successful student learning experience and contributes to the legal and ethical protection of faculty and students alike.

ESTABLISHING CLINICAL CONTRACTS

A wide variety of settings are used as practicum experiences for student nurses. Not all of these are health care agencies; community settings such as day care centers, senior residential communities, and neighborhood community centers are also used for the practical education of student nurses. Regardless of the setting, a formal contract must be in place for each one, delineating the expectations and obligations of each party.

Affiliation agreements between the academic institution that houses the nursing program and the sites at which students are placed are carefully designed and involve appropriate legal consultation. Using a template assures that key components of the agreement are consistently addressed. Details that are subject to change from term to term are best covered in a separate document. Although novice clinical faculty are unlikely to be responsible for initiating contracts with clinical settings, it could be beneficial to them to obtain and review a contract template for their specific nursing program. Although the contract may specify that the beginning dates and duration of student experiences must be confirmed a certain amount of time prior to the initiation of the experience, the actual dates may be part of a letter directed to the agency. This letter would also typically address the number of students to be placed in the agency, the days of the week, hours, and specific locations within the agency to be used because these may change from term to term. The contract would likely require the nursing program to supply objectives for each course and information related to the skill and knowledge capabilities of the students. The letter could then provide course-specific information and the name of a contact person within the nursing program.

In the contract, the academic institution provides assurance to the agency that the faculty placed there are qualified to teach; in the case of nursing education, assurance is provided that faculty are appropriately licensed to practice. If agency personnel are to function as preceptors, or as part of some other model of clinical nursing education, the role of the academic institution in the provision of adequate preparation should be addressed in the contract. The role of each party in the task of student evaluation and grading should be defined. The academic institution agrees to provide relevant student information to the agency. Typically, in addition to the students' names, this would include CPR certification and documentation of the currency of immunizations and TB screening. Depending on the state statutes and the academic program, criminal background clearance also may be required. The nursing program is obligated to provide the agency with information regarding the overall curriculum and assures the agency that students will be expected to comply with their policies and procedures.

Clinical settings used by nursing programs are expected to provide students with access to the resources they will need for their learning. This may be detailed in the contract in terms of patient/client access, supplies, and equipment. Agencies may retain the right to enforce their own policies on students, such as mandatory drug testing or the prohibition of students with any prior history of criminal conduct. It should be clearly stated that students cannot be relied on for the comprehensive care of clients/patients and should never be taken into consideration for personnel staffing purposes. This is an important legal point, reinforcing the mandated responsibilities of licensed professional nurses employed by the agency. Safety is paramount, and agency personnel must reserve the right to remove students from any situation they perceive as compromising the safety of either students or patients. Because the nursing program encourages compliance with agency policies and procedures, the agencies may state compliance as an expectation of students and reserve the right to remove students who fail to do so. The clinical setting may require conformity with appearance and dress standards unique to the location, but both the nursing program and the site expect appropriate student identification badges.

An important component of affiliation contracts is the discussion of liability. A great deal depends on the applicable laws of the state and the liability coverage provided by the nursing program to its faculty and students. The parameters of the liability provisions should be clearly articulated in the contract.

Contracts may speak to other mutually pertinent issues, such as confidentiality of records, provision of emergency medical care to students in case of injury on site, training related to protection from and interventions following exposure to blood-borne pathogens, and the grounds for termination of the agreement. Authorized representatives of the nursing program and the agency sign the agreement, and both parties then retain copies of the contract. Contracts usually remain in effect until modified or terminated, so do not have to be routinely negotiated. Letters addressing only the term to term changes are adequate.

▦ AGENCY POLICIES AND PROCEDURES

Policies and procedures, developed in accordance with the mission and unique needs of each agency, are influenced by applicable accreditation and/or licensing standards; state, federal, and local legislation; and pertinent practice standards (Brent, 2001). Those appropriate to health care settings are often not applicable to day care centers or low-income residential hotels. Variance is expected between health care facilities catering to different patient populations, for example, long-term care as compared to outpatient clinics. Some policies and procedures followed in acute care facilities vary between units; all those germane to pediatric units are not suitable for labor and delivery.

Faculty teaching courses in clinical settings should have more than a passing knowledge of each agency's guidelines and courses of action in order to support them in regard to their students. For instance, a hospital may have a policy that whenever possible, urinary catheterization procedures are performed by a staff member of the same gender as the patient. Being aware of this policy, faculty can take it into consideration as they and their students seek learning opportunities. Some policies, based on legislative mandates, are consistent across health care settings but vary in terms of the procedural mechanisms applied. This is true, for example, in the policies regarding the use of physical restraints. Health care agencies all have to follow the same general requirements but may differ in precisely how the policies are carried out procedurally. In some cases, agency policies require faculty preparation in advance of the initiation of any patient contact by students. This may include requirements such as the submission of student data related to immunizations, TB status, and results of drug screening; photos or identification numbers for issuing student and faculty nametags that are agency specific or passes for parking in staff parking lots; and student and faculty names needed for access to agency computers and databases. Knowing such policies exist allow faculty to make advance arrangements and thereby avoid delaying student contact with clients. Such documentation has been beneficial in court cases (Brent, 2001).

Formal agency orientation often includes important procedures related to fire and disaster management and to documentation in patient records. When students attend these orientations, faculty should document in their own records the content covered. They can then hold students accountable in relation to these procedures and reinforce them appropriately during the term.

Although implementation of both policies and procedures still requires the judgment of the individual health care worker, and are not meant to be followed blindly (Brent, 2001), deviations by student nurses should occur only in consultation with faculty and/or agency personnel. "When deviation from established policies and procedures occurs, liability may result..." (Brent, 2001, p. 78) and both faculty and students may be included in the liability.

REGULATORY LAWS

Health care agencies, and many other types of settings used in the clinical education of nursing students, are tightly regulated by laws emanating from the federal, state, and local judiciary (Brent, 2001). Day care centers for children and adults, for example, must comply with certain standards in order to be licensed at the state level and must conform to local zoning regulations. A general familiarity with those laws applicable to the site is beneficial for both faculty and students.

Ethically, confidentiality is to be protected in all instances of student-client interaction. In health care facilities, students and faculty alike should understand the implications of the Health Insurance Portability and Accountability Act (HIPAA). Additionally, in all settings there are applications to student clinical practice derived from the recommendations of the Occupational Safety and Health Administration (OSHA) of the Department of Labor.

Confidentiality and HIPAA

The protection of private, personal information by health care workers is supported by codes of ethical conduct and a number of state and federal laws.

From the position of clinical settings, the concern is student access to this information and its protection from inappropriate dissemination. HIPAA was passed in 1996 and became fully effective in the spring of 2003 (Waldo, 2000; Calloway & Venegas, 2002; Maddox, 2002; Maddox, 2003; Ziel & Gentry, 2003). HIPAA is a federal law whose confidentiality regulations supercede prior federal laws and all less stringent state laws (Calloway & Venegas, 2002; Maddox, 2002).

HIPAA came into being in response to a number of national public and professional concerns (Calloway & Venegas, 2002). Patients reported escalating distress about breaches in confidentiality and the erosion of public trust in the protection of private health care information. According to the preamble to the privacy rules, Congress had data indicating 20% of Americans believe information about their health is used inappropriately, and one of six acknowledge providing false information to health care providers out of fear that confidentiality would not be maintained (Calloway & Venegas, 2002). The burgeoning application of Internet technology in the health care industry generated further apprehension in the ability of the multiple systems in use to protect the veracity and security of health information communicated electronically (Waldo, 2000). Congress saw HIPAA as a means of addressing a plethora of problems in health care.

HIPAA's many goals include decreasing expensive overhead in health care by simplifying health insurance administration; offering improved access to health insurance by allowing it to be portable between employers; generation of more powerful provisions for the investigation and prevention of Medicare fraud; improving access to long-term care services and coverage; and enhancing standards for the security and privacy of health information (Waldo, 2000; Calloway & Venegas, 2002; Maddox, 2002). HIPAA legislation applies to any group that handles individually identifiable health care information (Maddox, 2002). Essentially, four entities are required to comply with HIPAA: health care clearinghouses, health plans, health providers, and the business associates of these three groups. Compliance by these groups is not optional; this is federal law, and compliance is mandatory (Calloway & Venegas, 2002).

Noncompliance with HIPAA mandates by health care providers can result in the imposition of major criminal and civil penalties including liability (Calloway & Venegas, 2002; Maddox, 2002; Maddox, 2003; Ziel & Gentry, 2003). Health care personnel in inpatient and outpatient settings that serve as clinical sites for nursing education are understandably committed to enforcing student compliance with HIPAA's privacy and security regulations. Faculty teaching these courses also must understand these requirements and know how to direct students in accordance with this compliance. If students begin their first clinical course armed with the basic knowledge related to the applicable standards, clinical agencies will need to address only *how* they will specifically enforce the standards.

For the health care providers working with nursing students, the privacy and security of all patient records and other individually identifiable health information in any electronic, written, or oral format is the significant issue associated with HIPAA standards. As differentiated by HIPAA, *security standards* deal with measures taken to keep patient health information safe, whereas the *privacy standards* deal with the actions taken related to how the information obtained is used (Calloway & Venegas, 2002).

Occurrences termed "incidental disclosures," such as discussing patients at the nurses' station, in the hallway, or in the patients' rooms, are permitted, provided the facility ensures these are kept to the "minimum necessary" (Calloway & Venegas, 2002). Security standards are maintained when personnel avoid talking about patients in public areas where they may be overheard, such as in elevators and the cafeteria of the facility (Calloway & Venegas, 2002; Ziel & Gentry, 2003). Security standards also apply to the patient's health information if it is shared anywhere it might be overheard by a third party, such as outside a classroom or in the school library.

Nursing students must be alert to avoid inappropriately sharing patient information, and they also must know what information may be shared under the appropriate circumstances. The patient's medical record, now to be termed *protected health information (PHI)*, contains individually identifiable health information (IIHI) (Calloway & Venegas, 2002). If these IIHIs are removed from a medical record, the de-identified patient data are no longer covered by HIPAA requirements and can then be disclosed (security) in specified situations (privacy). Information considered to be IIHI is detailed in Box 5-1. Gender, race, ethnicity, marital status, and age are examples of information that can remain in the record, although if the patient is older than 90, age must be reported as 90+ (Calloway & Venegas, 2002).

BOX 5-1
Individually Identifiable Health Information

- Patient name
- Names of patient's relatives
- Name of patient's employer
- PHI (medical record) number
- Date of birth
- Address
- Street name and number; apartment number
- City
- County
- Zip code (unless ≥ 20,000 people live there)
- Photographs
- Fingerprints
- Voiceprints
- Telephone and FAX numbers
- Numbers of any accounts, including Social Security
- Driver's license number
- Names of any health beneficiaries

When students collect information in advance of or during patient care, it must be de-identified. It should be presented in that de-identified format verbally, electronically, or in writing in logs or journals, care plans or concept maps, papers, projects, presentations, or any other assignment sanctioned by faculty for their courses. Students should not read the charts of patients for whom they are not providing care (Calloway & Venegas, 2002). Such approaches maintain HIPAA standards for both security and privacy and protect the interests of the health care facility while helping students learn professional practice expectations for maintaining the confidentiality of patient information.

Student Safety and OSHA

The mission of the Occupational Safety and Health Administration (OSHA) is to "...assure the safety and health of America's workers by setting and enforcing standards; providing training, outreach, and education; establishing partnerships; and encouraging continual improvement in workplace safety and health" (OSHA, http://www.osha.gov/). The power to accomplish this mission is derived from the Occupational Safety and Health Act of 1970. This federal law is designed to provide a safe environment for workers in the states and territories of the United States (Brent, 2001). OSHA enforces the Act through the promulgation of standards, workplace inspections, and the review of complaints. The standards are far reaching, even contributing to the protection of privacy and information management. But the primary focus is the protection of worker safety (OSHA, http://www.osha.gov/).

It was through OSHA that the universal precautions for blood-borne pathogens originated, following the recommendations of the Centers for Disease Control and Prevention (CDC) (Brent, 2001). Students should be taught, and have the opportunity to practice, universal precaution protocols prior to any patient or client contact in their first clinical course. Reinforcement is then provided in the clinical setting as needed.

OSHA also provides guidelines related to protection from and management of exposure to hazardous materials. Much of this information can be provided to students at the specific time they need it in relation to a clinical experience (e.g., precautions related to radiation exposure when observing or participating in procedures that involve radiation). Certain clinical experiences cannot be provided for students because they require additional OSHA-mandated training (e.g., administration of parenteral chemotherapy). Some other workplace safety issues that may not be addressed by OSHA may be regulated instead at the level of state law. If an appropriate OSHA standard has been mandated, federal law trumps that of the state (Brent, 2001).

ACCREDITATION

A variety of private organizations provide accreditation for compliance with their established standards. Although not legally mandated, the standards of some of these accreditation bodies are used in court cases (Brent, 2001).

JCAHO

The Joint Commission on the Accreditation of Healthcare Organizations (JCAHO) is a private health care accreditation body that monitors and evaluates patient care for quality, utilization, and risk management according to standards established by health care professionals (Joint Commission on the Accreditation of Healthcare Organizations [JCAHO], 2004; Brent, 2001). More than 15,000 health care organizations, both in the United States and abroad, are accredited by JCAHO (JCAHO, 2004). From hospitals, home care, and long-term care facilities to ambulatory care facilities and laboratories, organizations requesting accreditation agree to be measured by these JCAHO standards, to the identification of their strengths and weaknesses, and to accept the resulting education and consultation proffered in order to improve the quality of care provided. Accreditation confers a wide variety of other benefits, including expedited third-party payments and assistance in personnel recruitment (JCAHO, 2004). Trained surveyors make "site visits" to accredited organizations on routinely scheduled and occasionally unannounced bases. The scheduled visits are preceded by a flurry of activity by the facility which often engenders an undercurrent of tension. If such a visit will occur while students are assigned to the agency, they should be provided with an understanding of the purpose and significance of the inspection. Since surveyors may query students if they are present on site simultaneously, faculty should discuss with students in advance the types of questions they are likely to be asked. Most commonly, students are asked what they should do in the event of a fire, how to "call a code," or other questions regarding similar topics they should be familiar with as a result of their orientation and experience with the agency.

SUMMARY

The sites used for practicum courses have a variety of ethical and legal obligations of which academic faculty and their students should be aware. All these sites should have an affiliation contract with the academic institution, delineating the rights and responsibilities of each in relation to the other. Policies and procedures of each clinical site will vary, depending on its singular charge and requirements, whether or not accreditation or licensing standards are applicable, and the legislation or other standards that may be relevant. Federal, state, and local laws closely control many different types of facilities used for nursing student education. Regardless of the setting, there are implications for student safety based on the standards of the Occupational Safety and Health Administration (OSHA). The Health Insurance Portability and Accountability Act (HIPAA) imposes special confidentiality standards on health care facilities, their employees, and by extrapolation, nursing students. Finally, many agencies are impacted by accreditation requirements. Student nurses are very likely to be involved in visitations by surveyors for the Joint Commission on the Accreditation of Healthcare Organizations (JCAHO) during their clinical experiences in health care facilities. Faculty who understand the rights and responsibilities of the clinical settings in which their students are placed can share and bolster them in their students. Having such an approach will foster a more positive learning environment and will afford additional legal and ethical safeguards for all concerned.

Clinical Agency Policies and Procedures*

Reflect back on your experiences in clinical practice.

◆ If you were to teach a clinical course using one of those agencies as an example, what policies and procedures do you think would be essential for students to know from the beginning of the course?

◆ Are there other policies and procedures that could wait? Why? When would it be appropriate to introduce them?

*NOTE: Legal and ethical issues discussed in Chapters 5-7 will be specifically applied to clinical nursing education in Chapter 8. For now, consider the topics presented in isolation.

References

Brent, N.J. (2001). *Nurses and the law: A guide to principles and applications* (2nd ed.). Philadelphia: Saunders.

Calloway, S.D. & Venegas, L.M. (2002). The new HIPAA law on privacy and confidentiality. *Nursing Administration Quarterly, 26*(4), 40-54.

Joint Commission on the Accreditation of Healthcare Organizations (JCAHO). (2004). Retrieved November 28, 2004, from http://www.jcaho.org.

Maddox, P.J. (2002). HIPAA: Update on rule revision and compliance requirements. *Nursing Economics, 20*(2), 88-92.

Maddox, P.J. (2003). HIPAA: Update on rule revision and compliance requirements. *Medsurg Nursing, 12*(1), 59-63.

Stokes, L. & Kost, G. (2005). Teaching in the clinical setting. In D.M. Billings and J.A. Halstead (Eds.). *Teaching in nursing: A guide for faculty* (2nd ed.). (pp. 325-346). Philadelphia: Saunders.

Waldo, B.H. (2000). HIPAA: The next frontier. *Nursing Economics, 18*(1), 49-50.

U.S. Department of Labor Occupational Safety & Health Administration (OSHA). Mission statement. Available at http://www.osha.gov.

Ziel, S.E. & Gentry, K.L. (2003). Ready? HIPAA's here. *RN, 66*(2), 67-70.

CHAPTER 6

Rights and Responsibilities: The Student

- LEGAL AND ETHICAL ORIGINS OF RIGHTS AND RESPONSIBILITIES
- STUDENT RIGHTS
- DUE PROCESS
- PRIVACY
- NONDISCRIMINATION
- FIRST AMENDMENT LIBERTIES
- STUDENT RESPONSIBILITIES
- CODES OF CONDUCT
- LEGAL RESPONSIBILITIES IN CLINICAL SETTINGS
- SUMMARY
- *REFLECTION EXERCISE 7: CONSIDERING STUDENT RIGHTS AND RESPONSIBILITIES*

Nursing students must conform to the policies and procedures of the agencies to which they are assigned for their practicum experiences (Chapter 5). Abiding by these clinical agency guidelines is the responsibility that accompanies the right granted to use the sites to further their educational learning experiences. The laws governing nursing practice in the state in which they are enrolled engender additional student responsibilities. Student privileges are primarily afforded through the rules of their academic institution. Rights and responsibilities are intimately interrelated and are separated here merely for clarity of presentation. Box 6-1 illustrates the principal student rights and responsibilities with which both students and clinical nursing faculty should be knowledgeable.

BOX 6-1
Major Rights and Responsibilities of Nursing Students

Student rights	Student responsibilities
Due process	Adhering to rules of clinical agencies
Privacy	Conforming to codes of conduct
Nondiscrimination	Complying with documented academic policies
First Amendment liberties	Protecting patient safety
	Maintaining patient confidentiality

LEGAL AND ETHICAL ORIGINS OF RIGHTS AND RESPONSIBILITIES

Legal and ethical issues are often intertwined (Aiken, 2004). Societies develop and approve laws to provide direction and order for their people (Box 6-2). These laws incorporate a scheme of enforcement approved by the public through their state and/or federal governmental mechanisms (Aiken, 2004). Laws are primarily based either on the United States/Federal Constitution or those of the individual states (constitutional law) or on statutory laws that are passed by the legislative bodies at the national, state, or local level (Davis, 2002; Brent, 2001). There are also decisions, rules, and laws determined by agencies whose power is delegated to them by one of the legislative bodies (administrative law) and common or case laws derived from judicial decisions. Executive orders emanating from the President or state governors comprise the final source of laws (Davis, 2002; Brent, 2001).

Ethics is a discipline that addresses good and bad, right and wrong, in terms of moral values and principles of conduct. There is no universal mechanism for the enforcement of codes of ethics, but issues of law and ethics may overlap (Aiken, 2004). A society may choose to legislate a social agenda by providing the force of the legal system to enforce particular moral postures. Discord between legal and moral rights is common. Moral rights are often considered to be separate from legal rights, while at the same time creating grounds for mitigating or disparaging them (Brent, 2001).

STUDENT RIGHTS

Academic institutions develop regulations and processes, primarily drawn from state and federal laws, to meet their specific needs (Brent, 2001). These regulations and processes should be made available to students upon enrollment. Public schools, sometimes called *state schools*, are those affiliated with a state government and supported by state revenues. These academic institutions are subject to the applicable laws of the given state and the federal government. Postsecondary private institutions are subject to the same laws if they receive

---

BOX 6-2
Sources of Law

Constitutional law	**Administrative law**
U.S Constitution	Agencies empowered by legislative body
State constitutions	**Common law (Case law)**
Statutory law	Judicial decisions
Federal legislative body	**Executive orders**
State legislative body	President of the United States
Local legislative body	State governor

any state or federal funding, and today most of them do. If they receive no such funds, they are still required to abide by the United States Constitution and avoid any actions that may be deemed as "…arbitrary, capricious, or discriminatory when making decisions about students or faculty" (Brent, 2001, p. 428). Some academic policies are based on ethical codes or values associated with institutions of teaching and learning and may not have a foundation in law. And in other cases, rules and the processes for addressing their violation are a combination of both legal and ethical mandates.

DUE PROCESS

The legal right of due process is afforded to students and faculty alike, as assured by the Fourteenth Amendment of the Constitution of the United States (Johnson & Halstead, 2005; Brent, 2001). This right of due process is built into the procedures associated with a wide variety of policies at the institutional and nursing program levels. Due process is normally defined as what would be considered to be fair treatment in a given situation and is described in terms of the measures taken to make certain that fairness predominates (Brent, 2001).

It has been recommended that due process protocols for matters related to student misconduct (e.g., dishonesty) be more rigorous than those afforded academic issues of grading in light of their relative seriousness (Osinski, 2003). Such an approach is consistent with that used in the judicial system in which someone accused of a crime that carries the potential of imprisonment is afforded a greater degree of due process than one who is charged with an offense associated with a monetary fine or community service (Brent, 2001).

The right of due process is divided into procedural and substantive components (Osinski, 2003). Procedural due process entails the actions associated with the notification of those involved and the provision of a hearing in which they both can present their positions. In contrast, substantive due process concerns the quality of the decision ultimately made. Violation of this aspect of due process would occur if it could be shown that the decision itself was determined to be impulsive, frivolous, or demonstrated enmity toward the student (Osinski, 2003).

Although there may be variations in the process in terms of the timeline, composition and deportment of the hearing, and the appeals process, due to the circumstances and institution, the major components are standard and often predicated on the law (Johnson & Halstead, 2005; Boley & Whitney, 2003; Brent, 2001). It is essential that students be made aware of this right and where they can access the procedure. A general format for the due process course of action in terms of student rights is presented in Box 6-3.

The process may be initiated by the student in situations such as grade disputes or by the academic institution in circumstances such as violations of academic integrity. If initiated by the institution, student notification of the allegation should be presented in writing. Students may choose to not take advantage of aspects of their due process rights, but those aspects must be offered and properly documented if rejected. The membership of the hearing

BOX 6-3
Students' Rights of Due Process

- Right to initiate the process in selected circumstances
- Right to notification of the allegation
- Right to remain silent and avoid self-incrimination if criminal liability is possible
- Right to a hearing
- Right to adequate notification of the hearing
- Right to present their position at the hearing
- Right to review materials supportive of the allegation in advance of the hearing
- Right to be present at the hearing
- Right to an appeal of the decision

board or committee often includes students who are enrolled in the nursing program or the larger institution. The students' right to present their position in the matter includes the right to speak during the hearing and may include presentation of documentation and/or witnesses. The protocol may allow the student to bring another person to the hearing for moral support, but this person usually does not have the right to verbal involvement in the proceedings. In some cases, students may be allowed to challenge the composition of the hearing committee, and even request removal for cause. The policy may include the right to obtain documentation of the hearing, in written or audio format. Options for appeal depend on the specific circumstances, but appeals may be made to the chief nursing executive of the program or another administrator of the institution.

■ PRIVACY

The right to privacy for students in postsecondary academic institutions is protected through state and federal constitutional law, as well as statuary law (Johnson & Halstead, 2005; Brent, 2001). Federal law affords the right of privacy to students enrolled in all schools that receive funds under an applicable program of the United States Department of Education (U.S. Department of Education). These rights are provided to students over the age of 18; prior to that time, they are afforded to the students' parents. The Family Educational Rights and Privacy Act (FERPA) and its later Buckley Amendment essentially guarantee students the right to inspect and review their academic records and request amendment of records they believe to be inaccurate or misleading. If students believe that their academic records are inaccurate or misleading, they can request they be amended. If the school declines to do this, students have the right to request a formal hearing. Following the hearing, if the school still declines to make the desired changes, FERPA permits students to place a statement in their records presenting their positions. It also prohibits the release of personally identifiable information from student records, excepting for directory information. Schools are permitted to release directory information such as names, addresses and telephone numbers, honors and awards, and date and place of birth. Major and minor fields of study and other relevant data also may be published. Students must have the option of filing a request that the school withhold all such "directory" information and be notified of their other rights under FERPA annually. Finally, the Act allows students to file complaints regarding FERPA violations with the Department of Education (U.S. Department of Education).

Health information also may be kept with nursing students' records in a setting with controlled access (locked files in administrative offices). Nursing programs typically require documentation of immunization currency, a current physical examination, and other personal health information. In addition to being protected under FERPA, this information is also protected by the privacy and confidentiality guidelines established by the Health Insurance Portability and Accountability Act (HIPPA) discussed in Chapter 5 (Calloway & Venegas, 2002). Students are encouraged to share any information that might impact their clinical performance with faculty, but faculty are legally and ethically obligated to maintain the confidentiality of that information.

The students' legislated right to privacy is reinforced by both the codes of ethics of professional nursing and those created by academic institutions (Johnson & Halstead, 2005; Morgan, 2001). Students must be able to trust that information about their clinical performance or personal matters will be kept confidential by their faculty. Permission to release any information should be requested whenever possible, and faculty decisions to do so should be firmly grounded in first, the protection of patient safety and second, the well-being of the student (Morgan, 2001).

Routine and random drug and alcohol testing in nursing programs is a matter of increasing concern (Brent, 2001). In some cases, such testing is a requirement of the clinical agency prior to accepting student placements. Nursing programs continue to struggle with the legal ramifications of the need to protect public safety and the privacy rights and other constitutional rights afforded to students. Whatever policies are established must conform to legal parameters and be fairly implemented (Brent, 2001).

▓ NONDISCRIMINATION

Nondiscrimination policies of academic institutions are founded in state and federal constitutional law and in executive orders (Brent, 2001). They broadly address civil rights, equal opportunity, and affirmative action. The common wording is a prohibition of discrimination based on race, gender, religion, age, national or ethnic origin, marital status, sexual orientation, or disability. This general policy is echoed in those created to address the fair and equal treatment of students in matters ranging from violations of codes of conduct to access to school services (Brent, 2001).

For some students in clinical nursing courses, the most important aspect of the nondiscrimination policies is related to disabilities. Titles II and III of the Americans with Disabilities Act of 1990 prohibits discrimination and requires "reasonable accommodations" for students in public and private postsecondary institutions who self-identify as having a disability (U.S. Equal Employment Opportunity Commission, 1997; Sowers & Smith, 2004). The policies address the full range of disabilities, from sensory issues related to vision and hearing to learning disabilities and physical limitations. Efforts to design accommodations for clinical experiences are initiated when students provide notification of their disabilities to the academic institution according to the established procedures that should be documented in the student handbook. The creation of clinical accommodations is discussed in Chapter 8.

FIRST AMENDMENT LIBERTIES

The guarantees provided to United States citizens through the First Amendment of the Constitution include freedoms of religion, speech, press, peaceful assembly, and the right to petition the government to rectify wrongs (Brent, 2001). Everyone values these rights, students included. How these rights are acted on is often addressed by ethical codes established by the institution. Respectful dissent then becomes the responsibility associated with these rights.

STUDENT RESPONSIBILITIES

Student responsibilities, in addition to those associated with clinical agency policies, are drawn from the Nurse Practice Act of the state in which the student is enrolled and a variety of ethical codes of conduct. Clinical faculty need to be knowledgeable regarding these responsibilities and assure that their students are aware of and have access to them. They should be included in the student handbook and reviewed with the students as they are oriented to their clinical courses.

CODES OF CONDUCT

Nursing students are typically answerable to two codes of conduct—one for all students enrolled in the academic institution and a second one for the nursing program. Codes of conduct need to be included in student handbooks. Again, it is most desirable that faculty review them periodically with the students.

Many nursing programs have accepted the National Student Nurses' Association's Code of Academic and Clinical Conduct (2001) as an ethical code to which their neophyte students are introduced and held accountable during their educational process (see "Clinical Toolbox," Chapter 20, p. 357). This code incorporates many of the aspects found in those generally applicable to all students enrolled in the academic institution with the added benefit of addressing issues specific to the profession of nursing. Patient confidentiality is addressed here and also protected by HIPPA legislation. Violations of the students' code of ethics may be addressed through documented procedures established by the nursing program.

Academic institutional codes of conduct may be presented as a single document or a series of discrete policies. The ramifications of violations of codes of conduct also must be clearly documented and made available for students. Codes of conduct may incorporate an honor code, making students not only accountable for themselves but also responsible for reporting the misconduct of their peers. At a minimum, policies should address academic integrity and may also cover other topics such as student responsibilities related to discrimination, harassment, assault, alcohol and drugs, and respect for institutional property.

For students in clinical courses, the issue of academic integrity is very important. Students are expected to comply with these standards or be subject to disciplinary procedures. Academic dishonesty may be addressed even within state laws (Johnson & Halstead, 2005). Broadly defined, academic dishonesty includes lying, cheating, plagiarism, and contriving academic work. Types or degrees of plagiarism are often differentiated in terms of intent. The literature is rife with reports of not only an increasing incidence of academic dishonesty but also an escalating trend of acceptability of such behavior among students at all educational levels (Johnson & Halstead, 2005).

In clinical courses, some common examples of academic dishonesty range from cheating on math or skills exams, submitting another student's work as one's own, and inadequate referencing on a paper to documenting medications not given and interventions not performed. Dishonesty in direct patient care situations results in not only violations of institutional codes of conduct but also exposure of the nursing student to liability in the form of professional negligence (Brent, 2001). The consequences of academic dishonesty in the clinical setting should be clearly spelled out in writing in the student handbook or the course syllabus, or preferably in both. If the consequences are not specified in the syllabus, they should be referenced there. Placing them in the syllabus makes them readily available for students, and they can then be reviewed with faculty during course orientation. Violations of academic integrity policies may result in the student receiving a failing grade for an assignment, the day's performance, or for the course. Depending on the policies of the nursing program and the individual circumstances, expulsion may be an option. Due process and fair and equal treatment must be incorporated into any procedures established.

Appearance standards, or dress policies, may be included along with conduct codes or presented separately. A variety of factors impact the determination of the appropriate attire for clinical courses. Although some programs require consistency throughout the program as a reflection of professionalism, this is most often not a feasible option. In some cases, the clinical setting determines what these will be (e.g., labor and delivery, operating rooms, psychiatric units, day care centers). Safety, for student and client, and cultural awareness, as well as personal hygiene, is also important to consider. Standards should be clearly delineated for each clinical course, in as much specificity and detail as possible.

■ LEGAL RESPONSIBILITIES IN CLINICAL SETTINGS

Nursing students are often unaware that they are legally accountable for the care they provide in the clinical setting and, frankly, so are many faculty and clinical staff! Nurse Practice Acts are applicable to licensed practical/vocational nurses, registered nurses, advanced practice nurses, and student nurses. Each Nurse Practice Act is composed of a collection of state statutes designed to direct certain facets of nursing practice within that state (Mikos, 2004). These Acts are developed for the purpose of providing for the protection of public safety through the determination of requirements for licensure and the regulation of practice and education (Brent, 2001). The practice of student nurses is typically addressed in terms of both the academic setting and their employment outside of school. Until they are licensed as Registered Nurses, students and graduates are required to comply with the tenets of their state Nurse Practice Act pertaining to the provision of patient care while a student as opposed to a Registered Nurse (Brent, 2001). Nurse Practice Acts determine that patient care provided by student nurses "...can be given only pursuant to a recognized nursing education program that meets faculty and clinical supervision requirements" (Brent, 2001, p. 452). These are the programs that have been approved by the state, as stipulated in its Nurse Practice Act. The issue of professional liability for negligent student action or inaction is a concern often voiced by faculty, and by nurses working with students in clinical sites (Brent, 2001). Negligence is defined as "The failure to exercise the standard of care that a reasonably prudent person would have exercised in a similar situation" (Davis, 2002, p. 191). The standard applied to students is the same as that of a graduate professional nurse under the same or similar circumstances. This means that the student is legally obligated to:

> ensure that he or she is well prepared for any patient care assignments being undertaken, must ask for supervision or additional instruction when unsure of the care to be provided and must ask for a change in assignment if not able to carry out the patient treatment in a safe manner (Brent, 2001, p. 450).

This legal obligation should be emphasized in every clinical nursing course concomitant to a discussion of safe practice. It has even been suggested that nursing students carry professional liability insurance to afford a degree of fiscal protection (Brent, 2001).

SUMMARY

Nursing students are afforded rights and responsibilities of both a legal and ethical nature. Clinical faculty must be aware of these in order to protect students' rights while holding them accountable for their responsibilities. One of the obligations faculty carry with them into the clinical setting is to assure both students and agency personnel are cognizant of these rights and responsibilities and function in such a fashion as to preserve them.

REFLECTION EXERCISE 7

Considering Student Rights and Responsibilities*

◆ How has your understanding of student rights changed after reading this chapter?

◆ How might this new knowledge affect how you interact with students in the clinical setting? In group conferences? In one-to-one conferences?

◆ How could you communicate to students their rights and responsibilities in a meaningful way?

*NOTE: Legal and ethical issues discussed in Chapters 5-7 will be specifically applied to clinical nursing education in Chapter 8. For now, consider the topics presented in isolation.

References

Aiken, T.D. (2004). *Legal, ethical, and political issues in nursing,* (2nd ed.). Philadelphia: F.A. Davis.

Boley, P., & Whitney, K. (2003). Grade disputes: Considerations for nursing faculty. *Journal of Nursing Education, 42*(5), 198-203.

Brent, N.J. (2001). *Nurses and the law: A guide to principles and applications* (2nd ed.). Philadelphia: Saunders.

Calloway, S.D., & Venegas, L.M. (2002). The new HIPPA law on privacy and confidentiality. *Nursing Administration Quarterly, 26*(4), 40-54.

Davis, S.H. (2002). Glossary of legal terms. *Plastic Surgical Nursing, 22*(4), 188-193.

Johnson, E.G., & Halstead, J.A. (2005). The academic performance of students: Legal and ethical issues. In D.M. Billings & J.A. Halstead (Eds.). *Teaching in nursing: A guide for faculty* (2nd ed.). (pp. 41-66). Philadelphia: Saunders.

Mikos, C.A. (2004). Inside the Nurse Practice Act. *Nursing Management, 35*(9), 20-22, 91.

Morgan, J.E. (2001). Confidential student information in nursing education. *Nurse Educator, 26*(6), 289-292.

National Student Nurses' Association. (2001). Code of academic and clinical conduct adopted at 49th Annual Convention in Nashville. Retrieved from http://www.nsna.org/press/pr_code.pdf May 4, 2005.

Osinski, K. (2003). Due process rights of nursing students in cases of misconduct. *Journal of Nursing Education, 42*(2), 55-58.

Sowers, J.A., & Smith, M.R. (2004). Nursing faculty members' perceptions, knowledge, and concerns about students with disabilities. *Journal of Nursing Education, 43*(5), 213-218.

U.S. Department of Education, Family Educational Rights and Privacy Act. Retrieved November 8, 2004, from http://www.ed.gov/policy/gen/guid/fpco/ferpa/index.html.

U.S. Equal Employment Opportunity Commission. (1997). Facts about the Americans with disabilities act. Retrieved January 4, 2005, from http://www.eeoc.gov/facts/fs-ada.html.

CHAPTER 7

Rights and Responsibilities: The Faculty

The rights and responsibilities of faculty involved in teaching clinical nursing courses are considerable. Faculty are legally and ethically obligated to be knowledgeable of the legal policies and procedures pertinent to the clinical settings in which their students are placed (Chapter 5). They also must be mindful of the rights and responsibilities afforded nursing students in their particular academic setting (Chapter 6). And finally, faculty are required to understand and adhere to the guidelines and systems that are applicable to the roles of clinical nurse educator and academic faculty in their particular institution.

Broadly speaking, the policies and procedures that apply to nursing faculty in the clinical setting are derived from the policies of the individual academic institution, professional codes of conduct, and the legislation applicable to nursing practice (i.e., the Nurse Practice Act of the given state and legal obligations common to all health care professionals). To responsibly fulfill the role of clinical nursing faculty, it is essential that faculty understand these policies and procedures and know whereto find the pertinent documentation.

ACADEMIC INSTITUTIONAL POLICIES AND PROCEDURES

Faculty rights and responsibilities are primarily supported by federal and state laws (Brent, 2001) and often are also grounded in ethical codes of conduct. They are documented in institutional faculty handbooks and should be made available to new faculty at the time of initial employment. Increasingly, handbooks are being posted on college, university, and/or department web pages. This practice makes them easily accessible and facilitates management and disbursement of revisions. Any revisions should always be documented by date and faculty

---

BOX 7-1
Nursing Faculty Rights and Responsibilities

Faculty Rights	Faculty Responsibilities
Academic freedom	Abide by faculty code of professional ethics
Freedom of expression	Treat colleagues ethically
Freedom of inquiry and the obligation to seek truth	Respect confidentiality in faculty-student interactions
Protection from discrimination	Protect and promote academic integrity
Due process and confidentiality in disciplinary actions	Protect student rights
	Protect patient safety

---

should be routinely notified of substantive changes. Although the focus of attention is typically directed toward faculty responsibilities relative to matters of teaching and student deportment, other rights and obligations are afforded to faculty by virtue of their position in academe (Box 7-1).

Faculty Rights

One of the most treasured faculty rights is that of academic freedom. Developed in 1940 by the American Association of University Professors, the *Statement of Principles on Academic Freedom and Tenure* continues to be revised and updated through interpretive comments (American Association of University Professors [AAUP], 1940) (see "Clinical Toolbox," Chapter 20, p. 317). According to this document, academic freedom affords faculty the right to full freedom in their research and writing in that they are not subject to institutional censorship. They also have freedom in discussing their subject matter in dialogues with students but are urged to be cautionary when introducing controversial material that is unrelated to the subject at hand. Any topical limitations due to religion or other institutional objectives must be provided to faculty in writing at the time of appointment. In interactions with the public outside of the academic setting, faculty have the constitutionally granted rights of the First Amendment, including the right of free speech. But they are reminded by the AAUP that they represent their specific educational institution and the teaching profession in general and are therefore urged to be accurate and respectful in the opinions they express (AAUP, 1987).

The same rights of privacy, protection from discrimination, and due process that are guaranteed to students are also assured for faculty, although there may be some difference in the legal and ethical bases. Constitutional and statutory laws protect the right to privacy (Brent, 2001). Academic institutions conform to all legislation that prohibits discrimination in the hiring, promotion, and general treatment of faculty. These nondiscrimination policies generally speak to civil rights, equal opportunity, and affirmative action. Faculty disciplinary procedures related to violations of codes of conduct must preserve due process as assured by the Fourteenth Amendment of the U.S. Constitution (Brent, 2001). Fair treatment is supported by adequate notification, a hearing in which faculty may offer their own perspectives, and an appeal procedure. Imposed sanctions vary with the seriousness of the offense, ranging from warning to termination.

Faculty Responsibilities

Faculty job descriptions specify their role in the institution and are defined in their letters of appointment. Within the parameters of their assignments, faculty have a considerable amount of latitude. As members of an academic community, faculty are expected to conform to certain standards of deportment, which are often presented as an institutional code of conduct. These codes typically describe obligations associated with faculty rights, such as furthering the scholarship of their discipline, demonstrating integrity in their teaching and scholarship, respecting one another's opinions, ideas, and rights. Faculty responsibilities specifically associated with the nursing program often include maintenance and documentation of license to practice and certifications, immunization status, and Basic Life Support certification. Faculty are also expect to conform to any established dress/appearance clinical policies, and any requisite confidentiality statements, and inservice education (e.g., safety programs required by OSHA, AIDS/HIV education). Finally, faculty have the legal and ethical responsibility to protect the rights of their students.

■ PROFESSIONAL CODES OF CONDUCT

Nursing faculty may be bound by one or more codes of conduct. These ethical codes are designed specifically to address educational issues that apply to the teacher-student relationship in the clinical setting (Morgan, 2001), to the academic role, and to relationships with peers and the community. One such code is the National Education Association (NEA) Code of Ethics of the Education Profession, originally adopted in 1929 and most recently revised in 1975 (see "Clinical Toolbox," Chapter 20, p. 355). The NEA addresses public education through the graduate level and promotes both quality education and the education profession itself. As presented by the Association, this code "indicates the aspiration of all educators and provides standards by which to judge conduct." In two parts, this code reiterates commitments to the student and to the profession, emphasizing nondiscrimination, privacy, and respect of both students and colleagues.

The American Association of University Professors (AAUP) is an organization specifically for faculty teaching in higher education settings (colleges and universities), regardless of whether they are public or private. Committed to shared governance and the advancement of academic freedom, AAUP also provides a code of professional ethics (AAUP, 1987) (see "Clinical Toolbox," Chapter 20, p. 324). This code speaks to the various roles of faculty as scholars, teachers, professional colleagues, and members of the academic community and the community at large. Intellectual honesty in the pursuit of knowledge is supported, as is ethical behavior with peers and the right of free speech. Again, privacy, confidentiality, nondiscrimination, and respect are common themes.

Nursing faculty are most likely to recognize and have a personal copy of one or more of the ethical codes of conduct developed by their nursing organizations (American Nurses' Association, Canadian Nurses Association, International Council of Nurses). These codes are designed for use in the process of decision making and to guide the conduct of nurses and nursing students in research, education, practice, and management (Aiken, 2004).

The Ethical Code for Nurses of the American Nurses' Association (2001) was developed to delineate the profession's ethical standard by formally identifying the ethical obligations and duties of nursing and to present the profession's understanding of its societal commitment. Nurses are familiar with the tenants of the Code and its broad spectrum of moral and ethical positions regarding patient safety, confidentiality, and respect and the professional obligations associated with addressing questionable nursing practice. But nurses are often unaware that this code also speaks to nursing education. According to the Code, it is the nurse educator's responsibility to ensure that only those students with the essential knowledge, skills, and competencies are permitted to graduate (American Nurses' Association, 2001). This is the profession's mandate to nurse educators, and nowhere is it more keenly felt than in the clinical setting.

▪ LEGAL GOVERNANCE OF CLINICAL NURSING EDUCATION

Legislation related to nursing practice provides direction for clinical nursing faculty. These statutes are found in the Nurse Practice Acts and regulations for each state or U.S. territory and in broad-based laws applicable to all health care professionals.

Nurse Practice Acts

Even though they may not be formally labeled as nurse practice acts, each state and U.S. territory has statutes that provide the legal basis for nursing practice (Mikos, 2004). Nurse practice acts affect all licensed nursing groups and their prelicensure students. The National Council of State Boards of Nursing has designed a "Model Nurse Practice Act," available on the Internet at http://www.ncsbn.org/regulation/nursingpractice_nursing_practice_model_act_and_rules.asp that illustrates the typical components. Copies of individual state/territory Nurse Practice Acts can be found on the web (e.g., http://www.the-travel-nurse.com/nursepracticeacts.html), through state boards of nursing or at public libraries. All clinical faculty should obtain the one for the state in which they teach and review it for more specific detail than is provided here.

Although there may be some variation in what each state legislature determines should be included, nurse practice acts commonly address many of the same subjects (National Council of State Boards of Nursing [NCSBN], 2004; Mikos, 2004). These topics include the definition and scope of practice for each nursing group and their licensure requirements, the formulation and span of authority of the given state board of nursing, the grounds and processes for disciplinary action, and the delineation of standards and processes established for the approval of schools of nursing within the state. Initial licensure then requires documentation of graduation from an approved school (NCSBN, 2004; Mikos, 2004). The individual state boards of nursing are empowered to interpret and apply the laws pertaining to nursing within that state. The Board of Directors of the National Council of State Boards of Nursing provides oversight of these diverse state boards (Crawford, 2004).

According to nurse practice acts, the scope of registered nursing practice includes that of academic clinical instruction, specifically as related to the roles of supervision, delegation, and evaluation (NCSBN, 2004). One aspect of supervision is reflected in adherence to the maximal ratio of faculty to students in clinical settings; this is legislated in the state Nurse Practice Act. The liability of faculty and staff nurses is based on the appropriateness of each nursing student's assignment and the adequacy of supervision provided (Sullivan, 2001). Staff nurses legally share in the responsibilities associated with delegation to students, but faculty routinely assume the primary weight of this responsibility. As licensed registered nurses, it is the responsibility of faculty and nursing personnel to assure student competency in the tasks delegated to them. This means that they (primarily faculty and less so the staff) must be sure students have the knowledge and proficiency to perform their assigned nursing activities and must provide the supervision necessary to assure patient safety. Students are often unaware that they also have legal obligations that require them to be sufficiently prepared for their assignments, to request supervision or additional instruction when they are uncertain of their course of action, and to ask for a change in assignment if they feel that they are unable to provide care in a safe manner (Brent, 2001). Assuring patient safety is both an ethical and legal onus shared by students, faculty, and agency nursing personnel.

Statutory and Constitutional Law Applicable to All Health Care Professionals

Some of the laws applicable to nursing practice may not be located within the state's Nurse Practice Act. Statutes that are broadly applied to licensed health care professionals within a given state also encompass registered nurses (Mikos, 2004). As licensed health care professionals, clinical nursing faculty are required by law to report instances of elder or child abuse or neglect, suspicious or unnatural deaths, injuries due to lethal weapons, and injuries potentially associated with criminal conduct (e.g., rape/criminal sexual assault, battery, or other forms of assault) (Brent, 2001). If any such injuries are observed in the clinical setting by nursing faculty, or described to them by their students, reporting is legally mandated.

One of the most far-reaching legal concepts is the right of privacy, which is afforded by several of the protections of the Bill of Rights and in amendments that were subsequently ratified (Brent, 2001). The right of privacy is not absolute and some applications have been legally challenged, but it provides the legal basis for confidentiality requirements in health care. This is most recently evident in aspects of the Health Insurance Portability and Accountability Act (HIPAA). HIPAA legislation and its clinical educational implications are discussed in Chapter 5.

SUMMARY

Rights and responsibilities of faculty teaching clinical courses have both legal and ethical origins. In order to meet society's expectations for the preparation of competent nurses, faculty must understand the policies and procedures that impact students, clinical agencies, and their role as nurse educators. Faculty teaching clinical nursing courses must protect clients, students, and themselves as they endeavor to foster affirmative learning environments.

REFLECTION EXERCISE 8

Considering Faculty Rights and Responsibilities*

◆ Are there rights or responsibilities associated with faculty who teach clinical nursing that you were unfamiliar with before reading this chapter? If so, what does this new information mean to you? How will it change how you think or what you do?

Consider a social health care issue you feel strongly about, for example, stem cell research, assisted euthanasia, a woman's right to choose (abortion).

◆ How will knowledge of faculty rights and responsibilities affect what you might say about this issue to students?

◆ If the issue were not specifically related to nursing or healthcare (e.g., school prayer, or amending the Pledge of Allegiance), would your approach in discussion with students be any different in light of your knowledge of faculty rights and responsibilities? Why or why not?

*NOTE: Legal and ethical issues discussed in Chapters 5 to 7 will be specifically applied to clinical nursing education in Chapter 8. For now, consider the topics presented in isolation.

References

Aiken, T.D. (2004). *Legal, ethical, and political issues in nursing*, (2nd ed.). Philadelphia: F.A. Davis.

American Association of University Professors (AAUP). (1940). Statement of principles on academic freedom and tenure. Retrieved November 4, 2004 from http://www.aaup.org/Com-a/index.htm

American Association of University Professors (AAUP). (1987). Statement on professional ethics. Retrieved November 19, 2004 from http://www.aaup.org/statements/Redbook/Rbethics.htm

American Nurses' Association (ANA). (2001). Code of ethics for nurses with interpretive statements. Retrieved from http://www.nursingworld.org March 7, 2005.

Brent, N.J. (2001). *Nurses and the law: A guide to principles and applications* (2nd ed.). Philadelphia: Saunders.

Crawford, L.H. (2004). Perspectives of schools of nursing on nursing regulation. *Nursing Education Perspectives, 25*(5), 220-224.

Mikos, C.A. (2004). Inside the Nurse Practice Act. *Nursing Management, 35*(9), 20-22, 91.

Morgan, J.E. (2001). Confidential student information in nursing education. *Nurse Educator, 26*(6), 289-292.

National Council of State Boards of Nursing (NCSBN) (2004). Retrieved November 2, 2004 from http://www.ncsbn.org/

National Education Association (NEA). (1975). Code of ethics of the education profession. Retrieved November 19, 2004 from http://www.nea.org/code.html

Sullivan, E.J. (2005). *Effective leadership and management in nursing* (6th ed.). Upper Saddle River, N.J.: Prentice-Hall.

CHAPTER 8

Legal and Ethical Implications in the Clinical Education Setting

- THE FACULTY-STUDENT RELATIONSHIP
- PROBLEM PROPHYLAXIS
- UNSATISFACTORY CLINICAL PERFORMANCE
  Due Process
  Safety Concerns
- CLINICAL GRADE DISPUTES
- VIOLATIONS OF CONDUCT
  Academic Dishonesty
  Impaired Practice
  Due Process in Disciplinary Misconduct
- REASONABLE CLINICAL DISABILITY ACCOMMODATIONS
- CLINICAL NURSE EDUCATOR LIABILITY
- SUMMARY

The rights and responsibilities previously discussed come under consideration as nursing faculty teaching clinical courses deal with a wide variety of situations. It is important to remember that if faculty are employed at the clinical sites where they also teach, when they are there as academic faculty, they are obligated to function in that role only. Teaching clinical nursing courses, faculty face some challenges more often than others. At one time or another, most faculty teaching in clinical settings will have to deal with unsatisfactory clinical performance, grade disputes, and deviations from approved appearance standards. Unsatisfactory clinical performance may be associated with issues of safety such as insufficient preparation, difficulties with skills performance or knowledge transfer, and even student health problems. Less often, faculty may encounter problems related to chemical impairment, academic dishonesty, and breaches of conduct. Violations of this nature are legally subjected to a different process than those relating to clinical performance and the resulting grades (Osinski, 2003). Clinical accommodations for disabled students are usually addressed in concert with the administration of the nursing program and institutional support services, but faculty should be aware of the mandate for reasonable accommodations (see Chapter 6). Faculty in the clinical setting also have liability concerns, some of which are common to faculty in all disciplines and others that are unique to clinical nursing education.

Other legal issues related to higher education, both in public and private institutions, are not discussed here because they are not specifically applicable to the role of faculty teaching practicum courses. Academic decisions related to student admission, dismissal, and readmission are primarily addressed at an administrative level. The same can be said of certain matters pertaining to academic advancement in the program, such as catalog and curricular changes and student safety on campus. However, none of these topics are explored here; the focus remains specifically on nurse educators teaching clinical courses.

THE FACULTY-STUDENT RELATIONSHIP

The closer, more intimate learning environment found in clinical courses intensifies interactions between faculty and students. Students are more likely to share personal difficulties with their clinical faculty, and even turn to them when they are having problems in other courses. Emotions run high when students are involved in patient care, regardless of the clinical setting. Student anxiety in the clinical setting is ubiquitous. Whether they are nervous about starting a new clinical experience, afraid of making a mistake or performing clinical skills, feeling a lack of confidence, or fearful of being evaluated (Bozich Keith & Schmeiser, 2003), anxiety lowers the emotional barometer in the clinical site; storms are always on the horizon.

There is little doubt that a relationship with students that is characterized by openness, mutual respect, and a collaborative approach to learning will reduce the potential for problematic or adversarial experiences (Johnson & Halstead, 2005). But despite their best efforts to be clear and straightforward concerning expectations and feedback and to be egalitarian and caring in their interactions with students, faculty will inevitably encounter arduous situations involving students. An inherent imbalance in power is unavoidable as long as faculty are obligated by their institutions and accountable to their profession to determine the adequacy of student learning through the satisfactory attainment of course objectives. The reality is that nursing faculty are the gatekeepers of the profession, and they retain the ultimate responsibility for determining whether students are sufficiently competent to graduate and enter the profession. At the same time, they must honor student rights and allow every opportunity for success.

PROBLEM PROPHYLAXIS

Some basic steps can be taken by faculty that will both reduce the likelihood of problem development and provide the legal and ethical groundwork for the protection of the student and the faculty if problems do occur (Box 8-1). Primary prevention is the best approach in clinical practice and in clinical education!

Faculty must treat each clinical course independently, reviewing general institutional student responsibilities as they review specific agency and course materials. Review of the guidelines of the nursing program regarding student conduct should include appearance standards related to the clinical site, unsatisfactory clinical performance, and academic integrity, including the ramifications associated with problems in each area. It is best, from both a legal and an

---

BOX 8-1
Primary Prevention of Student-Based Clinical Problems

During student orientation to the clinical course:
- Review institutional policies related to student conduct including clinical performance and academic integrity
- Review student obligations regarding clinical agency policies
- Review course requirements written in the syllabus
- Review the evaluation tool, procedures, and data sources to be used
- Provide students with the opportunity to ask questions and seek clarification
- Provide orientation to clinical site and specific unit/area
- Assure evaluation tools used are reliable and valid
- Create opportunities for student self-evaluation
- Provide ongoing, regular feedback regarding progress in the course
- Assure all students are treated equally in terms of evaluation
- Assure privacy in interactions with students when sharing negative evaluative data
- Maintain anecdotal notes

---

ethical position, if these are provided in writing in the course syllabus. Use this opportunity to provide examples of academic dishonesty in the clinical area, and define plagiarism with and without intent. Explore in advance some of the resources available, such as the Center for Academic Integrity (http://www.academicintegrity.org). The Center offers a meeting place for the identification, affirmation, and promotion of the values of academic integrity. The site has a public tier that includes an Academic Integrity Assessment Guide for use in the development of an action plan for assessing learning climate and evaluating academic policies and procedures (Center for Academic Integrity). This is also the time to review the legally mandated student expectations for the protection of patient safety.

Students need to be introduced to the course expectations and evaluation criteria at the beginning of the course (Smith, McKoy, & Richardson, 2001). An in-depth discussion of evaluation is provided in Chapter 18. It is essential that this aspect of the course be internally and externally consistent. Within the course, faculty should not change the course expectations or grading criteria during the term. The written syllabus is essentially a contract between the faculty and the student (Brent, 2001; Boley & Whitney, 2003). In terms of external consistency, the same course expectations and grading criteria must be used in all sections of the same course. This does not mean all faculty teaching a specific clinical course must function identically. What needs to be communicated to students is that the outcome of attaining the course objectives is the same, but each faculty is free to use a variety of methods to reach that point. This not only allows faculty a degree of academic freedom but also permits adjustments based on the experiences and opportunities provided in differing clinical settings. For example, an objective related to demonstrating an understanding of the effects of chronic disease on activities of daily living could be addressed by students in one clinical group through a patient interview and written paper, while in another group the students might do a panel presentation.

In all cases, the data to be used in evaluation must be shared with students in advance. Sharing the methods faculty plan to use to collect data is important to avoid student distress later. For instance, if faculty routinely listen to student-patient interactions without self-exposure in order to obtain more valid data, this practice needs to be acknowledged and presented to students at the start of the course. In addition to direct observation and interaction with students, evaluative data may be obtained from a multitude of other sources, including written work such as student papers and journals, agency personnel, student presentations, and the first-hand accounts of patients and families with whom students work.

The beginning of the course also affords an excellent opportunity to communicate to students that faculty assess and evaluate students' *patterns of behavior*. A single isolated unsatisfactory performance is not sufficient to result in a failing grade any more than accomplishing one outstanding feat will assure passing the course (Johnson & Halstead, 2005). They are students after all, and students must have the chance to learn and grow, and that includes making mistakes. What students must demonstrate is an increasing self-awareness and a relatively consistent pattern of growth toward the attainment of course objectives.

Orientation to the clinical site as a whole and to the individual unit(s) where the students are to be placed has been deemed a legal requirement of assuring safe practice of nursing students (Smith et al., 2001). Specifics of care and terminology unique to the setting must be addressed. Providing a simple checklist, or perhaps using a site-specific scavenger hunt as a means for students to discover this information and "mark it off" the list during their orientation time, provides written documentation that this requisite has been met. Reducing procedural and logistical obstacles at this time permits faculty and students to focus on meeting the course objectives and maximizing learning during the term.

Every effort should be taken to assure that the methods and instruments used in evaluation are reliable and valid. "The closer we come to requiring real-world performance on an assessment task (authenticity), the more difficult it is to objectively rate the performance" (Tanner, 2004, p. 435). Clinical student evaluations will always include some degree of subjectivity (Scanlan, Care, & Gessler, 2001). Clarity regarding the successful attainment of course objectives is essential for both students and faculty. Group norming activities with all faculty teaching a given clinical course is an excellent way to accomplish consistency between faculty. Objectives are often so broad and general that they are open to too much variance in interpretation. One way to reduce this problem is to provide the students with exemplars of satisfactory attainment for each course objective. This can be done broadly for a pass-fail course, or levels of performance can be specifically differentiated for one that is graded. An example of each approach is provided in the "Clinical Toolbox" (see Chapter 20, pp. 369-370). A copy of the evaluation tool should be included in the course syllabus (Smith et al., 2001).

It is important that the students be included in the evaluation process. This self-assessment is essential to their developing professional practice. They can accomplish this in a variety of fashions, from journaling to filling out a daily or weekly self-evaluation form. If self-assessment is a course requirement, whether or not it is done should be noted. Students should receive guidance in how to carry out a self-assessment, and faculty may comment regarding students' degree of self-awareness. But students need to be assured that they have full freedom to expose their feelings and thoughts without risking some sort of grading penalty and that their confidentiality will be fully protected. Faculty need to pay close attention to students' perceptions of their performance to prevent a later dichotomy in grading.

Faculty must provide clear, specific feedback to students regarding their performance on a routine basis, ideally every week, in addition to midterm evaluations. This is informally done through assignments and daily interactions with students. More formal, brief written feedback along with specific suggestions for improvement gives students concrete direction, and the process of doing so furnishes faculty the chance to plan how to best help meet each student's learning needs. To assist nursing students in learning the discipline, faculty are obliged to provide guidance through honest assessment and stalwart feedback (Tanner, 2004). Document the feedback given, recommendations provided, and the timeline for accomplishing improvement in personal anecdotal notes (Smith et al., 2001).

Endeavor to perpetuate equality in student interactions and evaluations. Students may complain that faculty discriminate in these areas based on age, gender, ethnicity, and even personality. Thoughtful reflection on educational practices can be of great benefit in providing an internal check and in maintaining equilibrium when dealing with students. Discrimination is often found in the eye of the beholder. By making a conscious effort to be equitable and by analyzing behavior, faculty are kept alert to even the perception of discrimination.

Students are very sensitive to receiving any criticism from their faculty in a situation where others might overhear it. Anyone would naturally feel embarrassed under such circumstances, and those feelings could block reception of even the most well-structured constructive criticism. Students have both a legal and ethical right to confidentiality and privacy. If they perceive what is occurring as public humiliation, the antipathy generated can add fuel to an already difficult situation. Students are then less likely to accurately hear what is said and therefore less likely to make the suggested changes, and they may carry their resentment into future interactions with their faculty. Such experiences contribute to student accusations of unfair treatment and tend to surface in student-faculty disputes regarding overall performance and grading. In the clinical setting, find a private location, away from patients, staff, and their peers, to convey feedback the student may construe negatively. If a student's overall performance is unsatisfactory and there is a risk of failing the course, it is best to have a meeting away from the clinical site, in a private office.

Anecdotal notes are written documentations of all conferences with students, their daily clinical experiences, and their performance. These notes are of value in constructing routine feedback, preparing formal student evaluations, and providing documentation of any problematic performance areas (Zuzelo, 2000; Smith et al., 2001; Johnson & Halstead, 2005). Anecdotal notations should be sufficiently detailed as to present the most accurate picture of the situation at hand. It is imperative that faculty record both positive and negative aspects of each student's work as objectively as possible, (Smith et al., 2001) as it relates to course objectives, the source of the data, and actions they may have taken in regard to any student deficiencies. Care should be taken to avoid the appearance of bias by focusing only on negative aspects of performance. Comments related to personality traits should be avoided (Johnson & Halstead, 2005). If referrals are made to other individuals or services provided by the nursing program, these should be documented also (Zuzelo, 2000). Creating a method to keep track of student performance during a busy day is a challenge for the best of faculty. Here is another situation in which faculty can learn from their peers. All faculty teaching a specific clinical course can share both their methods and their tools for anecdotal note taking during a course meeting. What is most useful for an acute care setting is not necessarily of value in a community-based clinical course. Typically faculty must spend additional time embellishing notes made during the day in order to make them sufficiently detailed. These notes are the property of the faculty and are not a part of the student's academic record (Brent, 2001). They cannot be subpoenaed and serve only to enhance a faculty member's memory. Although the specific timeframe may vary based on the type of claim being made, students generally have up to 2 years to file lawsuits (Zuzelo, 2000). Should problems arise, memory alone is insufficient. Faculty should retain anecdotal notes in a secure file to protect confidentiality for at least 2 years after students complete the course (Zuzelo, 2000). Some nursing programs require keeping them until students graduate or for 2 years following graduation. Many faculty keep them even longer to facilitate preparing letters of recommendation at a later time. When they are destroyed, the method should be shredding, or some other method that assures complete destruction. An anecdotal notation example is provided in the "Clinical Toolbox" (see Chapter 20, p. 359).

UNSATISFACTORY CLINICAL PERFORMANCE

Unsatisfactory clinical performance is a rather general term because student performance may be deemed unsatisfactory for a variety of reasons. Students may be unable to transfer knowledge from their concurrent or prior courses into the current clinical course. They may have problems with one or more patient safety issues, such as difficulties with technical skill performance or inadequate preparation. Absenteeism and tardiness and late submission of written work are also common problems. Occasionally students violate appearance standards, warranting written notice of unsatisfactory performance. Violations of conduct (behavior) are usually handled separately. The faculty management of each of these problems varies, but the mandatory due process is identical in each case (Osinski, 2003).

To determine whether student performance is unsatisfactory, the standard for adequate performance must be clearly established and communicated to the students from the beginning of the clinical course. Determining that performance on a given day or with a specific assignment or skill is unsatisfactory is not usually a problem for faculty teaching in clinical settings. Actually deciding when the student's overall abilities relating to one or more objectives are *unsatisfactory* has historically been more challenging (Johnson & Halstead, 2005). Nurse educators struggle to determine how many occurrences constitute unsatisfactory performance (Scanlan et al., 2001).

Faculty are often caught between wanting to be sure they have sufficient data reflecting substandard functioning, providing early remedial intervention, and following through with failing a student in the course. This would be an excellent topic for discussion at a faculty retreat. Attaining consensus not only provides clarity for individual faculty but also may result in the determination of policies that could protect faculty and the nursing program from accusations of unfair and inequitable actions.

Due Process

With routine feedback, faculty can identify unsatisfactory aspects of performance and provide direction to the student to encourage improvement. If the student continues to be unsatisfactory in that area the following week, the behavior is inconsistently improved, or additional deficiencies present themselves, it is always best to formally follow the academic institution's procedural due process protocol. Due process policies and procedures should be reasonable and consistent (Boley & Whitney, 2003). The specific institution's procedure may vary, but the components are legally delineated (Box 8-2). Within these parameters, the nursing program's policies and procedures may provide guidance in (1) terms of remediation options, (2) when students must be removed from clinical sites, and (3) grounds for dismissal from the program. It is essential that all faculty follow any documented institutional policies consistently to avoid any suggestion of bias or discrimination and assure respect for the dignity of the student.

Notification of unsatisfactory performance may occur once, or a student may be notified multiple times over the course of the term for differing problems. Such notification can be seen as placing the student on clinical probation. The process is intended to provide additional support to the student and encourage success, while reinforcing that course failure will occur without significant and consistent improvement (Zuzelo, 2000).

The nursing program may have a specific form to be filled out that becomes part of the institutional documentation of due process. A sample notice of unsatisfactory performance is provided in the "Clinical Toolbox" (see Chapter 20, p. 368). Both student and faculty should sign the form. The student's signature

---

BOX 8-2

Assuring Procedural Due Process in Cases of Unsatisfactory Performance: Sample Policies and Procedure

At any time the student's performance or progress is unsatisfactory:

- Written notification is provided (Notification of Unsatisfactory Performance form)
- A plan for addressing deficiencies is provided, which includes an opportunity for satisfactory improvement within a specified time
- Specific ramifications are described that will be enforced if satisfactory improvement does not occur
- If the student believes the assessment of his or her performance is inaccurate or unfair after meeting with the faculty member, the student may discuss the matter with the faculty member's immediate supervisor
- Notification of unsatisfactory performance is to occur in a private, face-to-face meeting between faculty and student.

---

simply indicates the form was read and is not to be construed as an agreement with its contents (Zuzelo, 2000). One signed copy may be placed in the student's academic record; students must receive a copy, and the faculty member should retain one.

Students may choose to share their perceptions of what has occurred with others; whether this information is accurate or inaccurate is moot as far as faculty are concerned because they are legally required to protect student confidentiality. For faculty to address the issue with other students, the student's parents, or spouse requires the student's consent, preferably in writing (Morgan, 2001). Faculty may seek advice and guidance from a colleague or supervisor, in effect, discussing the situation without the student's consent, if it is presented as a hypothetical scenario without significant identifiers and the other person agrees to hold the information in confidence (Morgan, 2001). Otherwise, confidentiality must be maintained at all times.

A plan providing the student with direction for remediation, a specific point in time when satisfactory performance is to be attained, and the consequences if this does not occur should all be documented in records maintained by the faculty member. Except for the most dire of circumstances, usually those related to academic dishonesty or repeated unsafe clinical behaviors, notification should permit a period of time of at least one clinical day to allow the student to demonstrate correction of the behavior. If the student's performance is safe thereafter, the student must be permitted to work toward completing the course requirements until the end of the course, even if course objectives are not being met (Johnson & Halstead, 2005). The plan should be tailored to address the specific unsatisfactory behavior demonstrated by the student and may include such activities as written assignments or additional time in the skills laboratory.

Safety Concerns

Faculty would like to spend the bulk of their time with students in the clinical setting actively facilitating learning, assisting students as they bring theory from the classroom into the real-life learning laboratory. But, charged with protecting the patient from injury, a significant amount of time and energy must be delegated to the task of "Safety Officer." Probably the most common reason for student notification of unsatisfactory performance is failure to practice safely. In addition to efforts made to protect patients and to recognize unsafe behavior when it occurs, faculty teaching clinical courses must determine the course of action to take when they deem the student to be unsafe.

Protecting patient safety as nursing students learn poses different challenges depending on the level of the student and the clinical setting. Obviously, beginning students require closer supervision and more circumscribed practice guidelines than those further along in the curriculum. If beginning students are placed in community-based settings where faculty are unable to directly supervise their activities, agency personnel should be readily available and specific detailed instructions provided for both students and staff. In all settings, faculty should clearly state in their syllabi what students can do without supervision and what activities require prior notification of or consultation with faculty. The same information must be provided to the agency personnel. Faculty should determine the minimal amount of written and/or verbal competency students must demonstrate before beginning their patient care. It is always best to start the term with tight reins, allowing students more freedom as their competency can be individually assessed.

Both faculty and students should know what constitutes unsafe behavior in their clinical setting. A general definition should be included in their respective handbooks. Sample broad definitions of safe and unsafe student clinical practice are provided in Box 8-3. The definition of unsafe practice for nursing students in each clinical course then becomes their failure to conform to the preparatory and practice parameters documented in the course syllabus.

One single episode of unsafe practice should result in formal notification of unsatisfactory performance. This approach provides documentation and communicates to the student the gravity of safety violations. Repeated safety transgressions should be grounds for removal from the site and course failure. When students do not perform safely, patients' well-being may be jeopardized. It is the duty of faculty to recognize incompetent nursing care, to apply grading standards consistently, and to confer a failing grade if it is justified (Boley & Whitney, 2003). This policy should be documented in student and faculty handbooks and must be consistently applied to avoid accusations of capriciousness, which would be a violation of legal mandates for fairness and equity in student treatment (Brent, 2001). Box 8-4 illustrates a sample policy for removing students from the clinical site.

In some programs, because grades cannot be given until the end of the term, faculty keep repeatedly unsafe students in the clinical setting by limiting their scope of practice and/or providing closer supervision beyond the point

---

BOX 8-3

Definitions of Safe and Unsafe Student Clinical Practice

Safe student clinical practice

- Students are expected to demonstrate growth in clinical practice through application of knowledge and skills from previous and concurrent courses.
- Students are expected to demonstrate growth in clinical practice as they progress through courses and to meet clinical expectations outlined in each clinical course evaluation tool.
- Students are expected to prepare for clinical practice in order to provide safe, competent care. Adequate preparation to assure safety generally means being prepared to carry out all skills and having all requisite knowledge that is necessary and available in advance to execute the activities associated with the clinical assignment. Preparation expectations are detailed in each clinical course syllabus.

Unsafe student clinical practice

- Unsafe clinical practice is behavior that places the client or staff in either physical or emotional jeopardy.
- Physical jeopardy is creation of the risk of causing physical harm.
- Emotional jeopardy means that the student has created an environment of anxiety or distress that puts the client or staff at risk for emotional or psychologic harm.
- Unsafe clinical practice is an occurrence, or a pattern of repeated behavior, involving unacceptable risk.

Adapted from Scanlan et al., 2001.

---

in time when academic success is possible. By "building a box" in which the student's practice is tightly constrained, limited to what the faculty knows the student can safely do, the student has the opportunity to experience some degree of exposure to the clinical experience. This intervention seems rational and supportive of the student. Unfortunately, closer supervision of the unsafe student increases anxiety, which heightens the risk for error, and leaves the other students in the course with fewer faculty-facilitated learning

---

BOX 8-4

Sample Policy for Student Dismissal From a Clinical Site

Faculty may remove a student from a clinical site for unsafe practice, violations of clinical agency policies, or breaches of academic or professional codes of conduct documented in this handbook. The student also will have earned a failing grade in the course.

opportunities (Scanlan et al., 2001). Additionally, leaving a habitually unsafe student in the clinical area in any direct patient care capacity exposes faculty to a liability risk.

▓ CLINICAL GRADE DISPUTES

Clinical faculty have the final word in the evaluation of their students' clinical performance. Clinical courses are commonly graded as pass or fail. In those cases where letter grades are awarded, students may dispute the validity of one passing grade level versus another. Nursing students have the expectation of obtaining high grades; if their expectations are not met, they may dispute the criteria used and/or charge faculty with partiality (Tanner, 2004). This discussion, though focused on the dispute of failing grades, is applicable to those situations as well.

Novice faculty, uncertain of their judgments and possessing limited experience with students in the clinical setting, are hesitant to fail students (Scanlan et al., 2001). They are often torn between wanting to give students ample opportunity for success and their sense of obligation to the profession and the public. Seeing nursing as a caring profession and wanting to exemplify that quality in their interactions with students, novice and seasoned faculty alike may perceive failing a student as uncaring behavior "…when, indeed, it may be more caring to fail students than allow them to continue" (Scanlan et al., 2001, p. 26).

Although fear of litigation may inhibit faculty from failing students in the clinical setting, the legal system has overwhelmingly supported faculty grading decisions, provided that the process of their determination was neither arbitrary nor capricious (Brent, 2001; Boley & Whitney, 2003; Johnson & Halstead, 2005) and due process was provided in the case of disputes (Brent, 2001). Legally, the burden of proof that either criterion was not met falls to the student (Boley & Whitney, 2003). Faculty are seen by the courts as the experts in their field and courts are disinclined to become involved in grade disputes for fear of intruding on the sovereignty of the academic institution and the scholarly veracity and academic freedom of faculty (Boley & Whitney, 2003).

A failing final grade should never come as a surprise to the student; notification of unsatisfactory performance and the opportunity to address deficiencies is legally and ethically essential up until the last day of a clinical course. Exceptions to this policy are made only in specifically delineated areas, most often related to recurrent breaches of safety and violation of codes of conduct or academic integrity. When a student does not agree with the grade the faculty believes has been earned, a grievance action must be available to facilitate resolution of the disagreement. It is the faculty's responsibility to assure that students are aware of this option as part of the due process procedure and to direct them to the written document that delineates the steps involved in grieving a grade (Box 8-5).

Having applied evaluative standards consistently to all their students and documented their observations and actions, clinical faculty will have met the requirement for fairness and equity in grading decisions. Following well

---

BOX 8-5

Student Grievance Policy for Grade Appeal Due Process

If, at the end of the term, the student believes a course grade is inaccurate or unfair, after meeting with the faculty for the given course, he or she may:

- Meet with the faculty's immediate supervisor (lead faculty, course coordinator, administrator), and/or
- Request an appeal hearing

---

designed due process procedures and affording students the grievance option addresses the final judicial requirements faculty must meet. Failing students and dealing with grade disputes are never easy experiences for faculty, regardless of their years of experience. Administration and colleagues can provide the needed support along the way.

VIOLATIONS OF CONDUCT

Institutions of higher education take their role in enhancing the development of students' value systems and supporting those of society at large very seriously. Educational programs for the preparation of many professional disciplines, including nursing, use the time students are under their direction to instill in them their own standards of practice. These are usually expressed as a listing of principles, or codes of conduct. Codes of conduct for nursing students prohibit, among other things, acts of aggression that include harassment, breaches of privacy and confidentiality, misuse of institutional property, and drug and alcohol abuse. Additionally, academic institutions take the maintenance of student integrity as it relates to the learning process very seriously. Academic integrity violations are defined by the academic institution, but typically include cheating, lying, falsification of documents, fabrication, plagiarism, multiple submissions, abuse of academic materials, and complicity or misconduct in research.

Academic Dishonesty

Of all the disciplinary issues academic faculty may be involved in, violations of academic integrity are second only to grade disputes in frequency. Issues of academic dishonesty bring to the fore an applicable moral standard that extends beyond the perspective of ideology (Solomon & DeNatale, 2000). In clinical courses, academic dishonesty may occur as plagiarism, submission of an assignment already completed for another course, falsification of patient records, lying about an action or inaction, or cheating on a test. Chapter 6 provides a discussion of student codes of ethics, and the National Student Nurses' Association Code of Academic and Clinical Conduct is found in the "Clinical Toolbox" (see Chapter 20, p. 357).

It is essential that clinical faculty assure the accuracy of their data before making an allegation of academic dishonesty. Documentation of incidents of lying or falsified records may include statements from agency personnel, patients, or other students. Consultation with colleagues when suspicions are raised can be especially valuable. Although it does require additional time for faculty, at least spot-checking references cited in student papers is beneficial. Even knowing that this is being done can function as a deterrent to intentional plagiarism by students. There are organizations that evaluate papers for evidence of plagiarism. If the nursing program subscribes to such a service, it could be used by all faculty, including those teaching clinical courses. Turn It In is one such service (http://www.turnitin.com/), but there are others available.

Impaired Practice

The most common violation of the code of conduct in clinical courses is probably the inappropriate use of drugs or alcohol by students. Chemical dependency is documented to be the most common cause of impaired practice (Spier et al., 2000). Even so, suspicions that illicit drugs or alcohol are responsible for impaired practice must be validated and other potential etiologies ruled out in most cases. Obviously, if faculty directly observe a student imbibing or taking drugs or smell alcohol or marijuana, they can proceed from that point, but often only impaired cognitive or physical performance is noted and warrants further investigation.

A number of disorders such as depression, anxiety, diabetes, thyroid dysfunction, seizure disorders, asthma, migraines, and even the flu or a cold may present intermittently or continuously as impaired function (Spier et al., 2000). Students who skip breakfast and try to function through a busy morning commonly develop hypoglycemia, resulting in both impaired cognition and poor skill performance. Adverse effects of over-the-counter (OTC) antihistamines, or prescribed anticonvulsants or corticosteroids may be responsible for students' slowed information processing or skill performance (Spier et al., 2000). Numerous studies have demonstrated the role of sleep deprivation in negatively affecting visual acuity, verbal skills, problem-solving abilities, and producing emotional lability and increased errors (Spier et al., 2000). Pain medication taken for an injury, menstrual cramps, or migraine headaches also can be responsible for students' altered capabilities.

Although it is not the responsibility of the faculty to diagnose the etiology of the impairment (Spier et al., 2000), an underlying cause other than illicit drug or alcohol use may be readily identified and addressed without necessitating further formal action. Discuss the situation with the student and explore appropriate options. Eating breakfast and carrying packets of cheese and crackers can take care of hypoglycemia. Dosages or frequency of administration of OTC medications may be altered, or substitutions may be made. For routine prescribed medications, students may be told to consult with their health care provider about their problems with iatrogenic drug effects. If faculty believe they have solved the problem of impaired student performance, and that it is not related to illicit drugs or alcohol, they should carefully document their assessment and intervention and continue to monitor the student closely. If the

---

BOX 8-6

Student Due Process in Disciplinary Actions

- Oral or written notification of the violation is given to the student.
- Notification of the violation provides sufficient detail of the allegations.
- A hearing is conducted in which the student may hear/see the evidence against herself and present a defense.

---

problem persists, it may be necessary to remove the student from the clinical setting and follow institutional policies regarding impaired function.

When a clinical faculty member makes the professional judgment that a student is chemically impaired, the specific course of action established by the nursing program should be followed. The student should be removed from the clinical setting on the grounds of being unsafe to practice. Liability for the student, the faculty, and the nursing program may be attached if an impaired student provides patient care that is unsafe (Brent, 2001). Faculty should then provide their evidentiary documentation to the person designated by the policy as responsible for carrying out the policy, typically an administrator of the program. The clinical faculty member is excused at this point, and other personnel manage further assessment and intervention. The student should not be permitted to return to the clinical setting until assurance can be obtained that chemical impairment due to illicit drug use is not substantiated. Dismissal from the nursing program may occur.

Due Process in Disciplinary Misconduct

Violations of academic integrity and breaches of established codes of conduct by nursing students must be addressed according to guidelines that support students' due process rights (Brent, 2001; Osinski, 2003). The policies may vary, depending on the situation. If occurring within the context of a specific course, transgressions of this type may be grounds for immediate course failure. Disciplinary action for some infractions is dismissal from the nursing program. Due process for course failures and dismissals related to disciplinary actions differs from that of other grade disputes (Brent, 2001; Osinski, 2003) (Box 8-6). The courts require that institutional interventions meet the criteria of fairness and equity and that students are allowed to speak on their own behalf. The documented policies and procedures must be reasonable, clear, and specific (Brent, 2001).

REASONABLE CLINICAL DISABILITY ACCOMMODATIONS

Accommodations in clinical courses begin with student-initiated disclosure of the disability. Unless the student has notified the appropriate agency within the academic institution, there is no legal obligation to provide accommodations. A separate resource center may be in place to deal with disability issues, or the matter may be addressed within the administration of the nursing program itself. For clinical courses, adequate planning time is not only desirable, it is essential. The Americans with Disabilities Act requirement for nondiscrimination mandates the creation of reasonable accommodations for students with disabilities. This is most challenging for the clinical courses of a nursing program. Disabled students must meet the established standards for the course—the course objectives. The accommodations made should allow the student to attain the same competencies and require the same number of clinical hours. The emphasis is on the reasonability of the accommodations, so creating something entirely new and different for one person does not meet the expectations of the law (Frank & Halstead, 2005). Depending on the disability, faculty may find that one specific clinical section is most desirable for a particular student because of its geography or clientele. A "clinical buddy" may be selected, using an interested and motivated work-study student in the program, to provide physical assistance in the clinical or skills laboratory setting. Being naturally creative and caring, nursing faculty will most likely be able to design clinical experiences that meet the reasonable accommodation standard in a meaningful way.

CLINICAL NURSE EDUCATOR LIABILITY

Nurses, in education as in practice, are most often involved in violations of civil rather than criminal law (Professional law and liability). Criminal law is concerned with the protection of society, and violations are punishable at federal, state, county, and city levels. The two classifications of criminal law are misdemeanors (minor offenses) and felonies (major offenses). Nurses may become involved in criminal law scenarios by not renewing their license and continuing to practice anyway, by illegally diverting drugs, and by being a party to patient deaths, intentional or unintentional (Professional law and liability).

Civil laws are related to the rights of the individual, as opposed to society as a whole. Civil, noncriminal decisions are known as *tort actions* (Davis, 2002); these are the most common in education (Brent, 2001). Tort cases are those relating to civil injustices or injuries unrelated to breach of contract. For a tort charge to be brought, three essential requirements must be met. First, the accused/defendant must have a demonstrable responsibility to the plaintiff; second, it is alleged that this responsibility was not met; and third, damage or injury occurred as a direct result of this breach of responsibility (Goudreau & Chasens, 2002).

Negligence is defined as "the failure to exercise the standard of care that a reasonably prudent person would have exercised in a similar situation" (Davis, 2002, p. 191). In nursing education, as in nursing practice, the standard applied is that of the registered professional nurse: what an ordinary, prudent, and reasonable nurse would do in the same or a similar situation. If a nurse educator is found to be negligent, that is, not to have met this standard in a particular situation, liability may be attached. Liability is assigned when a person is found to be legally accountable, responsible to another person or society at large, and the action is enforceable by civil or criminal penalty (Davis, 2002).

BOX 8-7

Common Areas of Negligence and Liability for Nurse Educators

- Failure to properly delegate duties to a student
- Failure to properly document students' nursing skills
- Failure to require students to obtain more education in areas of poor performance
- Failure to adequately notify students of areas of failure/poor performance: the faculty member fails to discuss or present a plan for improvement to the student, outlining areas that need improvement such as behavior, skills, or knowledge base
- Failure to facilitate student due process
- Failure to protect student safety

From Goudreau & Chasens, 2002; Aiken, 2004.

Nurse educators and staff nurses alike have often fallen victim to the urban myth that students are "working on my license" in the clinical area. It is a fallacy that either the nurse or the nurse's license to practice is in jeopardy if the student nurse commits an error. As is shown in Box 8-7, only the nurse's actions or lack thereof put a license to practice at risk.

Most of the areas delineated in Box 8-7 have already been discussed. The topic of protecting student safety is a new one. The courts have insisted that educators must do more than give safety instructions through assigned readings; they must provide supervision, guided practice, and personal warnings regarding potentially unsafe situations (Goudreau & Chasens, 2002). Students must be taught and supervised in adequate hand washing, handling used needles, appropriate use of protective barriers, lifting and transferring patients, handling potentially hazardous materials, managing violent patients, and assessing community situations for safety. Adequate preparation of students for actual and potential risks to their safety in all health care settings should be documented to protect faculty from accusations of negligence (Goudreau & Chasens, 2002).

Nursing faculty may be involved in legal actions with students in a number of ways (Brent, 2001). They may be named as co-defendants, along with the school or college, or they may be sued as individual faculty. Depending on the statutes of the state, some public academic institutions provide faculty protection from involvement in tort cases according to what is known as *sovereign*, or *charitable, immunity*. Such protection may not be complete, however. In some states with sovereign immunity, certain actions are not covered, and/or the faculty may still be sued individually. It would behoove faculty teaching in nursing programs to explore whether their state provides charitable immunity, and if so, to what degree. Although covered to a certain extent by insurance carried by the academic institution, faculty teaching clinical courses should carry their own liability insurance. Such a policy can be obtained through a variety of professional organizations at a nominal cost and can be part of the professional expenses deducted from income taxes.

In addition to negligence, clinical nursing faculty also may be held legally accountable for the adequacy of their teaching. Students alleging that one or more faculty breached their duty to teach effectively file what are called *educational malpractice suits*. Such suits have not been successful against educators in general and nursing faculty specifically (Brent, 2001).

SUMMARY

Academic faculty teaching in clinical settings are faced with a number of situations that have potential legal ramifications. A proactive approach is best. Doing everything possible to engender a positive teacher-student relationship and supportive learning environment will go a long way in reducing the likelihood of misunderstandings and litigation. Precautionary activities begin with the orientation to the clinical agency and to the course itself and continue through the term in the provision of adequate student preparation, supervision, and evaluation. Under these circumstances, faculty are unlikely to be exposed to legal action but should always carry individual professional liability coverage. There are likely to be situations in which the rights and/or responsibilities of the clinical site or the academic institution require clarification. Under these circumstances, faculty are advised to seek assistance from the leadership of the specific organization.

References

Aiken, T.D. (2004). *Legal, ethical, and political issues in nursing,* (2nd ed.). Philadelphia: F.A. Davis.

Boley, P., & Whitney, K. (2003). Grade disputes: Considerations for nursing faculty. *Journal of Nursing Education, 42*(5), 198-203.

Bozich Keith, C.L., & Schmeiser, D.N. (2003). Student issues: Anxiety—What's in a word? *Nurse Educator, 28*(5), 202-203.

Brent, N.J. (2001). *Nurses and the law: A guide to principles and applications* (2nd ed.). Philadelphia: Saunders.

Center for Academic Integrity. Available at http://academicintegrity.org

Davis, S.H. (2002). Glossary of legal terms. *Plastic Surgical Nursing, 22*(4), 188-193.

Frank, B., & Halstead, J.A. (2005). Teaching students with disabilities. In D.M. Billings & J.A. Halstead (Eds.). *Teaching in nursing: A guide for faculty* (2nd ed.). (pp. 67-84). Philadelphia: Saunders.

Goudreau, K.A., & Chasens, E. R. (2002). Negligence in nursing education. *Nurse Educator, 27*(1), 42-46.

Johnson, E.G., & Halstead, J.A. (2005). The academic performance of students: Legal and ethical issues. In D.M. Billings & J.A. Halstead (Eds.). *Teaching in nursing: A guide for faculty* (2nd ed.). (pp. 41-66). Philadelphia: Saunders.

Morgan, J.E. (2001). Confidential student information in nursing education. *Nurse Educator, 26*(6), 289-292.

Osinski, K. (2003). Due process rights of nursing students in cases of misconduct. *Journal of Nursing Education, 42*(2), 55-58.

Professional law and liability. Retrieved November 30, 2004, from http://www.bakerstuff. com/new_page_18.htm

Scanlan, J.M., Care, W.D., & Gessler, S. (2001). Dealing with the unsafe student in clinical practice. *Nurse Educator, 26*(1), 23-27.

Smith, M., McKoy, Y., & Richardson, J. (2001). Legal issues related to dismissing students for clinical deficiencies. *Nurse Educator, 26*(1), 33-38.

Solomon, M.R., & DeNatale, M.L. (2000). Academic dishonesty and professional practice: A convocation. *Nurse Educator, 25*(6), 270-271.

Spier, B.E., Matthews, J.T., Jack, L., Lever, J., McHaffie, E.J., & Tate, J. (2000). Impaired student performance in the clinical setting. *Nurse Educator, 25*(1), 38-42.

Tanner, C. (2004). Practical issues in measurement and evaluation. *Journal of Nursing Education, 43*(10), 435.

Zuzelo, P.R. (2000). Clinical issues: Clinical probation—Supporting the at-risk student. *Nurse Educator, 25*(5), 216-218.

UNIT III

Setting the Stage

Preparing the Clinical Learning Environment

As the classroom teacher must prepare for the first class, so too must faculty teaching clinical courses prepare for their first clinical day. Faculty who teach only in the classroom may not realize the amount of time their colleagues in the clinical arena devote to what can be termed "public relations." Cultivation of agency relations is required to maximize the quality of student learning environments and maintain that level over time. Adequate advance preparation can avert many difficulties. Furthermore, once rapport and respect are established, problems that may later develop can be addressed much more straightforwardly. Returning to a clinical agency previously used will not require as much time and effort, but some preliminary contact is still essential. For novice faculty, everything is new, and time should be set aside before the students arrive to permit a thorough orientation to each site where students will be placed. If the clinical course being taught or the clinical teaching model used demands less direct supervision of students by faculty, the need for adequate preparation of the learning environment is even more essential.

SELECTING CLINICAL PRACTICUM SITES

Eventually, faculty teaching clinical courses will likely be involved in the selection of new practicum sites. But even tried and true settings should be periodically reevaluated for their appropriateness and quality in light of the needs of the given clinical course. Not all clinical settings are capable of offering students a positive learning atmosphere (Chan, 2002). Whether opening a new site or evaluating a current one, the litmus test is the same: is the site appropriate to the goals of the specific clinical course, and are the learning experiences available in the setting of the highest possible quality? The challenge of selecting clinical locations that can provide optimal learning milieus for students is an arduous one.

Curricular outcomes or objectives of the course provide direction in site selection. It should be asked, Will this location provide the students with opportunities to develop the distinct clinical knowledge and skills required for this course? If a site cannot meet all of the course needs, more than one setting may be needed, and students will have to be rotated between them in order to achieve all of the desired competencies. Multiple sites also may be required for a single group of 8 to 10 students if a clinical setting has restrictions on the number of students that can be accepted or has limited numbers of appropriate patients. Adequacy of supervision to assure patient safety and facilitate student learning assumes increased importance when students in one clinical group must be scattered across several sites.

Given all of the available sites that will accomplish the goal of meeting course objectives, which is the best selection? In reviewing prior research, Birx and Baldwin (2002) found students preferred structured settings that offered practical active learning experiences and caring relationships and also fostered the development of both assertive and nurturing behaviors. It is not possible to overemphasize the importance of the student learning environment. "Experiential learning is enhanced in supportive communities and organizational climates" (Benner, 2001, p. *xi*). Although many nurses and other staff welcome students to their agencies, there are those who are "frosty" toward them; they are annoyed by the stress of working with learners and fail to see helping to educate future nurses as a part of their role (Birx & Baldwin, 2002). If the overall sense is that personnel are not receptive to students, may be rude and demeaning to them, or serve as poor role models, that clinical agency should not be used until time can be spent creating a better learning environment. Students are very sensitive to the attitudes of those around them. A caring and supportive faculty member will not be enough to offset the negativity engendered by a cynical learning environment. Working with staff who are not friendly or accommodating produces one of the greatest stresses nursing students can experience (Birx & Baldwin, 2002). The ordeal can be so detrimental as to cause some students to consider other career options. Additional considerations for clinical site selection may include congruency of the agency's mission and philosophy with those of the academic institution, appropriateness of the practice model employed, and whether or not the facility is accredited or licensed appropriately (Stokes & Kost, 2005).

Many sites used for the clinical education of nursing students have other educational commitments that may impact the nursing practicum. This is especially true of the acute care settings, but with current economic constraints and personnel shortages, even community-based settings may be affected.

When new staff orientees are being precepted by agency personnel, the number of satisfactory role models available to work with nursing students may be decreased, or there may be insufficient numbers of patients available. Student assignments become a real challenge when nursing students from multiple academic programs use the same clinical setting. Even using different shifts or days of the week, patients seen as providing the best learning experiences often tire of having student nurses. Other disciplines such as Physician Assistant or Emergency Medical Technician programs also may use the clinical site for the education of their students. Although there may be opportunities for interdisciplinary learning experiences in these situations, agency personnel may weary of the demands of nurturing neophytes.

Once clinical sites have been selected, it is necessary to be prepared for adjustments that may be required over the course of the term. Students may have to be removed from agencies for a wide variety of reasons, and being aware of alternative sites in advance is advantageous. Time spent in course meetings can be devoted to the discussion of potential options that might be drawn on at a later time. Nursing programs sometimes have faculty or staff assigned to the exploration and establishment of clinical sites as a part of their role responsibilities.

■ THE ROLE OF FACULTY EXPERTISE

Should the specific practice background of each faculty member influence the selection of clinical sites? Should the nurse with many years of experience in labor and delivery place students in that department only, to the exclusion of community-based clinics, or the nursery and postpartum departments? Obviously, this would not be conducive to the students' overall learning. As previously discussed, site selection for clinical courses should be primarily governed by the course objectives and the quality of the learning experiences available. An effort is usually made to match faculty expertise and site, but the interpretation of expertise changes when clinical practitioners return to the academic setting to teach beginning nursing students.

Following graduation and licensure, new nurses turn to the enhancement of their practice skills and decision-making abilities by choosing an area of focus. From the academic foundation of a generalist, nurses choose to specialize in more narrow fields such as neonatal intensive care, pediatric oncology, or geriatric psychiatric nursing. Moving back into the academic world to teach beginning nursing students in clinical settings requires stepping back into the generalist knowledge base of the broader practice fields such as maternity, pediatrics, or medical-surgical nursing. Returning to the care of patients in venues such as orthopedic traction, interpretation of laboratory values, or management of dialysis catheters after years of teaching cardiac rehabilitation, for example, can be very daunting! A common assumption of novice faculty is that they have to know it all—have the answer to every question students might ask. Because this is impossible, faculty are left feeling humiliated when the limits of their knowledge are exposed (Siler & Kleiner, 2001).

The research of Benner (2001) in examining skill acquisition in nursing practice provides both insight into and recommendations for the education of student nurses. Her findings support the idea that...

> Probably it is not necessary for instructors of the novice to be able to perform clinically at the advanced levels. *They need to be expert, however, at making visible the explicit guidelines and principles that will get the novice into the clinical situation in a safe and efficient way* (p. 186).

For faculty, being able to share with beginning students the thinking involved in conceptualizing and processing clinical problems is ultimately more valuable to their learning than knowing the normal range of systolic pulmonary artery pressures!

MEETING WITH AGENCY LEADERSHIP

Numerous studies have identified the important role nurse managers assume in creating and sustaining an atmosphere beneficial to student learning (Chan, 2002). Well before the term begins, faculty should arrange for a private meeting with the person who is in charge of each site, or the area within the site where students will be placed. It is advisable to also schedule several brief meetings with this person over the course of the term to discuss how the students' experience is progressing and share any concerns. Who this person is and the position held will vary with the agency. In acute care facilities, there may be a courtesy visit with the Chief Nurse Executive, but most often faculty meet with the manager of each unit in which students are to be placed. In community-based settings, faculty may need to meet with the head of the agency and the person overseeing staff. The manager's commitment to student learning is an essential component of a positive clinical learning environment (Birx & Baldwin, 2002).

During this meeting, clinical faculty should be prepared to provide general information related to the nursing program and the specific clinical course (Box 9-1). There should be an opportunity for discussion, and the information

---

BOX 9-1

Information to Provide Agencies in Advance of Clinical Practicum

- Name of the academic program
- Name and contact information for the assigned faculty member's supervisor
- Name and contact information for assigned faculty person
- Dates and times students will be present
- Skill and experience level of students
- Course objectives (syllabus)
- Desired learning experiences
- How confidential information will be protected
- Personnel role in student learning
- Personnel role in providing student feedback

also should be provided in writing. Try not to supply an overwhelming amount of information or paper; be thorough while still being succinct. During the meeting, identify any additional information related to the course or the overall nursing program that may be required.

The agency director also may be the person responsible for arranging a general agency orientation for the students. Time constraints and agency needs for student orientation vary considerably, so the earlier orientation can be scheduled the better, for both the agency and the faculty.

GETTING TO KNOW THE SITES

Before bringing students into a clinical site, faculty need to spend some time orienting themselves to the agency. This is a step often skipped, which can result in problems later on for both students and faculty. Knowing such things as where supplies are kept or the format used to document a home visit will be very useful. Faculty may excel in their content area both practically and theoretically, but not knowing the site-based idiosyncrasies of dealing with even the most mundane aspects of care can bring a student's learning activity to a grinding halt.

If at all possible, plan to spend at least half a day at the chosen agency, preferably during the same timeframe students will be working with the patients. Actually shadowing a staff member is the fastest and most efficient learning activity for faculty. This experience will give faculty the opportunity to see the routine, gain a general understanding of procedures, policies, and documentation, and know the location and types of resources available for students. Observing the staff at work is also an ideal occasion to determine who might work best with students, which will help with the identification of the best role models.

In some cases, faculty are assigned to bring their students to a clinical site at which they have previously been employed, or are currently employed, as a practicing nurse. Orientation to the agency itself can be eliminated or markedly reduced under these circumstances, but both faculty and agency staff must be prepared for the significant role transformation. Expectations of the two roles differ significantly.

REFLECTION EXERCISE 9

Teaching in a Practice Setting

Consider a specific clinical site in which you have practiced as a nurse.

- If you were to return to that setting as a faculty member teaching nursing students, what would you do and say to help staff understand the change in your role?
- How would your interactions with them change?
- How would they remain the same?

▨ PREPARING AGENCY PERSONNEL

The quality of students' clinical experiences is highly dependent on the personnel in the site. Before the students even arrive, the relationship faculty develop with staff does a great deal to pave the way for them. If faculty have been employed as practitioners in the agency, they must help personnel relate and interact with them in accordance with their new academic role.

Establishing Trust and Communication

The orientation time spent working side-by-side with agency personnel is a first step in establishing trust and opening lines of communication. From the perspective of the staff, a faculty member having competency as a practicing nurse is very important and anchors the cornerstone of their respect for one another. The agency site personnel must first trust in the faculty member's judgment as a nurse. This does not mean clinical faculty must be expert clinicians in every practice area in which they are teaching students. What is important is that faculty have an awareness of the limits to their knowledge and skill, know the location of resources, and are able to verbalize to students the critical thinking that guides clinical decision making.

During this orientation time, observe the various personnel roles, their functions, and communication among personnel. Get to know as many of the staff as possible by name. As a general rule, people are more responsive when addressed by name. Be friendly and respectful. Ask questions and solicit opinions, compliment the expertise observed, be enthusiastic about bringing students to the site, and the learning opportunities provided there.

Teambuilding

Teambuilding is an effective approach for blending the talents of individuals into a unified, goal-oriented whole. Teams are work groups that share a common goal and work toward its attainment while embracing the core values of trust, interdependence, and effective communication (Ohler, 2004). American businesses have used teambuilding as an organizational approach for enhancing productivity and employee satisfaction for a number of decades. In clinical nursing education, faculty and the personnel in each clinical site work as a team with the goal of facilitating quality clinical education for nursing students. The challenge for clinical faculty is to create that sense of common commitment among individuals with diverse personalities and skill sets, whose primary responsibility is the provision of the services offered by their agency.

The seeds of teambuilding are planted during the time faculty spend orienting to the agency. Once oriented to the site, learning a few names, and knowing something about the roles and abilities of the personnel within the agency, it is time to enlist them as colleagues in the clinical education experience.

If at all possible, arrange to meet with the staff as a group for a few minutes, perhaps prior to report or another scheduled meeting. The information presented previously in Box 9-1 needs to be shared with the staff, and then posted for reference in their common space. This is all important certainly in facilitating smooth functioning over the term, but the real purpose of this group meeting is the generation of team spirit. Much like a sports coach, faculty need to instill personnel with enthusiasm and motivation for their role in student learning. A little inspiration can go a long way. These students will be the nurses of the future, caring for us and for our loved ones. Each interaction with students is an opportunity for staff to participate in the molding of those practitioners.

Fostering Staff-Student Relationships

There are two sides to any relationship, and the initial orientation period is the time to work on the staff aspect of the staff-student relationship. Remind staff that the students are watching and listening; urge them to communicate a positive image of professional nursing. Encourage them to think back to their own student days, to get in touch with the feelings of the novice, the vulnerability and anxiety associated with being a learner. Students need to feel that they belong and are accepted and will be allowed to function as autonomously as possible, given their knowledge and experience (Chan, 2002). Simple courtesy, a friendly word or smile can go a long way toward making students feel more comfortable. Efforts made by agency personnel to socialize students into the clinical setting are of tremendous value. Students need to feel they belong to a group and are supported, despite their short residence in the agency.

SUMMARY

The investment faculty consign to getting to know clinical sites and cultivating working relationships with agency staff before student arrival can ultimately result in more satisfying student learning experiences. Staff need to know that they have a significant role in the quality of the overall student learning environment. They must have access to faculty if questions or concerns come to mind and be able to contact faculty directly and promptly if problems arise. Establishing a sense of being a part of a caring community and a contributing member of the team allows students to maximize their learning potentials.

References

Benner, P. (2001). *From novice to expert: Excellence and power in clinical nursing practice.* Upper Saddle River, NJ: Prentice-Hall Health.

Birx, E. & Baldwin, S. (2002). Nurturing staff-student relationships. *Journal of Nursing Education, 41*(2), 86-88.

Chan, D. (2002). Development of the Clinical Learning Environment Inventory: Using the theoretical framework of learning environment studies to assess nursing students' perceptions of the hospital as a learning environment. *Journal of Nursing Education, 41*(2), 69-75.

Ohler, L. (2004). Building effective teams in a high-tech world. *Progress in Transplantation, 14*(1), 7-8.

Siler, B.B., & Kleiner, C. (2001). Novice faculty: Encountering expectations in academia. *Journal of Nursing Education, 40*(9), 397-403.

Stokes, L. & Kost, G. (2005). Teaching in the clinical setting. In D.M. Billings & J.A. Halstead (Eds.), Teaching in nursing: A guide for faculty (pp. 325-346). Philadelphia: Saunders.

Preparing for the Students

In addition to learning as much as possible about the agencies in which students are to be placed, faculty teaching clinical courses should allow sufficient time to prepare their materials and themselves for the first encounter with their students. However, keep in mind that it is not possible to plan for every contingency; clinical courses are infamous for their spontaneity! But some anticipatory planning will allow faculty to consider how they might best present their course and themselves to their students. It is more than a matter of preparing the syllabus; the first meeting with the students requires emotional and mental preparation as well.

■ KNOW WHERE YOU ARE GOING

From the beginning of any course, faculty need to be clear about the anticipated endpoints of student learning. The curricular outcomes/objectives provide direction, a map with the general destination marked. The learning experiences are the mile markers along the way. Without a clear destination in mind, the learning activities may fail to progress the students in the desired direction. The issue is even more complicated for faculty teaching clinical courses. In clinical courses, there are multiple sections, groups of students, typically placed in a number of different clinical settings and supervised by diverse faculty.

Novice faculty, and any faculty new to a course, need assistance in attaining clarity regarding the course destination.

A meeting with all faculty teaching a given clinical course before the beginning of the term can facilitate both the sharing of ideas and the norming of expectations. New faculty can gain a great deal from such a meeting, not the least of which is a sense of comfort that they are seeing the course from the same perspective and operating within the same parameters as faculty teaching other sections of the course. Consensus regarding the cognitive and technical skill expectations can be attained, sparking discussion about common assignments and the use of reference materials and resources. It might be decided that some of this information would be beneficial to the students and could be placed in the course syllabus.

■ KNOW WHAT THE STUDENTS BRING

Part of effective teaching is holding students accountable for their prior learning and facilitating the application and enhancement of that knowledge. Take the time to review the program curriculum, identifying prerequisite and co-requisite courses for the clinical course being taught. What technical skills can reasonably be expected to have been mastered? What theoretical foundations have been established? Contemplate how this information can be best used at this point. A different approach would be needed for students in a pediatric clinical course who have already had a course in growth and development than would be used if students were concurrently enrolled in such a class. Expectations for the proficiency of assessment skills for students in their first clinical course are markedly different from those for students in the program's final clinical practicum.

If it will not be possible to attend the theory companion class for the clinical course, there are ways to strengthen the connection of theory to practice. Ask for a copy of the course outline. Knowing that the maternity theory course begins with fetal development and knowing when the topic of high-risk pregnancy will be addressed can have a major influence on the structuring of a maternity clinical course. If all faculty have access to e-mail, the theory instructor might be asked to circulate a weekly update of what has been covered and what might be explored in the clinical course. If chronic respiratory disease is the current topic in the medical-surgical nursing theory course, clinical faculty will have different expectations of the student caring for a patient with emphysema, and employ teaching techniques at a different level. This might be the best time to work on blood gas analysis, explore modes of oxygen administration, or apply discharge-planning principles to chronic disease management.

Remember to consider the other classes students may have had or may be taking presently. Consider how management skills, ethical decision making, research skills, or fiscal planning, for example, might be applied in clinical practice. It is here, in the practicalities of practice, that previously ephemeral knowledge becomes relevant.

▨ SYLLABUS DESIGN

The amount of control faculty have over clinical course syllabi varies widely among nursing schools. In some cases, one syllabus is used by all faculty teaching a particular course, and it provides all general course information. Individual faculty members then supply the students in their groups with materials pertinent to their own clinical sections. Or there may be a common syllabus that all clinical groups use, and then faculty add pages to address their section's unique needs, thereby giving students a cohesive but specialized syllabus. Regardless of the approach, the following topics are some important considerations to bear in mind as syllabi are constructed. A sample generic syllabus is provided in the "Clinical Toolbox" (see Chapter 20, p. 365).

Address All Contingencies

The courts view course syllabi as an agreement, or contract, between faculty and students (Brent, 2001; Mann, 2004).Despite the considerable administrative costs of producing a syllabus, it must be as long as necessary to assure every likely contingency is addressed (Mann, 2004). The cost factor can be minimized in a number of ways, including having students purchase syllabi as they do other course materials or posting them online. An advantage of the online approach is that templates for recurring assignments can be included and printed by students as needed over the term. Depending on the course, this might include materials such as the formats for care plans, process recordings, patient information and clinical preparation, and discharge planning.

Students can always be referred back to relevant policies addressed in their student handbook, but regardless, the syllabus should include reminders to students that they are accountable to those policies and the consequences that will occur if they are violated. In clinical courses, appearance standards, safety parameters, and matters of academic integrity should be specifically addressed at the start. Expectations for attendance, submission of assignments, and the procedure for faculty and agency notification in case of illness all need to be spelled out, along with the ramifications if they are not met. For example, faculty cannot deduct points for late papers unless they have written this consequence into their syllabus or they can refer to a program-wide policy in such matters. Also, students need to be clear about what can be done independently and the circumstances under which they must contact their faculty person for approval or assistance; this should be documented in the syllabus. If these guidelines are expected to evolve as individual student capabilities are assessed and/or the term progresses, an addendum to that effect can be added. The educational application of the clinical practice doctrine of "if it isn't documented, *it wasn't done*," becomes "if it isn't documented, *it can't be done*."

It is also legally imperative that students know how they are to be evaluated and have the opportunity at the beginning of the course to ask questions regarding evaluative criteria and methods (Brent, 2001). It is expected, therefore, that a copy of the clinical evaluation tool will be included in the course syllabus. All assignments may not be fleshed out in detail, but the weight they are to be accorded in the course grade and due dates should be identified. Establishing expectations does not impose rigid adherence requirements for faculty. In fact, flexibility is often necessary and part of the faculty prerogative. Deadlines may be changed, with adequate notification, but additional assignments or evaluative expectations not covered in the syllabus should not be applied after the initiation of the course.

Establish the Ground Rules

Course expectations always need to be written in the syllabus and at the level appropriate for the curriculum. This is especially important in the area of student autonomy. It is always best to start the term with tight reins on students where safety is an issue. When individual students demonstrate satisfactory functioning in specific areas, independence can be permitted, within the parameters of the law and faculty comfort. Students may have to perform their first newborn assessment with faculty supervision; then once they have satisfactorily demonstrated their skills, they may be told they can do this unsupervised. The administration of intravenous (IV) medications may be a skill introduced early in a medical-surgical practicum; this requires direct faculty supervision. As the term progresses, some students may become skilled enough to give antibiotics independently, but they will still require supervision by faculty or staff for administration of IV push medication. Faculty can and should address each student's progress independently. Let students know what ground rules are the baseline and that progress and autonomy will be determined on an individual basis. A sample statement for a syllabus regarding this might be as follows: Students are expected to call faculty regarding X, Y, and Z and will be directly supervised in performance of these skills until faculty determine they can perform them independently.

One universal message should be included in all syllabi, whether they are for clinical or theory courses: expectations of civil student behavior. Luparell (2005) makes a powerful case for the need for nursing faculty to take an approach that deters student incivility as being a moral imperative. "Professional values are demonstrated in patterns of behavior and guide interactions with others; ... behaviors that are disrespectful to others, including faculty, indicate an essential lack of value for human dignity and altruism that are essential to professional nursing" (p. 25). One of Luparells's strategies is especially appropriate for inclusion within the course syllabus. Providing behavioral guidelines in writing communicates their importance and allows students to review and refer to them throughout the term (Box 10-1). This then serves as a reference for discussion at the first meeting of faculty and students.

Share Your Philosophy

The course syllabus is the students' first introduction to their faculty. More will be shared with them at the first meeting, but the syllabus is an opportunity to present personal thoughts, attitudes, and values about teaching and learning in

BOX 10-1

Sample Behavioral Guidelines for a Clinical Course Syllabus

Along with the learning of theoretical concepts and clinical knowledge and skills, development of professional behaviors is a key component of the nursing curriculum. Therefore, it is expected that students will demonstrate professional behaviors in all aspects of this course. Academic integrity and appropriate conduct are expected. Respect for one's colleagues includes considerate deportment in all settings. Inappropriate or disruptive behavior will not be tolerated, and students who disrupt the educational environment will be removed from class. Refer to the *Undergraduate Student Handbook* for specific details. The following expectations expressly address academic and behavioral conduct in this course:

- Treat other students, faculty, and staff with respect.
- Demonstrate ethical and professional behavior at all times.
  - Be prompt for clinical experiences and seminars and be prepared to participate.
  - In seminars, keep "sub-grouping" conversation to the bare minimum to avoid distracting others.
  - Turn off and put away cell phones.
- Students are expected to check their individual e-mails for course announcements on a regular basis.
- Consistent attendance and active participation are essential for effective learning. Absenteeism and tardiness can impact course grades. Faculty are to be notified a minimum of 2 hours before clinical experiences begin of anticipated absences, and as soon as possible if a student expects to be late.
- Any form of academic dishonesty is addressed as described in the *Undergraduate Student Handbook*.

the clinical environment. This written philosophy creates an impression of faculty that students will form before a word is spoken. Box 10-2 provides a sample. It is not necessary to write a treatise. There may even be one or two quotes that are applicable, or a simple statement such as "I am here to help you succeed" or "We will learn together." Such a straightforward philosophy communicates volumes to students.

ADVANCE INFORMATION

Typically, faculty collect information from the students in their clinical groups when they first meet with them. Whether to obtain information about them before that time should be carefully thought through. Some programs may have explicit policies regarding faculty access to student information, either from their academic records or from other faculty. Confidentiality of student information is always an issue for faculty, both legally and ethically (Johnson & Halstead, 2005; Morgan, 2001). Faculty want to assist each student to the very best of their abilities, and for some faculty, having some information about

---

BOX 10-2
Sample Teaching Philosophy for a Clinical Syllabus

Let's make every minute count! Learning is active, not passive. It is a process of inquiry—a search for information and understanding. No one can make another person learn. It requires a conscious choice and effort on the part of the student. What is available to be learned in this class is worth your time, effort, and attention.

A good teacher is one who helps the student think and learn. I will try to be impartial and consistent. I will try to be the best teacher and facilitator I can be. You will get out of this clinical experience exactly what you put into it. Ultimately, it is the student who does the work of learning.

Let's keep the communication open, direct, and honest. If either of us has a concern, we need to share it respectfully, and sooner rather than later.

There are no stupid questions; there are only questions to which we do not yet have answers. Work hard, have fun, ask "WHY?" frequently!

---

their students early on permits anticipatory preparation that they believe will ultimately benefit the students' learning, especially when formal warnings have been issued by previous faculty member or a student has been placed on clinical probation. This justification may be used as the grounds for obtaining information from student academic records and/or prior clinical faculty, but if permitted, it must be done prudently and not universally. It is not appropriate for faculty to peruse the records of all students in a clinical group in advance, but it can be helpful to know what the issues were for students who are repeating a clinical course or whether there are established problematic patterns such as chronic tardiness or safety concerns. Alternatively, knowing too much about students can result in faculty unconsciously altering expectations of student performance (Mann, 2004). Generally speaking, it is probably best for students and faculty to begin each term with a blank slate and no preconceived opinions that may even inadvertently morph into expectations. Then, if problems do arise, faculty may choose to explore whether they have occurred before and how they have been addressed previously.

■ FIRST MEETING: CREATING THE SET

Anticipatory set is a term used in education to describe what a teacher does that disposes students to view and approach a situation in a certain manner. Most often, a set is a brief activity used at the beginning of a class for the purpose of getting the students' attention and involving them in the specific learning objective to be addressed. The concept also can be applied in the introduction to an entire course. In the first meeting with the students in a clinical group, faculty create the set for the term by presenting the learning goals for the course, generating interest and motivation, and illuminating the knowledge and experiential bridge from what preceded this course to what will now follow. The fear of the unknown that precedes new clinical experiences can be reduced when a set is used. The set is created within the context of the student-faculty relationship that faculty begin to establish at this first meeting. It provides a foundation for the learning that will occur and for the environment in which that learning will take place.

Acknowledge and Assuage Anxiety

New clinical experiences generate anxiety in students (Bozich Keith & Schmeiser, 2003). Faced with uncertainties about themselves and their learning environments, nursing students experience and exhibit varying amounts of clinical stress (Oermann & Standfest, 1997). Acknowledging the discomfort is a significant step in assisting student coping (Bozich Keith & Schmeiser, 2003). In this first meeting with students, stress can be reduced if faculty provide structure, make sure the course expectations are clear, and encourage students to be open in discussing their feelings (Bozich Keith & Schmeiser, 2003). This means the course syllabus, with its expectations and methods of evaluation, should be reviewed, and students should be encouraged to ask questions. Discussion of expectations presented in the syllabus allows students to seek clarification; also students are more inclined to comprehend the importance of topics if faculty take the time to discuss them.

Feed the Masses

An offering of food seems to naturally generate a change in the environment, disposing people to be more receptive and conversational. And students, with their long days and busy lives, tend to skip meals and eat poorly. Arriving at the first meeting with the students with a plate of cheese and crackers or fruit in hand creates a positive ambience from the start! Question: In addition to exercising muscles, what body organ requires a continuous supply of glucose and can take it up into the cells without the presence of insulin? Answer: the brain. So, feeding the masses also energizes the brain!

Encourage Active Learning

Acknowledge the active learning that is the essence of clinical courses; find ways to involve the students at the first group meeting, and communicate that this will be the norm for the entire term. Actions speak louder than words, so rather than tell, show. Consider some creative icebreakers and getting-to-know-you activities. Avoid lecturing from the syllabus; instead, operate under the assumption the students have read it, and encourage discussion and questions. Pose questions to the students that move them from the content in the syllabus to the application level. For example, ask, What modifications in the school appearance standards will be necessary in this clinical site? Or, knowing the requirements of the state Nurse Practice Act and the school's safety policy, what can you do before coming to this clinical site to assure patient safety?

Get to Know One Another

There is some purely informational and pragmatic data that faculty and students need to have about one another. This can be exchanged efficiently, without consuming inordinate time. Faculty can then move on to interpersonal activities that will give them insight about the new students and create a much more enjoyable atmosphere.

Write faculty access information on the face sheet of the syllabus, so that students will know office hours, e-mail addresses, telephone and/or pager numbers to use, and any special circumstances under which they must contact faculty. In the meeting, draw students' attention to this information; then be sure they know where faculty offices and mailboxes are located at the school, ask for questions, and move on.

Create an information sheet for each student to fill out, pass them out, and set a later time and location for students to turn them in so that meeting time is not consumed with filling out forms. Some variance may be required, depending on the course, but a general sample information sheet that could be used is shown in Figure 10-1.

Activities that help faculty get to know the students do not have to be boring and mundane. Rather than going around the group with the usual "tell us all about you" format, consider using a technique that is fun and stimulates creativity. These activities help students relax and can foster the development of both trust in the group and openness to listening and contributing. Some examples are provided in the "Clinical Toolbox" (see Chapter 20, p. 352).

It is important for faculty to give some thought to the type and amount of personal information they will share with their students. Novice faculty, in their desire to be liked, may fail to establish adequate boundaries with their students. This is a student-teacher relationship, not one between peers or colleagues; it is not a social relationship in the traditional sense. There is a degree of inherent inequality, as between employer supervisor and employee, that is a part of the relationship. That is why it is best for relatives or friends of the faculty member to be assigned to another clinical section; trying to change the parameters of a relationship once it has been established can be very difficult. Bear in mind the purpose of the relationship: for the student to attain the requisite knowledge and skills associated with the course. With this in mind, consider what personal information to share that will facilitate the goal. Faculty must be caring and supportive while maintaining a certain degree of personal distance. Education and practice experience help establish credibility and respect with the students, but it is primarily through the act of teaching that these are engendered. Telling anecdotal stories from selected practice experiences can be a useful teaching technique, but commiserating with students by sharing personal divorce stories, for instance, is not appropriate. Parents are told not to try to be a friend or a pal to their children; children need their parents to be parents. The same is true of students; students need their teachers to be teachers.

Name: _____

Telephone number: _____

E-mail address: _____

Nursing career goals: _____

_____

Prior work or volunteer experience in health care: _____

_____

Commitments outside of school that you think I should be aware of: _____

_____

Any specific concerns about this course or your learning that I should be aware of:

_____

_____

Specific learning experiences that you would like to have in this course:

_____

_____

What can I do to best help you learn? _____

_____

FIGURE 10-1 ▤ Sample student information sheet.

Assess Clinical Group Dynamics

At this first meeting, initial impressions are made. As the students participate in the activities of the first meeting, their sense of the course, their peers, and their faculty merge and their overall initial notions are formulated. Likewise, faculty leave their first meeting with students with a feeling for the group as a whole, along with perceptions of each participant.

BOX 10-3
Clinical Group Role Behaviors

Does there appear to be a leader in the group? If so, what leadership
  characteristics are exhibited?
Consider each student in light of the following common group role behaviors.
  More than one may apply to each student.
Nonparticipant
Follower
Monopolizer
Aggressor
Blocker
Recognition seeker
Jokester
Harmonizer/mediator/smoother
Distracter
Information seeker

Each group has definable characteristics that are an amalgamation of the predominate characteristics of the individuals that compose it. As the term evolves, the group's personality becomes increasingly clear. A group culture of ideas and values emerges. And a social structure, defined by the interactions among the members, also evolves. One faculty may have a quiet group of students, another a young and inexperienced group, and still another a divisive group.

The individual students in the group are unique. Although there may be some differences in later one-on-one interactions, initial observations of how each student interacts within the group can be very useful to faculty. After the first meeting, while thoughts are still fresh, record these impressions. The suggestions in Box 10-3 may provide a useful starting point. Then consider how these insights might be used to assist the functioning of the group and individual student learning.

SUMMARY

For faculty teaching clinical courses, preparing for the students requires advance effort in gathering information, designing a syllabus, and planning for the first meeting. Creating an anticipatory set that incorporates active learning opportunities effectively sets the stage for the entire course. Initial impressions of the students in the clinical group can be used to guide later teaching activities for both the entire group and the individual students.

Anticipatory Set

Imagine you are teaching a clinical course in nursing fundamentals, the first clinical course in the curriculum.

◈ What might you do and say to introduce yourself to the group?

◈ What might you do to create an anticipatory set?

◈ How would this differ from what you might say and do to create a set for a later course in your practice area (e.g., pediatric nursing, psychiatric nursing)?

References

Bozich Keith, C.L. & Schmeiser, D.N. (2003). Student issues: Anxiety—What's in a word? *Nurse Educator, 28*(5), 202-203.

Brent, N.J. (2001). *Nurses and the law: A guide to principles and applications* (2nd ed.). Philadelphia: Saunders.

Johnson, E.G., & Halstead, J.A. (2005). The academic performance of students: Legal and ethical issues. In D.M. Billings & J.A. Halstead (Eds.). *Teaching in nursing: A guide for faculty* (2nd ed.). (pp. 41-66). Philadelphia: Saunders.

Luparell, S. (2005). Why and how we should address student incivility in nursing programs. *Annual Review of Nursing Education, 3,* 23-36.

Mann, A.S. (2004). Faculty forum: Eleven tips for the new college teacher. *Journal of Nursing Education, 43*(9), 389-390.

Morgan, J.E. (2001). Confidential student information in nursing education. *Nurse Educator, 26*(6), 289-292.

Oermann, M.H. & Standfest, K.M. (1997). Differences in stress and challenge in clinical practice among ADN and BSN students in varying clinical courses. *Journal of Nursing Education, 36*(5), 228-233.

UNIT IV

Tools, Tactics, and Techniques

CHAPTER 11

Stimulating the Growth of Critical Thinking and Clinical Judgment

C linical judgment and critical thinking may indeed be entirely different constructs, if the analysis of current data is correct (Tanner, 2005). This interpretation is based on the incongruence of existing measures and differences in the definitions of the two constructs. At the same time, educators most often perceive clinical judgment in nursing as a discipline-specific reflection of critical thinking or reasoning skills in the practice arena (Alfaro-LeFevre, 2004). Outcomes of students' critical thinking are spoken of in broad terms. Although endeavors have been made to identify strategies that will develop and enhance critical thinking skills in the classroom and the clinical setting, in nursing, it is most obvious that the development of valid and reliable instruments to measure critical thinking has failed to keep pace with the evolution of the definitions of this construct (Tanner, 2005). Educational research and practice related to critical thinking in nursing are out of synch. As scholars endeavor to refine the theoretical basis for the decisions practicing nurses make in the clinical setting, educators must continue their efforts to produce graduates capable of displaying these skills.

Good clinical judgment may be interpreted as being one outcome of effective critical thinking in nursing; indeed, it is the praxis of critical thinking. The results of critical thinking in nursing practice can be seen in the skillful performance of a complicated dressing change, in sensitive and caring communication with an autistic child, in appropriate delegation of tasks to ancillary personnel, and in the analytical evaluation of the results of a teaching program

129

for new mothers. Once developed, critical thinking skills can be universally applicable. They can be applied to personal matters such as career development and financial management and to civic problems such as determining what organizations to support or what position to take on legislative issues (Lynch & Wolcott, 2001). Like other skills, skill in thinking requires practice if one is to learn and improve. In one way or another, every teaching activity and intervention students experience in the clinical setting has the potential to promote the development of critical thinking skills. The development of beginning practitioners who possess the skills and abilities to provide nursing care that is knowledge-based, intentional, and outcome-directed is the charge. How well this is accomplished is highly dependent on the judgment and skill of the faculty.

Some of the tools, tactics, and techniques presented in this unit are most appropriate for certain settings or for a particular type or level of student. But most are of broad value as far as assisting students to learn to think critically, and they can be easily modified depending on the circumstances. The literature exploring critical thinking is vast; an in-depth synthesis is inappropriate here. As critical thinkers themselves, readers are encouraged to further explore both the general literature and that which is specific to critical thinking and clinical judgment in nursing. This chapter provides a background and structure for critical thinking in clinical nursing education and is foundational to the use of the tools, tactics, and techniques presented in the subsequent chapters of this unit.

◼ CRITICAL THINKING: WHAT IS IT?

Teaching and learning today are evolving to be very different from what most faculty experienced during their own initial nursing education. The consensus opinion that people who go to college learn has been reexamined in terms of whether they learn to think (Halonen, Brown-Anderson, & McKeachie, 2002). The mere exposure to information through behaviorist pedagogies by content-centered faculty does not produce individuals prepared to deal with a world increasingly characterized by complexity and ambiguity. Graduates from all disciplines must demonstrate a contextual perspective and flexibility that will permit them to not only adapt but also excel. To accomplish this, the educational focus is now on the learner and how to foster effective thinking skills. Nearly every profession has spawned models for thinking, working through problems to result in improved professional judgments (Lynch & Wolcott, 2001). Educators have embraced the generation of critical thinkers as a panacea for societal adaptation in a swiftly changing world (Scheffer & Rubenfeld, 2000).

Critical thinking did not originate in either the education field or nursing. Its roots reach back to the Greek philosophers—Socrates, Plato, and Aristotle (Staib, 2003). Wherever its origins, discussions about thinking skills began to appear in the educational literature in the 1950s (Lynch & Wolcott, 2001), and since the early 1980s, the term has attained increased prominence (Staib, 2003).

Critical thinking is a construct, a theoretical entity. Those of a traditionalist perspective have viewed critical thinking as "...a rational approach...a means of knowledge acquisition...distinctly conscious mental operations that precede and guide human action" (Walthew, 2004, p. 408). Feminist writers since the early 1990s have imbued definitions of critical thinking with subjectivity in addition to its rational elements, acknowledging the role of curiosity, creativity, and intuition, as well as context (Walthew, 2004). Historically, scholars have debated whether critical thinking is discipline-specific, generic to all disciplines, or an amalgamation of the two (Staib, 2003). The lack of consistency in the definition of critical thinking has impacted both scholarship and practice within many disciplines.

Endeavoring to address this problem for higher education, the American Philosophical Association lent its support to a survey of experts in the arts and sciences conducted by Facione (1990). Using a Delphi methodology, the resulting interdisciplinary consensus definition of critical thinking was:

> the process of purposeful, self-regulatory judgment, which results in interpretation, analysis, evaluation, and inference, as well as explanation of the evidential, conceptual, methodological, criteriological or contextual considerations upon which that judgment is based (p. 2).

NURSING'S VIEW OF CRITICAL THINKING

Conceptualizations of the intellectual process aspects of the profession were subsumed in nursing's early definitions of critical thinking; affective components were added later but are often less emphasized and even ignored by some who perceive critical thinking as strictly a cognitive activity (Scheffer & Rubenfeld, 2000). Modern theorists have suggested that in addition to knowledge, attitudes, and skills, critical thinking is also a disposition, implying a propensity and desire to think critically (Youngblood & Beitz, 2001). Nurse scholars and educators have generated multiple definitions of critical thinking, all of which typically both define and operationalize the term since practitioners of nursing must act on their thought processes (Staib, 2003). Like beauty, critical thinking often exists in the mind's eye of the beholder. Unfortunately, the multiplicity of definitions has negatively impacted both nursing education and nursing scholarship. The development of a theoretical foundation has been impeded, as has the evolution of valid and reliable methods of assessment and evaluation.

Seeing the need for unanimity within the profession, Scheffer and Rubenfeld (2000) replicated the Facione study using an International sample of nurse researchers, educators, and practitioners. Their results included not only a definition of critical thinking with more than an 88% consensus but also the identification and description of its component subskills, termed *habits of the mind and skills* (Box 11-1). Although many others are available, this definition of critical thinking and those of the subskills will be applied throughout this text.

BOX 11-1

Consensus Definitions of Habits of the Mind and Skills of Critical Thinking in Nursing

Habits of the mind

Confidence: assurance of one's reasoning abilities.

Contextual perspective: considerate of the whole situation, including relationships, background, and environment, relevant to some happening.

Creativity: intellectual inventiveness used to generate, discover, or restructure ideas; imagining alternatives.

Flexibility: capacity to adapt, accommodate, modify, or change thoughts, ideas, and behaviors.

Inquisitiveness: an eagerness to know by seeking knowledge and understanding through observation and thoughtful questioning in order to explore possibilities and alternatives.

Intellectual integrity: seeking the truth through sincere, honest processes, even if the results are contrary to one's assumptions and beliefs.

Intuition: insightful sense of knowing without conscious use of reason.

Open-mindedness: a viewpoint characterized by being receptive to divergent views and sensitive to one's biases.

Perseverance: pursuit of a course with determination to overcome obstacles.

Reflection: contemplation upon a subject, especially one's assumptions and thinking for the purposes of deeper understanding and self-evaluation.

Skills

Analyzing: separating or breaking a whole into parts to discover their nature, function, and relationships.

Applying standards: judging according to established personal, professional, or social rules or criteria.

Discriminating: recognizing differences and similarities among things or situations and distinguishing carefully as to category or rank.

Information seeking: searching for evidence, facts, or knowledge by identifying relevant sources and gathering objective, subjective, historical, and current data from those sources.

Logical reasoning: drawing inferences or conclusions that are supported in or justified by evidence.

Predicting: envisioning a plan and its consequences.

Transforming knowledge: changing or converting the condition, nature, form, or function of concepts among contexts.

From Scheffer, B.K., & Rubenfeld, M.G. (2000). A consensus statement on critical thinking in nursing. (p. 358). *Journal of Nursing Education, 39*(8). Reprinted with permission from SLACK Incorporated.

The definition of critical thinking in nursing that resulted from the research of Scheffer and Rubenfeld (2000) is:

> an essential component of professional accountability and quality nursing care. Critical thinkers in nursing exhibit these habits of the mind: confidence, contextual perspective, creativity, flexibility, inquisitiveness, intellectual integrity, intuition, open-mindedness, perseverance, and reflection. Critical thinkers in nursing practice the cognitive skills of analyzing, applying standards, discriminating, information seeking, logical reasoning, predicting and transforming knowledge. (p. 357).

It has been noted that the cognitive skills named in this definition reflect the steps of nursing's rendition of the scientific method: the nursing process (Staib, 2003). A significant number of nurse educators are reported to perceive critical thinking to be the same as or at least closely related to the nursing process (Tanner, 2000; Staib, 2003; Walthew, 2004). However, the definition of Scheffer and Rubenfeld (2000), taken in its entirety, supports another position. From their perspective, critical thinking is seen as more than a cognitive activity because it also incorporates affective aspects (e.g., creativity and intuition), and the essential role that context plays in clinical decision making is acknowledged (Tanner, 2000). This broad interpretation of critical thinking is much more congruent with the realities of professional nursing practice (Staib, 2003).

Critical Thinking in Nursing Education and Professional Practice

Nursing practice today demands practitioners who are prepared to address extraordinarily complex health care issues. Educating nurses to provide that care demands more than requiring the memorization of facts and minutia. Today's nurses must have "... a sound knowledge base and cognitive skills for processing and analyzing information, weighing alternatives, and deciding on actions to take ... to solve clinical problems, (and) arrive at appropriate decisions after considering different alternatives" (Oermann, Truesdell, & Ziolkowski, 2000, p. 155). It has been postulated that if the majority of nurses who graduated were excellent critical thinkers, the resulting changes in practice settings would be revolutionary (Valiga, 2003). These nurses would be extremely capable in:

> managing conflicting information, examining the assumptions that underlie our practices and behaviors, making sound decisions despite incomplete information, questioning existing practices, searching for the evidence that underlies what we do in practice, making valid suggestions to change current practices, (and) functioning as leaders (Valiga, 2003, pp. 479-480).

Accrediting bodies have required evidence of critical thinking skills as an expected outcome of nursing education for more than a decade now and, in so doing, provide a degree of educational quality assurance (American Association of Colleges of Nursing [AACN], 1998; National League for Nursing Accrediting Commission, 2001).

Fortunately, the necessity of preparing student nurses for this ambiguous, context-dependent, multifaceted care environment has been accompanied by a reconceptualization of teaching to center on active, learner-focused strategies. The relationship between active learning and critical thinking is an intimate one (Youngblood & Beitz, 2001). The process of learning is heightened when students wrestle with ideas and teaching is focused on the learner (Halonen, Brown-Anderson, & McKeachie, 2002). During this educational transition, classroom teachers struggle to shift from traditional methods that relied extensively on covering content through lectures to approaches that depend on more dynamic student involvement. Students too are required to let go of the comfort of the familiar, prepare for class differently, and become participants in their educational experience in an entirely new fashion. Change is imbued with resistance for both groups.

■ DEVELOPING CRITICAL THINKING SKILLS IN THE CLINICAL SETTING

The documented resistance to classroom pedagogies that increase student critical thinking skills (Shell, 2001) does not seem to occur in the clinical setting. This may be related to the fact that learning in this environment is real-life and, by its very nature, active. Clinical instruction also provides faculty with the opportunity to interact with individual students and small student groups enabling a level of assessment, facilitation, and evaluation of critical thinking development not possible in the classroom.

Students must understand what critical thinking is, why it is so important for nursing practice, and what their role is in its development so that the strategies used in the clinical setting have meaning and are seen as part of a greater overall goal. The desired learning outcomes are generated through the interaction of faculty-designed learning strategies with the students' own application of motivation, learning skills, and self-awareness.

Many tools, techniques, and tactics designed to facilitate the development of critical thinking skills are explored in this unit. The use of the Learning Resources Center, the role of the clinical faculty as coach, the facilitation of critical thinking through group learning activities and written assignments, and in specific clinical situations and environments are presented. This is done with the educational goal of cultivating competent graduates with the requisite critical thinking skills to exercise clinical judgment at an entry level of practice and who are equipped to continue to grow and flourish. The teaching strategies presented in this unit are more effective when combined with reflection by the learner.

Although often cited as a freestanding strategy for developing critical thinking skills, reflection is far more than that. Reflection increases students' self-awareness of the effect of learning strategies, focusing their attention on their internal as well as external learning experiences. Furthermore, reflection is a skill first applied as a student and then as a practicing nurse in order to continue to learning effectively from experience and to grow as a critical thinker. Reflection can be incorporated into assignments and into dialogues with faculty, patients, and peer colleagues. The basics of reflection and its application to critical thinking are presented in this chapter.

▓ FOSTERING REFLECTION—THINKING ABOUT THINKING

Learning in the clinical setting occurs through preparation and then doing, thinking about what has been done, and receiving feedback about experience. The two major ways faculty help students learn the most from their clinical experiences are by (1) providing constructive, timely feedback about their work and self-assessments and (2) assisting them to effectively reflect on the experiences themselves (Westburg & Hilliard, 2001).

Link to Critical Thinking—Metacognition

As they develop, students become more knowledgeable about thinking in general and more aware of their own thinking. When they take action based on this awareness, they learn better (Anderson et al., 2001). Metacognition is literally thinking that is above or transcends thinking. Basically, metacognition is thinking about one's thinking. The resulting self-knowledge is crucial for learning. "A hallmark of experts is that they know what they know and what they do not know, and they do not have inflated or false impressions of their actual knowledge and abilities" (Anderson et al., 2001, p. 60). By practicing thinking about their thinking through reflection, students tap into metacognition and the skills of critical thinking are refined and honed.

Reflection to Monitor the Development of Critical Thinking

As students progress through their education, the courses they take should sequentially build on the thinking skills of the discipline until the desired level of the beginning professional is attained (Halonen, Brown-Anderson, & McKeachie, 2002). The knowledge of each discipline is highly contextual, and this profoundly impacts the thinking that occurs (Halonen, Brown-Anderson, & McKeachie, 2002). In nursing curricula, students' knowledge base expands, and their awareness of the impact of context on their practice progressively increases. Clinical experiences in any setting as beginning students are different from those at the end of the program because the students' knowledge and thinking skills, including their ability to respond to contextual differences, have grown. This growth is both mirrored in and facilitated by the students' reflections. If the skill of reflection is introduced in the first clinical course, and continues to be nurtured in successive practicum courses, a record of the development of each student's critical thinking abilities emerges. Both faculty and student can witness the student's transmutation into the role of a professional nurse who is prepared to enter practice as a critical thinker. Some approaches to the collection and use of such data are discussed in Chapter 18.

What is Reflection and Why Do It?

Reflection is the process of intentional contemplation on experiences and the accompanying thoughts and feelings. This is done purposefully in order to enhance self-discovery and personal meaning while practicing and refining critical thinking skills. Reflective practitioners examine the assumptions underlying their behavior, the knowledge brought to the situation, the choices made, and the effectiveness of their actions and words (Brookfield, 1995; Westburg & Hilliard, 2001). Reflection can occur during or following the experience (Westburg & Hilliard, 2001). For students just learning the practice of reflection, taking time after the experience to focus on it retrospectively will likely result in greater insights and quality of exploration. Reflection skills can be used broadly in clinical courses, with actual clinical experiences, in teacher-designed scenarios, and in reading and writing assignments. Westburg and Hilliard (2001) have identified a number of research-based reasons for fostering reflection in health care professionals (Box 11-2).

BOX 11-2

Research-Based Reasons for Fostering Reflection in Health Care Professionals

- Too many students in the health professions lack well-developed reflection skills
- Reflection skills can be learned
- Using reflection, existing knowledge can be identified and built upon
- Knowledge deficits and errors in thinking can be identified through reflection
- Reflection allows generalization from experiences and application of this knowledge to subsequent situations
- The integration of new knowledge is facilitated by reflection
- Reflection accelerates learning
- Assumptions and biases that may interfere with learning and patient care can be exposed through reflection
- Self-care and the provision of compassionate, comprehensive patient care are increased when students use reflection to understand their feelings
- Students obtain a sense of personal ownership in insights gleaned through reflection
- Self-identification of strengths and limitations increases students self-respect and confidence
- Students are able to attend accurately to their individual learning needs through reflection
- Encouraging student reflection enhances collaborative relationships with faculty
- Skill in reflection is essential for future competency and learning following graduation
- Better patient care is provided by reflective caregivers
- Incompetency and potentially unsafe practice can occur if health care providers are not reflective, self-governing, and self-critical

From Westburg, J., & Hilliard, J. (2001). *Fostering reflection and providing feedback: Helping others learn from experience.* New York: Springer Publishing. Used by permission from Springer Publishing Company, Inc., New York 10036.

Using Reflection in Clinical Nursing Education

The teaching activities and interventions presented in this unit have the potential of promoting the development of critical thinking skills, and incorporating reflection into their application enhances that process. Suggestions for how to accomplish this are appropriately incorporated into the discussion within subsequent chapters. The vehicle for recording and guiding reflection is most often some form of a student journal (Herrman, 2002; Kennison & Misselwitz, 2002; Kessler & Lund, 2004; Ruthman et al., 2004), so that approach is explored here.

Reflective journaling assists students in heightening their awareness of their thinking and decision making, and how this is echoed in their clinical practice. Retrospective analysis allows students to gain a deeper understanding of the multiplicity of factors involved within clinical situations. With the benefit of time and resources, students can analyze their experiences, incorporating variables not previously considered, and explore a wide variety of potential alternative approaches. Initiated in the first clinical course, journaling can become an increasingly familiar and useful tool as the student progresses through the curriculum. Faculty guide the process through the directions provided to the student.

In some cases, students may be given anticipatory guidance to help them focus during a clinical experience by determining what they bring to it, establishing learning goals (Westburg & Hilliard, 2001), or providing questions they are to direct to a patient. In journaling after the experience, students are provided general instructions or specific prompts that are directed toward the assignment or setting. These directives can become increasingly sophisticated over time, in the given course and across other courses in the program. Materials in the "Clinical Toolbox" (Chapter 20, pp. 351, 360) provide general guidelines for reflective journaling and some examples of how reflective journaling can be used in clinical courses.

Students should be provided with directions for reflective journaling, along with illustrative examples (Kessler & Lund, 2004). An emphasis on quality over quantity, context over content, and process over product is important. Guidance in how to write reflectively is essential for students beginning the practice. Extensive descriptions of a situation are not necessary; students should provide only as much background as is required to permit the reader to understand the context. Having students focus on their thoughts and feelings, explore and challenge preconceptions, and discover connections to prior learning encourages the development of self-awareness and insight (Kessler & Lund, 2004).

Reflective journals are a written dialogue between students and faculty. Providing feedback that recognizes and rewards critical thinking, helps guide students into areas that need further attention, stretches and/or refines their thinking, and engages and sustains their interest will maximize their learning and increase the development of self-awareness and mastery of reflection

(Westburg & Jason, 2001; Kennison & Misselwitz, 2002). At the same time, positive feedback for quality thinking and growth must be incorporated. Examples of this are "Good beginning. What did you think about . . . ?" or "This is a good observation. What factors did you consider in determining this was the best patient teaching approach?" When students identify limitations, faculty should congratulate them on their self-awareness and assist them to prioritize them, if necessary (Westburg & Jason, 2001). Ask rather than tell, but avoid questions that are so vague students would have to be mind readers to guess the answer. Encourage them to consider what others in the situation might have been thinking and feeling as a means of enlarging their perspective. Guide students to link current thoughts and feelings with those from past experiences (Westburg & Jason, 2001). The feedback provided should build on the teacher-student relationship, and to do that, trust must be engendered and openness encouraged through a nonjudgmental, caring approach. High-quality faculty participation in the dialogue must be sustained in order to maximize the educational value of reflective journaling.

Evaluating Reflective Journaling

The evaluation of reflective journaling as part of a course grade is a subject of considerable discussion; it reflects faculty assumptions about both grading and learning. Anecdotal evidence and personal experience has lead some faculty to generalize that grades are a primary impetus for learning and that students devalue assignments that do not contribute toward their grade in a class, expending little effort on the tasks (Kennison & Misselwitz, 2002). Opponents to grading reflective journals insist it quashes freedom of expression and creates anxiety in students that is counterproductive to the purpose of the assignment (Kessler & Lund, 2004; Kennison & Misselwitz, 2002). In one case, students were asked whether their entries would have been any different if they had been graded, and 94% of the sample (N = ?) responded that they would not (Kessler & Lund, 2004).

In many nursing programs, clinical courses are graded as pass/fail; completion of assignments under these circumstances is usually a requirement for receiving a passing grade, and a level of acceptability is established as a standard. Overall clinical evaluation and grading are the subject of Chapter 18. In those cases where reflective journal entries are graded, detailed criteria for evaluation should be established and consistently applied (Kennison & Misselwitz, 2002) and shared with students in advance. If reflective journaling is to be used throughout a nursing program, or in more than one clinical course, it would probably be advantageous for faculty to determine an overall position regarding grading in order to communicate clearly to the students how reflective journaling is viewed at a programmatic level. "Is reflection used to foster self-evaluation and critical thinking, or is it used to augment grade assignments in clinical practice?" (Kennison & Misselwitz, 2002, p. 240). Whether reflective journals are graded or not, the expectations for journal assignments should be explicit in order to enable students to maximize their learning.

SUMMARY

The ability to think critically is considered an essential educational outcome for today's college graduates. Critical thinking skills are not discipline-specific; they are seen as universally applicable life skills, enhancing the ability to be successful and proactive in today's complex global society. In nursing practice, these skills increase the quality of clinical judgments, and managerial and leadership acumen. The definition of critical thinking and its subskills by Scheffer & Rubenfeld (2000) are used in this text. It is incumbent on nursing faculty to teach and interact with students in such a way that these skills are developed and valued. The tools, tactics, and techniques described in this unit contribute to this goal. Used in conjunction with these methods, and as a part of the clinical learning experience, reflection augments the acquisition of critical thinking skills and contributes to their mastery.

REFLECTION EXERCISE 11

Thinking About Critical Thinking

Briefly describe a clinical situation from your practice experience in which you believe you practiced and demonstrated critical thinking. Read again the habits of the mind and skills of critical thinking in nursing and their definitions in Box 11-1.

◆ Which of these skills do you see within your scenario?

◆ Now that you have read the list again, are there some others that you feel occurred that you didn't mention before?

◆ Of the subskills that you did not use, how might the process or result differ had you done so?

◆ What were the contextual issues in this scenario? Did their consideration impact your thinking? If so, how did this occur?

References

Alfaro-LeFevre, R. (2004). Critical thinking and clinical judgment: A practical approach (3rd ed). Philadelphia: Saunders.

American Association of Colleges of Nursing (AACN). (1998). *The essentials of baccalaureate education for professional nursing practice.* Washington: AACN.

Anderson, L.W., Krathwohl, D.R., Airasian, P.W., Cruikshank, K.A., Mayer, R.E., Pintrich, P.R., et al. (Eds.). (2001). *A taxonomy of learning, teaching, and assessment: A revision of Bloom's taxonomy of educational objectives.* New York: Longman.

Brookfield, S.D. (1995). *Becoming a critically reflective teacher (Jossey Bass Higher and Adult Education Series).* San Francisco, CA: Wiley and Sons.

Facione, P.A. (1990). *Critical thinking: A statement of expert consensus for purposes of educational assessment and instruction.* Millbrae, CA, The California Academic Press (ERIC ED 315423).

Halonen, J.S., Brown-Anderson, F., & McKeachie, W.J. (2002). Teaching thinking. In W.J. McKeachie (Ed.), *McKeachie's teaching tips* (11th ed.). (pp. 284-290). Boston: Houghton Mifflin.

Herrman, J.W. (2002). The 60-Second Nurse Educator: Creative strategies to inspire learning. *Nursing Education Perspectives, 23*(5), 222-227.

Kennison, M.M., & Misselwitz, S. (2002). Evaluating reflective writing for appropriateness, fairness, and consistency. *Nursing Education Perspectives, 23*(5), 238-242.

Kessler, P.D., & Lund, C.H. (2004). Reflective journaling: Developing an online journal for distance education. *Nurse Educator, 29*(1), 20-24.

Lynch, C.L., & Wolcott, S.K. (2001, October). Helping your students develop critical thinking skills. Idea paper #37. The Idea Center. Retrieved January 14, 2005 from http://www.idea.ksu.edu/papers/index.html.

National League for Nursing (NLN) Accrediting Commission. (2001). *Accreditation manual and interpretive guidelines by program type for post-secondary and higher degree programs in nursing.* New York: NLN.

Oermann, M., Truesdell, S., & Ziolkowski, L. (2000). Strategy to assess, develop, and evaluate critical thinking. *Journal of Continuing Education in Nursing, 31*(4), 155-160.

Ruthman, J., Jackson, J., Cluskey, M., Flannigan, P., Folse, V.N., & Bunten, J. (2004). Using clinical journaling to capture critical thinking across the curriculum. *Nursing Education Perspectives, 25*(3), 120-123.

Scheffer, B.K., & Rubenfeld, M.G. (2000). A consensus statement on critical thinking in nursing. *Journal of Nursing Education, 39*(8), 352-359.

Shell, R. (2001). Perceived barriers to teaching for critical thinking by BSN nursing faculty. *Nursing and Health Care Perspectives, 22*(6), 286-291.

Staib, S. (2003). Teaching and measuring critical thinking. *Journal of Nursing Education, 42*(11), 498-508.

Tanner, C.A. (2000). Critical thinking: Beyond nursing process. *Journal of Nursing Education, 39*(8), 338-339.

Tanner, C.A. (2005). What have we learned about critical thinking in nursing? *Journal of Nursing Education, 44*(2), 47-48.

Valiga, T.M. (2003). Teaching thinking: Is it worth the effort? *Journal of Nursing Education, 42*(11), 479-480.

Youngblood, N., & Beitz, J.M. (2001). Developing critical thinking skills with active learning strategies. *Nurse Educator, 26*(1), 39-42.

Walthew, P.J. (2004). Conceptions of critical thinking held by nurse educators. *Journal of Nursing Education, 43*(9), 408-411.

Westburg, J., & Hilliard, J. (2001). *Fostering reflection and providing feedback: Helping others learn from experience.* New York: Springer Publishing.

Westburg, J., & Jason, H. (2001). *Fostering reflection and providing feedback: Helping others learn from experience.* New York: Springer Publishing.

CHAPTER 12

Role of the Nursing Learning Resource Center

- CURRICULAR APPLICATIONS
- PSYCHOMOTOR, COGNITIVE, AND AFFECTIVE SKILL DEVELOPMENT
- CLINICAL LEARNING RESOURCES
- LOW-TECH TOOLS
- HIGH-TECH TOOLS
- SUMMARY
- *REFLECTION EXERCISE 12: USING THE LRC*

Yesterday's nursing skills lab has metamorphosed into a multimedia focal point for teaching and learning. Known by a wide variety of names, the burgeoning educational technology and ever-expanding knowledge of educational pedagogies have combined to produce a setting for learning of nearly boundless potential. Depending on how it is conceptualized by the nursing program, and the fiscal and human resources available, the learning resource center (LRC) of today may encompass an assortment of services and fulfill many functions. In addition to supporting psychomotor, cognitive, and even affective skill acquisition, the LRC may provide an abundance of other supportive services to the nursing program (Hodson-Carlton & Worrell-Carlise, 2005). The LRC often also incorporates the program's multimedia and computer laboratories. It may provide technologic support services, and produce multimedia programs. The LRC can be used to enhance faculty development and consultation for teaching activities, coordinate distance-learning programs, and support continuing education for practicing nurses in the community (Hodson-Carlton & Worrell-Carlise, 2005).

New LRCs are being designed and old ones renovated to facilitate incorporation of technologic and educational advances and equip them to meet the needs of increasingly diverse student populations and community health care agencies (Snyder, Fitzloff, Fiedler, & Lambke, 2000; Ankele, Lohner, & Masiulaniec, 2001; Jeffries, Rew, & Cramer, 2002). Networks are being developed to further discussion, research, and scholarship regarding the teaching and learning environment in LRCs performance evaluation, and methods of operation of LRCs; these include national and international conferences, Listservs, and various publications (Hodson-Carlton & Worrell-Carlise, 2005). To maximize the use of the LRC in the support of clinical nursing education, faculty must become familiar with how this facility is used in their specific nursing

141

program, the equipment and supplies available, and the accessible personnel and technologic resources. This chapter serves as an overview of how the LRC and its resources may be used to assist teaching and learning in clinical nursing education.

■ CURRICULAR APPLICATIONS

Nursing programs use their LRCs to meet a variety of goals, and these, in combination with the resources available, determine how clinical nursing faculty integrate the centers into their teaching. Investigate how the LRC is used in your specific nursing program, meet the personnel, and explore the resources housed there with an eye toward the focus of the clinical course you will be teaching.

The role of clinical faculty in the LRC is highly dependent on the number and use of LRC personnel. In some nursing programs, LRC personnel provide direct skill instruction, supervision of student practice, evaluation of skill performance, and supervision of educational multimedia. Other programs limit the involvement of LRC employees in one way or another, most commonly by excluding their involvement in skills instruction and/or evaluation. The use of student-peers as instructors in the LRC also has been reported (Owens & Walden, 2001).

Time spent in the LRC may be incorporated into the total number of hours allocated for a clinical course, on a weekly basis or in blocks of time over the term. Alternatively, the time students spend in the LRC may be extracurricular, as is the time spent in the library or otherwise studying. A combination of these approaches may be used in which students have access to the facilities on their own time in addition to that spent as part of their clinical hours.

Nursing faculty must determine the essential skills (psychomotor, cognitive, and affective) to be required of their students, at what point in the curriculum they are to be mastered, and the desired competency outcomes to be attained at a programmatic level (Hodson-Carlton & Worrell-Carlise, 2005). Typically, some sort of checklist approach is used, with the applicable skills for each clinical course designated. The selection of essential skills may be derived from textbooks and clinical agency procedural manuals (Hodson-Carlton & Worrell-Carlise, 2005), surveys of health care agencies (Utley-Smith, 2004), and/or accrediting bodies (American Association of Colleges of Nursing [AACN], 1998). It is important that input from the service arena be obtained in order to attain congruency between clinical practice and educators' expectations. "The minimal research on skill competence, assessments, and expectations indicates disparate opinions between these two groups" (Miracle, 1999, p. 88). The need for independent practice will escalate with the continuation of current trends in health care in general and nursing in particular. This means that educators must continue to develop new methods of teaching skills efficiently while integrating critical thinking applications.

It may be that students are required to practice all or some psychomotor skills in the LRC before performing them in the clinical area. A designated level of competency may have to be demonstrated and documented in the LRC before skills may be performed on patients. Evaluation of some psychomotor skills may be done exclusively in the LRC. Understanding of theoretical aspects of some psychomotor skills also may be evaluated through other methods, such as paper and pencil or computer testing. Novice faculty need to be clear about these expectations before the beginning of the term.

Clinical faculty face many challenges today. Higher patient acuity levels, shorter lengths of hospital stay, shortages of nursing staff capable of assisting students, reduced faculty availability, increased faculty-student ratios, and limited access to some learning settings impede the ability to provide meaningful clinical learning opportunities for student nurses. LRC experiences may be used to replace selected clinical experiences such as those provided in labor and delivery, critical care, and the emergency department (Miracle, 1999; McCausland, Curran, & Cataldi, 2004; Medley & Horne, 2005; Tarnow & Butcher, 2005). Increasingly sophisticated technologies are available that are capable of creating realistic learning opportunities of a highly contextual nature.

The LRC may be a place where students can make up clinical absences, but more commonly it is used for remediation for students deemed to be inadequately prepared for clinical experiences or for students having difficulty transitioning theory from the classroom to the clinical setting (Haskvitz & Koop, 2004; McCausland et al., 2004). The amount of clinical faculty involvement in remediation in the LRC depends on the individual student's needs, the resources available, and the role and accessibility of LRC personnel. At a minimum, faculty should meet with the student to create a plan that will allow the student to repeat the skills or scenarios that have posed difficulty. The faculty, or the LRC personnel, depending on the philosophy of the nursing program, may carry out the implementation and evaluation. Such an approach to remediation may enhance student learning while protecting patient safety (Haskvitz & Koop, 2004; McCausland et al., 2004).

Depending on the nursing program, alternative experiences in the LRC also may be used in cases of faculty absenteeism. Although it may be possible to find replacement faculty in the case of an instructor with a protracted illness, rarely are additional faculty available who can take over clinical courses in the event of short-term absences of 1 or 2 days. And often neither is it possible to simply add a day or 2 to a clinical course to make up for lost practice time. Preplanned learning activities in the LRC may be one alternative to this dilemma; this and other options for overcoming faculty absences are explored in Chapter 17.

▥ PSYCHOMOTOR, COGNITIVE, AND AFFECTIVE SKILL DEVELOPMENT

Classically, the LRC has been used for the teaching, practice, and/or evaluation of technical psychomotor skills. In the LRC, the environment for learning clinical skills is far more controlled than it is in clinical settings. Extraneous variables can be eradicated, allowing the student to focus on the specific learning activity at hand, and then gradually these variables are reintroduced to add the complexity of typical clinical scenarios.

The major advantages of using the LRC for psychomotor skill acquisition are the promotion of patient safety and the opportunity for skill repetition (Miracle, 1999; McCausland et al., 2004). Students are able to perform skills over and over until they attain a certain degree of technical skill competency before performing the skill on actual patients. Assumptions also have been made that practicing in this not-quite-real setting has the added benefits of reducing student anxiety and increasing confidence. These assumptions are challenged by studies of learning, performing, and testing in lab settings, where nursing student anxiety and confidence levels have been variously reported as equal to, higher, and lower than those in the actual clinical setting (Miracle, 1999).

More specific discussion of the teaching of psychomotor skills is provided in Chapter 13. Generally, although psychomotor skills incorporate cognitive and affective dimensions, for optimal learning these aspects are separated during instruction for beginning students (Miracle, 1999). Skill development must progress to a certain point before more abstract skills may be introduced (O'Connor, 2001). Then, with the integration of cognitive and affective components, the full meaning of the performance of technical skills is truly learned. All three domains may be incorporated through the use of replicated clinical experiences such as vignettes, standardized patients, and multimedia simulations. Contextual perspective and critical thinking are thereby assimilated into the students' overall learning experience in the LRC. The art, as well as the science, of nursing can be introduced, modeled, and reinforced in this setting (Tarnow & Butcher, 2005).

Two broad, general approaches are used in LRCs for the instruction of psychomotor skills: a traditional approach involving direct faculty instruction and supervision and a student self-directed approach using applicable multimedia (Hodson-Carlton & Worrell-Carlisle, 2005). In comparative studies, such as that of Jeffries, Rew, and Cramer (2002), differences in learner satisfaction, self-reliance, cognitive gains, and self-efficacy in learning are the typical variables studied. Results of such research have been varied, affected by the designs and methodologies used as well as sample sizes (Miracle, 1999; Hodson-Carlton & Worrell-Carlisle, 2005). Depending on the circumstances, both approaches are commonly used in the LRC. Efforts also have been made to match learning style with teaching style, with insignificant outcome variation (Miracle, 1999). Today's Gen-X and Net-Gen students are increasingly competent and self-sufficient technologically and desirous of both independence and autonomy. This makes the multimedia approach increasingly more applicable and acceptable as a means of acquiring skills and bridging students into the clinical setting.

Several methods of skill evaluation have been employed in the LRC: peer evaluation, videotaping, direct instructor evaluation (Miracle, 1999). Both advantages and disadvantages of using the LRC setting for evaluation have been identified in the literature (Miracle, 1999). Positive aspects include the ability to control variables and specifically define criteria, to observe more than one outcome at a time, and to provide a setting that is more realistic than what would be found using written testing methods. Disadvantages, depending on the method employed, include the significant amount of time and resources required for the preparation and monitoring of skill performance and evaluation (Miracle, 1999).

As in peer instruction, peer evaluation requires that students have adequate preparation and clarity in expectations. Peer evaluation does have the advantage of helping evaluators mentally visualize the skill, which enhances their own procedural knowledge (Hodson-Carlton & Worrell-Carlisle, 2005) and may result subsequently in decreased student anxiety (Owens & Walden, 2001). Peers may directly observe skill performance or critique videotapes that have been made while other students carried out skills. Peer evaluation is most often used for formative evaluation as a part of obtaining skill mastery; responsibility for summative competency evaluation is most likely to be retained by the faculty or LRC personnel.

Videotaping of skill performance may be done for the purpose of engendering student formative self-evaluation or peer evaluation to provide a tool for enhancing skill mastery or a means for faculty to compose formative or summative evaluations of students (Winters, Hauck, Riggs, Clawson, & Collins, 2003). If the LRC has the necessary resources, this can be a time-efficient approach to skill evaluation. However, a preference for direct faculty evaluation has been reported by both faculty and students (Miller, Nichols, & Beeken, 2000), and some skills do not lend themselves to a videotaping approach (Winters, Hauck, Riggs, Clawson, & Collins, 2003). However, "Seeing themselves as their patients and others see them guides students in developing their caring, aesthetic behaviors, and in changing less effective behaviors" (Tarnow & Butcher, 2005, p. 381).

Depending on the nursing program, clinical faculty and/or LRC personnel may carry out direct evaluation in the LRC. In either case, the skill performance may be observed and questions posed in order to evaluate multiple domains of knowledge simultaneously. The process may be placed within the clinical context through use of scenarios or vignettes or through high-tech modalities such as multimedia simulations or virtual reality systems. Criterion-based checklists are commonly used for skill evaluation, but are usually reported as effective only anecdotally (Miracle, 1999). A simple list of skills may document the location of evaluation, be initialed when the skill is satisfactorily attained, and then used as a means of communicating such information to other faculty and students. A sample of this approach is provided in the "Clinical Toolbox" (see Chapter 20, p. 364). As with the use of differing instructional strategies, the evaluation of skill competency testing undoubtedly will benefit from future nursing research.

▇ CLINICAL LEARNING RESOURCES

Spend some time perusing your nursing program's LRC, in terms of materials and policies. Typically there are policies for the removal of supplies for use outside of the LRC, as well as for procedures students are permitted to perform on one another (e.g., IV starts, injections). The learning materials available in an LRC vary widely, commonly including patient teaching materials and other items for student use in the clinical setting, copies of agency procedure manuals, simulated patient records, and agency-specific equipment such as infusion pumps. In addition to these general materials, the LRC may have other learning tools available that use low-level or high-level technology.

LOW-TECH TOOLS

Exploration of the cupboards and cubicles in the LRC can reveal a wealth of low-tech, often inexpensive teaching tools that clinical faculty can use there or, in some cases, check-out for use elsewhere. Box 12-1 provides a summary list of potential applications of these effective and low-cost tools, tactics, and techniques.

The LRC setting itself is a valuable environment for learning. Typically, there are minimilieus within the LRC that provide backdrops for nursing practice. Hospital bedsides for adult and pediatric patients are recreated, medication rooms and nursing stations are replicated, sinks are designed for surgical scrub practice, and critical care cubicles are stocked with emergency equipment. The near replication of reality in terms of the environment and equipment is important for maximizing student learning. The clinical context can be further enhanced when students are encouraged to behave as they would in the actual settings (Medley & Horne, 2005), for instance, by using curtains and screens for privacy (Tarnow, 2005) and conforming their demeanor to be consistent with expectations for professional behavior.

These minimilieus can be very effective backdrops in which to develop successful and inexpensive teaching techniques based on role-playing or standardized patient scenarios. Role-play is typically less structured than standardized patient scenarios. In simple role-playing activities, students, and sometimes faculty, take on the roles of clients and nurses, enacting a given situation to facilitate practicing a variety of skills, especially those in the affective domain. Interview skills and other communication skills such as history taking, conflict resolution, group dynamics, patient teaching, and nurse-patient or

---

BOX 12-1

Low-Tech Tools, Tactics, and Techniques in the LRC

- Minimilieus as context for:
  - Role-playing with/without vignette/case study–based simulations
  - Standardized patient scenarios
- Simple models and mannequins with/without vignette/case study–based simulations
- Commercially prepared and faculty-designed posters, brochures, teaching kits, and games

nurse-physician interactions are commonly practiced in this way. Home visits and telephone assessments that simulate calls to suicide hotlines or poison control centers also can be role-played. Psychomotor skills can be practiced through role-play as well. Endeavoring to mimic the context of actual interactions with patients and teach critical thinking skills, faculty may design case vignettes to provide perspective (Staib, 2003) and add props to serve as environmental cues and/or require some sort of documentation during or following the role-play (Van Eerden, 2001).

Standardized patient scenarios are similar to role-playing but are more structured and more reflective of the clinical context. Before this technique can be used as a teaching or evaluation method, subjects are trained to act the part of patients as consistently and realistically as possible. In most cases, laypeople are used, usually nonnursing students and sometimes professional actors (Konkle-Parker, Cramer, & Hamill, 2002; Yoo & Yoo, 2003). Standardized patients are provided with scripts that include information relevant to the intended scenario. Depending on the situation, scripts may include germane history of a presenting problem, signs and symptoms, responses to likely questions, and "personal" details, all of which allow the standardized patient to portray the role as realistically as possible. Standardized patients may "be" a paralyzed patient needing mouth care or repositioning in a long-term care setting (Yoo & Yoo, 2003), a person in a clinic being assessed for HIV risk behaviors and taught risk reduction interventions (Konkle-Parker, Cramer, & Hamill, 2002), or any number of prototypical patients located in diverse LRC minimilieus.

Debriefing discussions with students immediately following role-playing or standardized patient scenarios provide faculty with opportunities to analyze the experience, emphasize key points, provide feedback, explore alternative approaches, and address questions. To build even more on these experiences, students can be provided with focused questions to address in their reflective journals following their role-play and standardized patient scenarios (e.g., what were you thinking when…; how do you think the "patient" felt when…; how did you feel when…; upon reflection, how else might you have responded/acted when…; how will you deal with similar situations in actual clinical practice based on what you have learned?).

Anatomic models and mannequins are common features in LRCs and are routinely used to teach and evaluate psychomotor and associated cognitive skills (Hodson-Carlton & Worrell-Carlisle, 2005). Simple anatomic models such as arms designed for practicing IV starts, injections, and arterial blood gases, and torsos for urinary catheterization, enemas, and abdominal wound management are available in most LRCs. Full-size scale mannequins are available as adults, children, and infants of both genders. Modifiable pregnant models for practicing Leopold maneuvers, pediatric and adult mannequins designed for practicing CPR techniques, torsos with ostomies, and models for breast exams are just a sampling of the products available.

Consistent with other efforts to make the learning experiences as realistic as possible, mannequins can be placed in the minimilieus of the LRC, given wristbands for identification, and individual names (Tarnow, 2005). A variety of other approaches can be used with mannequins in the LRC to add contextual perspective and foster critical thinking. Tarnow and Butcher (2005) suggest ways to simulate dried serous drainage, blood clots, and infected wounds to enhance the reality of the experience. Simple role-playing can be added to the performance of psychomotor procedures by having students introduce themselves, properly identify and address the "patient," explain the procedure (Tarnow, 2005), and communicate appropriately while carrying it out. Departing from the "one right answer" mentality, student learning is expanded when faculty ask higher level questions and encourage reflection on the contextual aptness of interventions (Snyder et al., 2000). Faculty can create scenarios or case studies of varying degrees of complexity in which skills are to be performed (Oermann, Truesdell, & Ziolkowski, 2000; Snyder et al., 2000; McCausland et al., 2004), or references can be used to guide scenario design (Hertel & Mills, 2002). Using scenarios with faculty direction, students can be guided to assess the patients before, during, and after carrying out procedures, with faculty providing the applicable findings (McCausland et al., 2004; Tarnow, 2005) (e.g., "You hear fine crackles in the bases of the lungs"). Faculty can respond to student questioning as the patient, as other members of the health care team, or as members of the patient's family (McCausland et al., 2004). As with role-playing and standardized patient scenarios, the provisions for a debriefing opportunity and focused questions for reflective journaling augment students' learning and critical thinking when mannequin-based scenarios are used.

Other useful low-tech clinical teaching tools are often stored in the LRC. Posters, brochures, and kits for teaching both students and clients such topics as nutrition and dental hygiene, and games that have been purchased or donated commercially or prepared by faculty may be found in the LRC. Posted on the walls of the LRC, photographs and illustrations from articles and advertisements taken from professional and lay publications can meet many educational goals. These reflect the diversity of health care providers and recipients, help students attend to nonverbal communication, and enhance their developing self-awareness (Tarnow & Butcher, 2005). Only by exploring the program's LRC will faculty locate many of these items and be able to then use them for clinical instruction.

▊ HIGH-TECH TOOLS

If the nursing program has access to the fiscal resources necessary to purchase them for the LRC, a large number of high-tech teaching tools are commercially available, and more are being designed and marketed every year (Box 12-2). Students have a preference for experiential learning (Medley & Horne, 2005), and faculty are constantly looking for opportunities to provide that type of learning as realistically as possible outside of actual clinical settings while maintaining contextual perspective and stimulating critical thinking. Technologic advances have permitted many educationally based businesses to rise to the challenge.

BOX 12-2
High-Tech Tools, Tactics, and Techniques in the LRC

- Computer-assisted instruction programs and simulations with/without interactive video
- Procedural simulators (task trainers)
- Interactive human simulators
- Immersive virtual reality simulations

In the 1980s, computer programs for educational instruction became commonplace in nursing programs (Hodson-Carlton & Worrell-Carlisle, 2005). Supporting the self-directed approach to skill acquisition, students seated in front of a computer screen in the LRC could be presented with learning modules. These were followed by terminal testing questions, or ones that advanced the student further into the content or looped back for remedial teaching. Initially modeled after programmed learning modules in textbooks and journals, computer assisted instruction (CAI) eventually evolved to the point that an interactive video component was added. This provided students with more data to work with and feedback on the accuracy of their responses. Computer simulations became increasingly sophisticated with the addition of touch sensitive screens to supplement keystrokes and the incorporation of sound. Now, students could touch the screen in the area of the heart or lungs and hear the normal heart and lung sounds; murmurs and adventitious lung sounds were added to reflect pathology. Highly contextual computer simulations are also now available. They "place" students in settings such as labor and delivery or the emergency department, where they must collect and analyze data, choose appropriate interventions, and evaluate their own actions, as well as collaborate with practitioners from other disciplines. CAIs evolved from computer discs (CD-ROM) to DVDs and now are increasingly Internet based (Hodson-Carlton & Worrell-Carlisle, 2005). Many publications are available that anecdotally present the impact of CAIs on the development of critical thinking skills and recount their use as a substitution for clinical experiences (Staib, 2003).

The next natural technologic step was to take the computer programs and place them physically within mannequins or connect the mannequins to external computer interfaces. This produces a much more realistic simulation experience for students as they perform selected assessments and procedures. Simulation technology has been used for educational purposes for some time; it has been applied in the training of pilots and astronauts, military personnel, personnel in nuclear power plants, and used in both the behavioral and social sciences (Rauen, 2004). In health care, physicians have used simulations to practice surgical techniques, including robotic surgery. In each case, the primary value of these simulations is that they permit a safe learning experience, with no potentially dangerous human ramifications.

The term *fidelity* is common parlance among those involved in designing and using simulation technology (Seropian, Brown, Gavilanes, & Driggers, 2004). Fidelity describes the degree to which a simulation is capable of accurately recreating clinical experiences for the learner and may be divided into two (Medley & Horne, 2005) or three categories (Seropian et al., 2004), depending on the reference. Low-fidelity simulations are usually inert and lacking in the specific features and lifelike qualities of the actual situation; these models are used for psychomotor skills development and testing (Seropian et al., 2004; Medley & Horne, 2005). The anatomic models and mannequins previously discussed are examples of low-fidelity simulations. For example, if a model used for practicing intramuscular injections had realistic skin texture and provided the student with the actual sensations associated with advancing the needle through the layers of epidermis, dermis, fat, and muscle, its fidelity would be increased. This force-feedback, called *haptics*, provides the tactile reality to the simulation (Seropian et al., 2004). High-tech simulators provide moderate- to high-fidelity learning experiences for nursing students.

High-tech simulation technology extends from procedural simulators, or task trainers, that provide heart and lung sounds to interactive human simulators that provide a range of verbal and nonverbal assessment and feedback cues to enrich learning experiences (Seropian et al., 2004; Medley & Horne, 2005). Models range from those providing practice and testing of specific skills, such as assessing the cardiovascular system or inserting intravenous access devices, to highly accurate and realistic models enabling problem solving and decision making based on fluctuating assessment results. Human simulators that are the most highly reflective of actual clinical situations provide such features as vocalization, coughing, vomiting, palpable pulses, cardiac rhythms, and respiratory excursion. They provide opportunities for blood pressure and pulse oximetry measurements and the auscultation of heart, lung, and bowel sounds. Phlebotomy, initiation of intravenous (IV) lines and the infusion of fluids, injections, catheterization, nasogastric tube placement, and ventilation methods can all be practiced with these sophisticated simulators (Laerdal SimMan; McCausland et al., 2004). This level of simulation is definitely reflective of high-fidelity, possessing both cosmetic fidelity in the outward appearance of reality and response fidelity by responding realistically to student interventions (Seropian et al., 2004). Students can assess "patients" and use the data to select interventions and obtain immediate feedback in terms of outcomes. Relevant theory from their course work is integrated into the process of care, including management and leadership skills. Care is action-oriented and theory-based, and faculty are able to assess students' thinking skills as well as their task performance (McCausland et al., 2004). There are simulators available for childbirth, trauma, and cardiac and ostomy patient care. Resuscitation models are obtainable to practice with preemie, neonatal, pediatric, and adult "patients."

Ravert (2002) reviewed studies addressing computer-based education in medical and nursing education, seeking those with outcome measures of knowledge and skill acquisition. She found that, although limited in number and design, 75% of the studies that met the review's inclusion criteria showed affirmative results (N = 9). An International survey of the use of human simulators in nursing education in the United States, Japan, Germany, Australia, and England (Nehring & Lashley, 2004) found human simulators are being used worldwide for undergraduate and graduate nursing education, continuing education for practicing nurses, and in nursing educational research. Among their other findings, they report that these simulators have been found to be useful for "…developing critical thinking skills, applying theory to practice, providing a better transition to clinical experiences, and providing safe, simulated experiences" (p. 247). Elsewhere, the literature reports numerous advantages of this technology: active, interactive student learning is supported as is the application of critical thinking, clinical problem solving skills. Human simulations result in improved retention of procedural knowledge, offer the opportunity to stop and review student performance during the simulation, enhance student self-confidence, and facilitate repeated skill practice (Feingold, Calaluce, & Kallen, 2004; McCausland et al., 2004).

Barriers to the application of simulation technology to nursing education are not minor, and their use demands a commitment from both faculty and program administrators. The time required for faculty to learn to use the technology and prepare learning activities is considerable, and the LRC must have the physical space to accommodate both the technology itself and the groups of students who will use it (McCausland et al., 2004). Human simulators are costly, both in terms of faculty time and organizational fiscal resources (Feingold, Calaluce, & Kallen, 2004; McCausland et al., 2004; Nehring & Lashley, 2004; Seropian et al., 2004). In addition to the cost of the equipment, long-term maintenance costs must be factored into any cost analysis (McCausland et al., 2004). Programs permitting regional sharing as one means of cost control are being explored (Nehring & Lashley, 2004).

From the perspective of the literature, simply using these high-tech human simulators augments critical thinking skills, and that does appear to be true. However, faculty can significantly enhance this process during and following the use of simulations. Because it is possible to pause the simulation, faculty may do so in order to help students clarify and articulate their thinking processes. Some questions might be more appropriate for discussion following the simulation in a debriefing session. The greater the quality of the simulation, the more unpredictable the experience becomes for both students and faculty (Seropian et al., 2004). Debriefing sessions should be respectful and constructive; the experience can be emotionally traumatic if improperly conducted (Seropian et al., 2004). Peer feedback and questions that require students to examine why they chose one intervention as opposed to another, and what other information they might have collected help students critically analyze their decisions. Asking students what they need to tell the "patient" humanizes the simulation technology even further. Students should be asked how they would evaluate their interventions and to critique their organization and delegation skills, if appropriate to the given scenario. Reflective journaling always has a place in student learning, and the use of human simulators is no exception. Again, focused questions give students guidance and avoid rambling entries. Some of the previous questions may be reserved for this venue, or students may build on what was discussed earlier. In their journals, students can be encouraged to analyze their feelings about the overall simulation experience and their thoughts and actions and to speculate about the feelings of a patient in such a situation. McCausland et al. (2004) provide detailed and specific suggestions for preparing and carrying out a scenario for undergraduate nursing students, as well as an inclusive sample learning activity that may be of particular value in helping faculty learn the basic principles involved in simulation technology.

Designating a simulation as representative of virtual reality technology also may be confusing, because differing interpretations exist in the literature. Some of the high quality human simulators previously discussed can be classified as virtual reality systems, as could the intramuscular injection model equipped with high-fidelity haptics (Hodson-Carlton & Worrell-Carlisle, 2005; Seropian et al., 2004). But in the classic interpretation, virtual reality systems immerse students into the learning experience, making them actually feel physically present in the simulation (Hodson-Carlton & Worrell-Carlisle, 2005). Although it is the most costly and technologically advanced simulation modality possible, the long-term impact of this type of immersive virtual reality on nursing education will likely be significant because of the degree to which it emulates clinical practice environments (Simpson, 2002). In this type of virtual reality, the student dons a body suit, augmented with a data glove, helmet, and hand controls, and experiences the simulation within an environment suffused with multimedia (Hodson-Carlton & Worrell-Carlisle, 2005). This level of technology is now more commonly used in areas such as surgical training for physicians, but will certainly be a part of nursing education in the future. Faculty will continue to have an important role in facilitating debriefing and guided reflection in order to maximize student learning experiences.

SUMMARY

Learning resource centers provide a wealth of resources to supplement and facilitate clinical nursing education. Nursing programs vary widely in both the content and use of their LRCs within the curriculum and in the role of clinical faculty in relation to them. Faculty teaching clinical courses must have a clear understanding of this in order to make the greatest use of the LRC. Diverse low- and high-tech tools for clinical nursing education are available through the LRC. Health care science fiction has become science fact (Simpson, 2002). Regardless of the tools used, faculty retain the responsibility for promoting a caring and contextual perspective and enhancing students' critical thinking skills beyond the activity itself.

REFLECTION EXERCISE 12

Using the LRC

◆ Identify the role of the LRC within your nursing program.

◆ Explore the resources and supplies provided by your LRC.

◆ Now, consider the clinical course you teach (or would likely teach).

    ◆ What available resources might you incorporate into your course?

    ◆ What course objectives/outcomes would they support?

    ◆ Would you use them to augment or replace clinical experiences?

    ◆ For each clinical application, think about how you could enhance students' critical thinking skills. Be specific.

◆ Now, in light of the goal of enhancing critical thinking, go back and reconsider the three questions. Did your answers change? Reflect on how the resources are designed to be used and on how they might be used differently. Would you make changes in your teaching methods with the use of LRC resources?

References

American Association of Colleges of Nursing (AACN). (1998). *The Essentials of Baccalaureate Education for Professional Nursing Practice.* Washington, DC: AACN.

Ankele, R., Lohner, L., & Masiulaniec, B.A.S. (2001). Innovative teaching within the nursing resource center: A blueprint for student success. *Journal of Multicultural Nursing and Health, 7*(3), 6-8.

Feingold, C.E., Calaluce, M., & Kallen, M.A. (2004). Computerized patient model and simulated clinical experiences: Evaluation with baccalaureate nursing students. *Journal of Nursing Education, 43*(4), 156-163.

Haskvitz, L. M., & Koop, E.C. (2004). Students struggling in clinical? A new role for the patient simulator. *Journal of Nursing Education, 43*(4), 181-184.

Hertel, J.P., & Mills, B.J. (2002). *Using simulations to promote learning in higher education: An introduction.* Sterling, VA: Stylus Publishing.

Hodson-Carlton, K.E., & Worrell-Carlisle, P.J. (2005). The learning resource center. In D.M. Billings & J.A. Halstead (Eds.), *Teaching in nursing: A guide for faculty* (pp. 349-375). Philadelphia: Saunders.

Jeffries, P.R., Rew, S., & Cramer, J.M. (2002). A comparison of student-centered versus traditional methods of teaching basic nursing skills in a learning laboratory. *Nursing Education Perspectives, 23*(1), 14-19.

Konkle-Parker, D.J., Cramer, C.K., & Hamill, C. (2002). Standardized patient training: A modality for teaching interviewing skills. *The Journal of Continuing Education in Nursing, 33*(5), 225-230.

Laerdal SimMan. Retrieved February 1, 2005, from http://www.laerdal.com/simman/simman.htm.

McCausland, L.L., Curran, C.C., & Cataldi, P. (2004). Use of a human simulator for undergraduate nurse education. *International Journal of Nursing Education Scholarship, 1*(1), Article 23. Retrieved August 23, 2005, from http://www.bepress.com/ijnes/vol1/iss1/art23

Medley, C.F., & Horne, C. (2005). Using simulation technology for undergraduate nursing education. *Journal of Nursing Education, 44*(1), 31-34.

Miller, H., Nichols, E., & Beeken, J.E. (2000). Comparing videotaped and faculty-present return demonstrations of clinical skills. *Journal of Nursing Education, 39*(5), 237-239.

Miracle, D.J. (1999). Teaching psychomotor nursing skills in simulated learning labs: A critical review of the literature. In K.R. Stevens & V.R. Cassidy (Eds.), *Evidence-based teaching: Current research in nursing education* (pp. 71-103). Sudbury, MA: Jones and Bartlett.

Nehring, W.M., & Lashley, F.R. (2004). Current use and opinions regarding human patient simulators in nursing education: An international survey. *Nursing Education Perspectives, 25*(5), 244-248.

O'Connor, A.B. (2001). *Clinical instruction and evaluation: A teaching resource.* Sudburg, MA: Jones and Bartlett.

Oermann, M., Truesdell, S., & Ziolkowski, L. (2000). Strategy to assess, develop, and evaluate critical thinking. *The Journal of Continuing Education in Nursing, 31*(4), 155-160.

Owens, L.D., & Walden, D.J. (2001). Peer instruction in the learning laboratory: A strategy to decrease student anxiety. *Journal of Nursing Education, 40*(8), 375-377.

Rauen, C.A. (2004). Simulation as a teaching strategy for nursing education and orientation in cardiac surgery. *Critical Care Nurse, 24*(3), 46-51.

Ravert, P. (2002). An integrative review of computer-based simulation in the education process. *Computers, Informatics, Nursing, 20*(5), 203-208.

Seropian, M.A., Brown, K., Gavilanes, J.S., & Driggers, B. (2004). Simulation: Not just a manikin. *Journal of Nursing Education, 43*(4), 164-169.

Simpson, R.L. (2002). The virtual reality revolution: Technology changes nursing education. *Nursing Management, 33*(9), 14-15.

Staib, S. (2003). Teaching and measuring critical thinking. *Journal of Nursing Education, 42*(11), 498-508.

Snyder, M.D., Fitzloff, B.M., Fiedler, R., & Lambke, M.R. (2000). Preparing nursing students for contemporary practice: Restructuring the psychomotor skills laboratory. *Journal of Nursing Education, 39*(5), 229-230.

Tarnow, K.G. (2005). Humanizing the learning laboratory. *Journal of Nursing Education, 44*(1), 43-44.

Tarnow, K.G., & Butcher, H.K. (2005). Teaching the art of professional nursing in the learning laboratory. *Annual Review of Nursing Education, 3,* 375-392.

Utley-Smith, Q. (2004). 5 Competencies needed by new baccalaureate graduates. *Nursing Education Perspectives, 25*(4), 166-170.

Van Eerden, K. (2001). Using critical thinking vignettes to evaluate student learning. *Nursing and Health Care Perspectives, 22*(5), 231-234.

Winters, J., Hauck, B., Riggs, C.J., Clawson, J., & Collins, J. (2003). Use of videotaping to assess competencies and course outcomes. *Journal of Nursing Education, 42*(10), 472-476.

Yoo, M.S., & Yoo, I.Y. (2003). The effectiveness of standardized patients as a teaching method for nursing fundamentals. *Journal of Nursing Education, 42*(10), 444-448.

Clinical Faculty as Clinical Coach

The analogy of teacher as coach has been a useful one in general education and translates well into the realm of nursing education too (Grealish, 2000). The dictionary definition of *coach* confirms the essential commonality between them: coach (noun)—"a private tutor; one who instructs or trains ..." (Merriam-Webster's Collegiate Dictionary, 2004, p. 236). The similarities between a coach and a teacher are especially noticeable in the clinical practice setting where interactions occur with individuals and small groups of students. When the word *coach* is used as a verb, the value of the analogy is amplified. It is through the motivating and facilitating activities of teaching that faculty, in effect, become coaches. In the context of clinical nursing education, coaching is exemplified in the reciprocal interactions between student and faculty member that occur while the student is acquiring the necessary behaviors and skills that are foundational to clinical nursing practice (Grealish, 2000). For clinical nurse educators, the concept of *coach* is a large part of both who we are (noun) and what we do (verb).

■ BEING AN EFFECTIVE TEACHER-COACH

A considerable body of knowledge has been amassed that identifies the qualities, characteristics, and abilities of effective teachers in the clinical setting (Stokes & Kost, 2005). Many of these likewise appear in other contexts describing successful

---

BOX 13-1

Characteristics of an Effective Clinical Nursing Coach

An effective clinical nursing coach is:

- Enthusiastic about the profession of nursing
- A role model of professional nursing
- Enthusiastic about clinical instruction
- Knowledgeable regarding theoretical foundations of practice
- A clinically competent practitioner
- Flexible
- A skillful communicator
- Fair, respectful, and consistent in interactions with others
- Able to create an environment conducive to learning
- Sensitive to the students' learning needs and styles of learning
- Motivational
- Facilitative

---

coaches (Blythe & Sweet, 2003). All too often, these aspects of the teacher and coach's character and personality are poorly differentiated from the teaching and coaching methods employed. Box 13-1 illustrates how the characteristics of an effective coach can be applied to faculty involved in clinical nursing instruction.

These broad characteristics subsume many others that can be intuitively extrapolated. For example, a teacher who is a *skillful communicator* is also a good listener. All teaching and learning are constructed on the underpinning of communication (Lichtman et al., 2003). Possessing the quality of *flexibility* allows faculty to alter teaching strategies as circumstances warrant, such as when there is an unexpected change in patient status. Faculty flexibility is also essential for assisting students with diverse learning needs. Students progress at different paces; some require more guidance in connecting theory to practice whereas others find mastering psychomotor skills to be especially challenging. *Fairness* implies that faculty are aware of their own biases and endeavor to control them while teaching and evaluating students. Faculty carry out innumerable activities in order to create environments that are conducive to learning. They strive to assure that learning experiences are appropriate and meaningful and to foster a positive relationship with agency personnel. They also enhance the learning environment through the judicious use of humor (Hayden-Miles, 2002).

As discussed in previous chapters, the appropriateness of humor depends as much on the social and interpersonal context as it does on the content itself. Faculty must work from a foundation of trust and respect, recognizing the individuality of the student and the situation. Honing in on a pearl of wisdom regarding clinical instruction, one expert clinical nursing coach deemed appropriately used humor to be a crucial device for teaching and reducing stress for both students and faculty (Lichtman et al., 2003). For example, when a student is anxious about performing her very first urinary catheterization on a female patient, faculty might decrease stress before entering the room, while providing the student with a useful clinical tool, by suggesting that when the student is trying to locate the urethra, the patient be asked to cough to make it "wink" back. When faculty laugh at themselves and the situations in which they find themselves, they enhance the learning environment and their relationship with students (Hayden-Miles, 2002).

Faculty teaching clinical nursing courses are expected to be skillful practitioners who are knowledgeable about the theoretical bases of their practice. Tantamount to their practice and theory expertise, they also must endeavor to motivate students while facilitating their learning. Motivation and facilitation are the crux of the teacher-coach role. When students are motivated to learn and engaged in the learning process, clinical faculty coaches are able to choose from a wide variety of pedagogical methods to facilitate that learning.

▓ MOTIVATING STUDENTS TO LEARN IN THE CLINICAL SETTING

In a study of Taiwanese nursing students, motivation was identified as the most critical factor in the successful transfer of theory to hospital clinical practice (Tsai & Tsai, 2004). The delineation of influences on students' willingness to learn has been a focal point of study for social psychologists and educational theorists for decades. Theories have been generated that connect learning and motivation, behavior and motivation, and behavior, learning, and motivation (Bastable, 2003). Every theory postulated is an effort to attend to some aspect of the complicated and rather intangible concept of motivation.

In clinical nursing instruction, student motivation is markedly influenced by the learning goals established and the feedback provided. Because faculty teaching clinical courses work with individual students, both the goals and the feedback can be somewhat tailored to meet the unique needs of each student. In order to maximize the effectiveness of the learning process, a clinical coach might consider carrying out a brief motivational assessment of each student.

Motivational Assessments

Both internal and external factors impact an individual learner's motivation; these factors can be positive, serving to encourage motivation, or negative, impeding it in a given individual. Redman (2001) sees motivational assessment of the learner to be integral to successful teaching. Such assessments draw heavily on the internal and uniquely individual elements of learning that are encompassed in cognitive learning theories (see Chapter 2). Some of the possible considerations in such a motivational assessment of a nursing student in a practicum course are listed in Box 13-2. The accuracy of this assessment is highly contingent on the degree of trust established within the student-faculty relationship. A trusting relationship is a key constituent of a positive learning environment. Seen as a continuum of degree, the bedrock of trust is laid on the first day of the course (see Chapter 10), and every interaction faculty have with students will affect it. From the students' perspective, the quality of the current

---

BOX 13-2
Aspects of a Student Motivational Assessment

■ Previous learning experiences (i.e., positive and negative outcomes and processes)
■ Personal attitudes and beliefs about learning
■ Readiness to learn (e.g., interest in the subject, impact of external factors such as demands of other courses or family life)
■ Availability of resources to support learning (e.g., library, lab, and computer access; social support; financial status)
■ Level of anxiety (moderate level enhances motivation; high or low levels impede it)

---

relationship also makes an important contribution to motivation in subsequent clinical courses.

Student motivation often waxes and wanes over the course of the term, so assessments might be done more than once, perhaps at the beginning and again at the midpoint of the term. One effective way to collect motivational assessment information is through the students' reflective journals (discussed in detail in Chapter 11). The aspects provided in Box 13-2 can be used to construct questions to be addressed in the students' first journal entries, after the first course meeting prior to the first clinical experience. This approach encourages reflection and provides ample time for students to offer considered responses. Reassessment of motivation could then be done as part of each student's formative midterm evaluation (Chapter 18). Guided by the results of the motivational assessment, while remaining within the parameters of the overall clinical course expectations, individualized learning goals are then prepared and feedback imparted.

Goal Setting

"Implicit in motivation is movement in the direction of meeting a need or toward reaching a goal" (Bastable, 2003). Murphy (2005) identifies specific learning goals as an essential tenet of "guided practice," her term for coaching by clinical faculty. The characteristics of student learning goals in clinical courses are summarized in Box 13-3. Cognitive learning theories have contributed significantly to the current application of student learning goals to enhance motivation. Goals established by faculty without student participation are less likely to be attained. Collaborative goal setting can minimize the deleterious effects of negative motivators for the student, bring to the foreground any hidden agendas, and diminish the possibility of learning activities being sabotaged by the student (Bastable, 2003). From a coaching perspective, setting goals in concert with students is seen as a pivotal activity (Grealish, 2000; Broscious & Saunders, 2001; Blythe & Sweet, 2003; Bastable, 2003).

BOX 13-3
Characteristics of Student Learning Goals

- Collaboratively established
- Clearly written
- Appropriate to the course and student
- Realistic (attainable but challenging)
- Performance-based
- Based on prior knowledge/experiences
- Short-term (for 1-2 clinical days)

As the learning goals are being collaboratively designed, the clinical coach provides students with the guidance to prepare goals that will be meaningful to them. To be meaningful, goals must be realistic; they should be attainable while still being sufficiently challenging to the student (Grealish, 2000; Westberg & Jason, 2001; Bastable, 2003). When goals are too easy or too difficult, they are not seen by the student as motivational and will most likely be discarded. Goals that are based on past learning are most likely to be realistic and therefore meaningful to a learner (Grealish, 2000). The teaching strategies that ultimately evolve from goals that link new to old learning are also presumed to best promote students' critical thinking skills (Youngblood & Beitz, 2001).

Performance-based learning goals can be cognitive, psychomotor, or affective in nature. The assumption that underlies these goals is that student learning can be inferred from student performance. Since the 1940s, educational objectives have been inexorably associated with the control and manipulation of learners subsumed by *behaviorism,* the dominant psychologic theory of the time (Anderson et al., 2001). Tyler, considered the father of educational objectives, had the perspective that the desired consequence of learning was simply a change in behavior (Anderson et al., 2001). Omitting the erroneous assumption of learner control and manipulation inherent in behaviorism, learning goals prepared in concert by faculty and students become the learning target and guide the selection of learning experiences.

Cognitive learning goals reflect an understanding of theoretical concepts, and their attainment can be conveyed by the student in many ways. By preparing concept maps, responding to clinical queries, applying theory in practice activities, reflecting in a journal entry, or completing a self-evaluation, students demonstrate their achievement of cognitive learning goals. A psychomotor skill performance goal addresses carrying out the skill with efficiency, safety, and accuracy and communicating in actions and words an understanding of the conceptual aspects of the skill. Performance-based affective goals describe behaviors reflective of caring, professional ethics, and self-awareness. Faculty can assess their attainment through direct observation, clinical queries, and written work such as process recordings and journaling. If this discussion or the

---

BOX 13-4
Sample Cognitive, Psychomotor, and Affective Student Learning Goals

Cognitive learning goals
- Prepare and carry out a balanced prenatal vegan nutritional teaching plan for Mrs. Smith.
- Create a time management plan to organize the provision of care for four patients.

Psychomotor learning goals
- Apply the 5 Rights during the preparation and administration of medications.
- Conduct developmental screening on four children of differing chronologic ages and accurately interpret the results.
- Correctly perform a central line dressing change.

Affective learning goals
- Record the interaction of an admission assessment in a process recording and indicate my verbal and nonverbal behaviors that are reflective of caring.
- Discuss in my journal the effectiveness of my collaboration with Mr. Jones and his wife in creating a plan for medication administration.

---

examples in Box 13-4 are not clear, refer back to the presentation of the domains of learning in the clinical learning context presented in Chapter 2. Evaluative data sources are explored in detail in Chapter 18.

There certainly is a place for long-term goals, which can be worked toward over the course of the term. But to maximize student motivation, breaking large long-term goals into smaller short-term ones will be most beneficial (Grealish, 2000). When goals are established for a single day or 2 of the practicum, both coach and learner can assess the degree of progress attained and modify goals and approaches accordingly. Students will benefit most from goals that are focused on their performance (Grealish, 2000) and worded in a fashion that will facilitate the evaluation of their attainment. Whether the goals are for manual (psychomotor), cognitive, or even affective skill development, clarity of the desired results is imperative.

The collaborative establishment of learning goals can be accomplished in several ways. Ideally, as students evaluate their learning for each day or week, they determine goals for their next clinical experience. Students may have a faculty-designed self-evaluation form to fill out or address their learning through journal entries, concluding with their learning goals for the next clinical experience, obtaining feedback from faculty. There may be brief weekly meetings with faculty for collaborative goal setting, carried out in person or via online discussion (with appropriate confidentiality parameters). In courses using the preceptor model, goals may be established between the students and preceptors while faculty assume a consulting role.

Providing Feedback: Oreos® and Helium Balloons

The second aspect of motivating students to learn in the clinical setting is the provision of faculty feedback. Feedback to learners is essentially reinforcement for behavior exhibited and is a defining feature of behavioral learning theories (see Chapter 2). In this text, feedback is differentiated from evaluation by virtue of its immediacy and informality. A more formal, written evaluation of learning within a clinical course is typically carried out at a midpoint in the term (formative) and at the end of the term (summative). Formative and summative clinical evaluations are addressed in Chapter 18. Box 13-5 lists techniques for providing feedback in the clinical setting that are discussed in this chapter.

The student's receptivity to faculty feedback is a critical aspect in the efficacy of clinical coaching. For long-term changes to occur, students must be receptive, comprehend, and attach importance to faculty suggestions (Westberg & Jason, 2001). Openness to feedback is highly variable, differing not only between students but also in the same student over time. The degree to which anyone is receptive to feedback is the result of both current and historical experiences (Westberg & Jason, 2001). How parents, peers, supervisors at work, and other faculty have provided feedback will affect how each student responds to their clinical coach's observations and suggestions. One of the most important contributors to students' receptivity to feedback is the quality of their relationship with their current clinical faculty. A trusting and collaborative relationship between faculty and students, one in which students feel supported in their learning, provides an open door to feedback. If that relationship erodes or was

---

BOX 13-5
Techniques for Providing Feedback in the Clinical Setting

- Assess student receptivity
- Work from within a trusting faculty-student relationship
- Provide feedback in close proximity to performance
- Assure privacy for constructive criticism
- Present balanced feedback
- Monitor nonverbal behaviors, emotional tone, and pacing
- Consider the careful use of touch
- Offer the student the opportunity to self-critique
- Begin with positive feedback
- Consider Oreos® and helium balloons
- Limit the focus; prioritize issues
- Be clear, direct, specific; provide descriptive examples
- Use questions to guide student self-evaluation
- Use partial affirmation to guide student self-evaluation
- Link feedback to current and future learning goals

never adequately established, students may believe their faculty are "out to get them," and the receptivity switch is flipped off. Under such circumstances, students will not hear feedback accurately or value it. Having established the tone for professional interactions and explained the feedback process at the first meeting (see Chapter 10), faculty may find it useful to refer back to their belief that students will accept the feedback provided as a vehicle for both professional and personal growth (Luparell, 2005).

In clinical coaching, feedback assumes a crucial function in motivating students' learning and needs to be provided as close in time to the students' performance as possible in order to be most effective (Grealish, 2000; Westberg & Jason, 2001; Weimer, 2003; Bastable, 2003). When feedback is provided in a timely fashion, students are more likely to remember the specifics of their performance and make the necessary modifications accordingly (Westberg & Jason, 2001). Meaningful feedback should be offered both during and following the task at hand, if possible and appropriate. Certainly, there are times when faculty should consider postponing feedback. If the feedback addresses issues that are quite sensitive or personal, the situation was highly emotionally charged or stressful, or the student is pressured and behind schedule, it may be best to defer it for a time (Westberg & Jason, 2001).

To be meaningful, feedback is provided based on the proximity of performance to predetermined guidelines, established standards, or past performance (Bastable, 2003). Feedback can be positive or negative in nature. Positive feedback serves as a reward to students, providing the impetus for continued learning efforts (Bastable, 2003). If students are rewarded for asking questions, stating ideas, and trying out new ways of thinking, they will tend to continue this behavior. The intent of negative feedback, often called "constructive criticism," is to redirect the learner's thinking or performance in a more desirable direction. Feedback of this sort must be given with care and be somewhat individualized for the particular student and circumstance. Even when provided with the best of intentions, constructive criticism can be devastating to some students. When providing feedback that could be construed by students as negative, it is always best to do so in a private location where it cannot be overheard by others and cause students embarrassment. Ideally, the feedback provided is rounded, a balance of positive and negative, and presented in a caring and respectful manner (Weimer, 2003).

Feedback is most often provided verbally to students in the clinical setting. Written feedback is discussed in connection with written assignments in Chapter 15. Delivery of verbal feedback encompasses more than just the words themselves; it includes the emotional tone embedded in the words, the pacing of what is said, and the accompanying body language (Westberg & Jason, 2001). The content and impact of verbal feedback is supported, heightened, or sometimes even replaced by faculty's nonverbal behavioral cues. Nonverbal behaviors must be congruent with the verbal feedback being provided or students are likely to be confused or distracted. As a student responds to questions or performs skills, the faculty coach can convey approval and encouragement by nodding, smiling, moving toward the student, gesturing in ways that communicate approval and attention, and perhaps by maintaining eye contact or using touch. When students are performing a skill during the provision of patient care, it can be beneficial to have a predetermined signal to communicate to the student it is all right to continue, that the correct injection site has been identified or the student's hand is correctly placed to palpate the fundus of the uterus.

This seems an appropriate time to address faculty's use of touch with students. Patients are generally comfortable being touched by a nurse because of the context; there is an understanding that carrying out the nurse's role requires touching patients. The context is different in teaching, and faculty must be astute regarding the feelings of the individual student and the circumstances involved. Given the complexity of human interactions, interpretations of sexual harassment, and the litigious propensity of American society today, faculty must use considerable caution in their use of touch. Circumstances do change, and the touch that was initially accepted and comforting to a student can be negatively reinterpreted at a later time. Some faculty are simply inherently disinclined to use touch beyond a handshake in their interactions with anyone outside of their nursing practice. This may indeed be the best approach. But if the clinical coach is comfortable and wants to use touch as part of communicating caring, conscientious consideration of the individual student's comfort level as well as the situation is essential. If the faculty member or student is not comfortable, other nonverbal or verbal approaches should be used. Faculty must also be sure their intent is clear and the touch is appropriate. Faculty often make it a policy to avoid touching a student of the opposite gender under any circumstances out of concern that their actions might be misinterpreted. As a caring gesture, a pat on the back or shoulder given as part of feedback or comforting solace at the appropriate time is generally not misconstrued, but it may be best to err on the side of caution.

Feedback sessions may be only a few minutes in length, but it is always important to begin by asking students to critique their own performance. Doing so reinforces the collaborative nature of the process, communicates respect and value, enhances self-awareness, and allows students to acknowledge aspects of their own performance before they are pointed out by faculty (Westberg & Jason, 2001; Weimer, 2003). This approach also can serve to alert faculty of upcoming areas of potential disagreement. Assure that students include their accomplishments, the things they feel good about, so that they will learn to balance their self-analyses. As the coach, affirm aspects of the student's assessment that are congruent with your own, positive or negative, then begin your feedback with a positive observation. Initiating a feedback session with an affirmation has been found to be especially valuable if students are ill at ease, distrustful, or markedly self-disparaging (Westberg & Jason, 2001). Providing negative feedback sandwiched between positive observations, like the layers of an Oreo® cookie, is a useful technique for creating balance and capturing students' attention. The downside of this technique, however, is that students recognize it if it is overused, ignore the positive in anticipation of the negative, and then focus on the negative and miss the closing positive feedback (Westberg & Jason, 2001). No single method of providing feedback should be used exclusively or excessively. Oreos® taste best when they are not the only food available but instead are an occasional treat!

It is best if a feedback meeting focuses on a restricted scope of behaviors (Weimer, 2003), that is, a single skill performance or patient interview. Overloading students with feedback limits their ability to pay attention to what is said and then process and incorporate it. Prioritizing the feedback to be provided by focusing on the most important features at the moment and postponing others might be most advantageous (Westberg & Jason, 2001).

Feedback should be unambiguous, straightforward, and as precise as possible (Weimer, 2003). Avoid long, meandering, one-sided commentaries. Be as objective as possible in describing behaviors and avoid labeling students. Sometimes subjective feedback is appropriate, but it should always be identified for what it is (Westberg & Jason, 2001). As experienced clinicians, observations are made and conclusions are drawn that are by their very nature subjective. Owning this type of feedback for what it is as it is given to students makes these selective perceptions and personalized interpretations clear for what they are. This can be done by prefacing comments with phrases like "I thought...", "It appeared to me...", or "From my point of view...". Students should be encouraged to see this type of feedback as an opening for dialogue with their coach, a time when they might explicate their thinking or behavior (Westberg & Jason, 2001).

Illustrative examples enhance positive feedback by making desirable behavior more visible to students (Westberg & Jason, 2001) and elucidate constructive criticism by identifying where problems lie. Telling a student, "You did a good job of clarifying Mrs. Smith's comment about her financial status when you reflected it back to her" is more meaningful than simply saying that good therapeutic communication skills were used. Pointing out to the student that the patient's hands were shaking and her voice was tremulous during preoperative teaching for a mastectomy helps the student see what was missed and is easier to accept than being told that observational skills are poor.

Clinical coaches may pose questions to guide students in the examination of their behavior and help them focus and draw their own conclusions, thereby increasing their self-awareness. For example, rather than tell a student what was wrong with a dressing change procedure, use guiding questions such as, "What did you notice about the wound when you removed the old dressing?" Whenever questions are posed, allow sufficient time for students to ponder and collect their thoughts. Using more adverbs than adjectives tends to increase the specificity of feedback (Weimer, 2003). The more descriptive the feedback is, the better it serves to guide learning. Students' most common criticisms regarding feedback about their clinical practice is that it is insufficient, unclear, and lacking in detail (Westberg & Jason, 2001).

Sometimes partial affirmation can be used to combine positive and negative feedback in a qualified approach. This is a useful method because it acknowledges student efforts and uses what was accurate and right (positive) as a springboard for the student to identify and correct errors. The clinical coach might say to a student, "You did a good job setting up your sterile field. Now, tell me what happened when you turned from the sterile field to the patient." The student can be guided to identify a problem or error, alleviating some of the distress that could be generated by negative faculty feedback. Other examples of partial affirmation include statements such as, "That's partially right" and "You're on the right track."

It seems to be a culturally derived aspect of human nature that learners generally attend more to criticism than to positive reinforcement. Part of the role of clinical faculty as coach is to endeavor to assure that students truly hear the feedback provided. To help students unaccustomed or uncomfortable with positive feedback, try using the analogy of a helium balloon. It can be used at any point in a feedback session, but starting with the opening positive observation, it can serve to focus students' attention during the entire feedback period. After proffering that initial positive comment, tell students that compliments are like helium balloons in that they have to be caught and cherished or they float away and are gone forever. Then, tell the students to "grab the string on the balloon" by repeating back the positive observation in their own words while really listening to the content and character of the words. Initially, often feeling embarrassed and reticent, students not only become accustomed to grabbing the string but also come to value the balloon!

To provide the maximal motivational effect, feedback to students should be linked to their learning goals when possible and appropriate. Increased receptivity to feedback has been connected to students' perceptions that the feedback being given relates to the goals they participated in creating (Westberg & Jason, 2001). Certainly unforeseen opportunities will arise in the clinical setting that were not part of the plan for the day. The student may not have had a previously established goal related to performing a urinary catheterization or participating in a group therapy session. Under those circumstances, a student may be asked to consider how this experience and the feedback provided could be incorporated into future learning goals. Negative feedback can press down on a student like dead weight, impeding the motivation to learn. When criticism has been given, students need assistance in reframing it into new learning goals and encouragement to begin to consider how these new goals might be attained. Students need to be helped to see this as a part of the entire learning experience. In fact, growth cannot occur without making mistakes. Perfection is not only unlikely, it is boring and stagnating!

▓ FACILITATING STUDENT LEARNING IN THE CLINICAL SETTING

Together, students' learning goals and clinical faculty feedback support the motivation to learn. The clinical coach's attention then shifts from the role of motivator of learning to that of facilitator of learning. The pedagogies clinical faculty use to facilitate learning are drawn from educational theories and philosophies (Chapter 2) and must be applied with consideration of the course, setting, and student, as well as the knowledge and abilities of the faculty. Like our students, faculty are individuals; some approaches "fit" better than others, and all of them are unique when they are applied by individual clinical coaches. As they teach, as they did in practice, clinical nursing faculty "... use themselves, their attitudes, tone of voice, humor, [and] skill... [and] offer ways of being, ways of coping, and even new possibilities" (Benner, 2001, p. 78).

Provision of Safe Patient Care

"Supervising experiential learning requires finding a balance between student independence and teacher control" (McKeachie, 2002, p. 247). Bevis (1988) told nursing faculty that protecting patient safety is but a minimal aspect of their role, yet clinical faculty routinely find this obligation consumes an inordinate amount of their time and effort, often to the detriment of their teaching. The concern for maintaining safety in the clinical setting has resulted in a faculty preoccupation with ensuring the supervision of students and high levels of anxiety when that is not possible. Some tactics clinical faculty may want to consider for facilitating the provision of safe patient care by nursing students are summarized in Box 13-6.

As an application of collaboration, the provision of safe nursing care should be a shared responsibility, with student and faculty contributing what each has to offer (Burst, 2000). Upon graduation, practitioners at the level of advanced beginner should reasonably be expected to provide safe patient care and assure that those they supervise are protecting patient safety. In order to attain that goal, students as novice practitioners must learn how to achieve safe practice with incrementally diminishing faculty guidance and support. By modeling an

---

BOX 13-6
Tactics for Facilitating the Provision of Safe Patient Care

- Approach safe patient care as a collaborative responsibility*
- Initiate dialogue about legal and ethical obligations for patient safety
- Assist students to incorporate the provision of safe care as a professional value
- Help students learn to assess dangerousness in each clinical course*
- Identify safe and unsafe behaviors*
- Anticipate potential safety breaches
- Determine when to ask for help*
- Name who to ask for help*
- Establish how to recognize important changes in patient status*
- Maintain a safe learning space by maintaining a safe distance*
- Carry out intermittent evaluations of safety assessments
- Monitor for situations where students risk unsafe care*

---

*From Diekelmann, N., & Scheckel, M. (2004). Leaving the safe harbor of competency-based and outcomes education: Re-thinking practice education. *Journal of Nursing Education, 43*(9), 385-388.

awareness of their own practice limitations, faculty communicate to students that this self-assessment is a part of professional nursing practice.

As discussed in Unit II, faculty need to discuss with students their legal and ethical obligations to promote patient safety beginning with the first clinical course. As a part of that discussion, faculty should assist students in incorporating the protection of patient safety to the level of a professional value. Once a disposition toward something or someone reaches this point, it is internalized and becomes a benchmark for guiding actions and judging oneself and others. Students must learn to value patient safety as a part of their nursing education. "To learn to be a nurse is to learn from Day 1 how to always worry about safety and how and where to go for help and when you need it and what back-up looks like" (Diekelmann & Scheckel, 2004, p. 386).

In the context of each clinical course, faculty must help their students understand what behaviors are safe and unsafe, anticipate possible threats to safety, identify when they need help, determine who to approach for assistance when they need it, and recognize what assessment data are indicative of significant changes in their patients' status. In an application of narrative pedagogy, Diekelmann and Scheckel (2004) discovered that students contemplate assessing dangerousness to a much greater degree than faculty appreciate. A reasonable assumption based on this knowledge could be that believing that only they are the bastions of patient safety, clinical faculty may excessively "hover" over their students or stress out when students are "on their own" in the community. Perhaps by helping students expand their skills in the assessment of danger clinical faculty can back away, relax a bit, and ultimately have more time and energy to teach! For Diekelman and Scheckel (2004), and the faculty and students who participated in this colloquial dialogue, the issue distills to a matter of distance: "Students need a safe space to learn nursing practice, which means teachers must keep their distance, yet still be close enough to protect the patient and student while ensuring students learn to figure out on their own the issues of safety in providing patient care" (p. 388).

Hovering over students and experiencing significant stress when students are not being closely supervised certainly are not the singular province of novice faculty, but these issues seem to be the most extreme for them. Believing it somehow assures patient safety, they may require their students to submit extensive written preparatory papers, and then try to review them as they dash from student to student and site to site. In the name of patient safety, they may pose lists of "factoid" questions about drug side effects and nursing responsibilities associated with treatments, losing opportunities to help students develop skills in critical thinking and clinical judgment. But if not these approaches, how can faculty evaluate students' danger assessments and determine the optimal distance to maintain? For novice faculty, their expertise in clinical practice holds the answer.

As with appraisals of students' knowledge base in the clinical setting, the accuracy and thoroughness of students' danger assessments may be determined through intermittent and random faculty review. Based on faculty's knowledge and experience of clinical practice in situations similar to those students are involved in, faculty can determine key safety issues and query the students regarding a sample of them. As with other clinical queries, questions should be posed at a level of complexity appropriate for each student's knowledge and experience, and tap into higher-level thinking skills whenever possible. Students should know in advance the components of their danger assessment and come to the clinical site prepared to address any aspect of it when asked. This is their part of a collaborative approach to patient safety. This week, Susan Student may be asked how she will recognize the most common adverse effects of one or two medications; next time she might be asked to speak to her patient's risk of falling.

At the beginning of the first clinical course, danger assessments might be discussed with the entire clinical group during a preconference so that students can better learn the aspects of the assessment. Danger assessment includes problem anticipation, and posing questions of a "what if" nature help students be more prepared if one of any number of common risks to patient safety occur. Questions such as, "What if the patient wants the side rail left down after you give the preop medication?" or "What if your patient becomes dizzy while you are ambulating him down that long hallway?" help the student develop skill in anticipating potential challenges to patient safety. In each course students may be assigned to evaluate their danger assessments periodically in their reflection journals following their clinical experiences so they can obtain faculty feedback. Danger assessments can be explored as a group activity in postclinical conferences as well. These tactics also can be used by coaches teaching clinical courses where decreased direct faculty availability and the concern for safety can generate high levels of faculty stress (e.g., community-based settings, independent learning experiences, or when collaborative or preceptor models of clinical instruction are employed).

Using their clinical expertise and their judgments regarding the student and the situation, faculty must determine the amount of supervision required. The common mistake novice faculty often make is to oversupervise, hovering over students, increasing student anxiety and the risk for errors, decreasing student confidence, and retarding the development of competent advanced beginner practitioners. Backing off can be difficult, but it can be done with the application of tactics for the provision of safe patient care.

Clinical Patient Assignments

The practice of nursing is learned within the general framework of patient care. Over the course of their academic programs, students learn about nursing by observing, participating in, or supervising the care of patients (clients) in a variety of settings.

Students need experiences in *acting like nurses*—experiences in which students are immersed in a clinical setting. They need enough time to discover the pace and rhythm of the setting and where and how to access information, and they need to understand that they practice as a member of the health care team. They need an opportunity to pull it all together (Tanner, 2002, p. 52).

BOX 13-7
Tools for Facilitating Learning Through Clinical Patient Assignments

Assignment selection
- Faculty directed
- Collaboration with faculty/agency personnel
- Student independent selection

Organization of the assignment
- Traditional (1 student:1 or more patients)
- Student teams (3 students:1 patient)
- Student pairs (2 students:1 or more patients; senior student/junior student)
- Student supervisor (1 student: agency personnel/junior students)
- Peer mentoring (1 student: several students in the same course)

Location of the assignment
- Consistent placements
- Multiple placements

Clinical assignments for students vary with the goals of the course and the resources of the clinical setting. From a faculty perspective, the primary determinants of student clinical assignments are (1) the role the student assumes in the selection of the assignment, (2) the composition of the assignment in terms of number and level of students to number of patients, and (3) the decision to place students in only one or a variety of settings over the term (Box 13-7).

Faculty may make assignments for their students; students may collaborate with faculty and/or agency personnel in determining their assignments; or they may select their own assignments independently. The degree to which students are involved in choosing their clinical assignments also may vary student to student within a course or clinical setting. Typically, clinical coaches assume a more active role in the choice of assignments when students are just beginning their clinical experiences, often making specific assignments for them. As students accrue more expertise and skill in establishing their learning goals, they usually become more involved in the process. Ultimately, the degree to which students self-select their assignments is governed by the programmatic and course outcomes, the beliefs and comfort level of individual faculty, the amount of assistance available within the clinical agency (Stokes & Kost, 2005), and the teaching model being followed. Congruent with the current educational philosophies and frameworks in nursing, student involvement in the learning process is fostered when opportunities for student choice are facilitated. When collaborative or preceptor models are used, students may work with agency personnel directly in assignment selection, and faculty assume a supervisory function. A cooperative approach, with faculty assuming some role in guiding student learning in light of the established learning goals, allows for more active student learning and the development of personal accountability and responsibility.

Students' learning goals within the context of the course and setting are integral to the selection of assignments. In some cases, this involves an assignment to a particular setting, such as labor and delivery or radiational oncology, where the student must come prepared with a specific set of goals, knowledge, and skills to be applied. If the student is to select an assignment with the assistance of agency personnel, both parties must be clear about the learning goals of the student and the expectations of the course.

The clinical assignment may be carried out in differing organizational patterns of students to patients. The pattern used depends on the course expectations and clinical setting, and additionally, the students' abilities, patient acuity, and the numbers of students, patients, and personnel available (Stokes & Kost, 2005). With the escalating demands on nursing education, faculty must consider new and creative patterns for meeting educational outcomes. Currently, the methods that follow are being used.

What has been termed the "traditional" method involves a single student assigned to one or more patients (Stokes & Kost, 2005). In this approach, students begin their practice education by providing selected aspects of care to a single patient. As students' skill levels develop, the assignment is expanded to the provision of total care to one and then to increasing numbers of patients.

Variations of this approach are created by altering the number of students involved with one or more patients, that is, students work in pairs or as teams of students. Student pairs or teams may be composed of students at the same or differing levels of experience. This technique can be used to meet many different learning goals while responding to environmental constraints.

When the selection of patients is limited, student teams composed of three beginning students in the same clinical group may be assigned to a single patient (Stokes & Kost, 2005). Responsibilities within the assignment may be divided (e.g., one student performs care, one does the necessary research, and one observes and evaluates the care provided). When this tactic is used, students must be clear about their individual responsibilities, which might rotate over a 2-day assignment period. Although the research was done more than 30 years ago, the multiple assignment method has been reported to be at least as and perhaps more effective than the traditional method (Stokes & Kost, 2005).

The use of student pairs is a more common alternative to the traditional clinical assignment. Beginning students can be paired together to address differing aspects of care for a patient. According to Stokes and Kost (2005), assigning two students to one patient with very complex care needs can have a number of benefits. It reduces student anxiety; facilitates student communication and collaboration; enhances the development of organizational and time management skills; reduces the number of patients faculty must attend to; and provides students the opportunity to obtain peer feedback. Again, clarity regarding role responsibilities is essential, and responsibilities may rotate between the two students.

Another approach to student pairs that is increasingly popular is its application with students who are at differing points in their education (Broscious & Saunders, 2001; Schmeiser & Yehle, 2001; Becker & Neuwirth, 2002; Bradshaw, Rule, & Hooper, 2002; Sprengel & Job, 2004). This pattern usually has been incorporated into the academic program and course requirements in most cases, but it also has been used to provide student work-study employment (Becker & Neuwirth, 2002). This "junior/senior"-pairing tactic has been selected as a means to reduce student anxiety and maintain safety in light of decreased acute-care clinical sites and preceptors. The more advanced (senior) student may demonstrate complex skills, guide and supervise a junior student in skill performance, assist in theory application, and even participate in the junior student's evaluation (Scheiser & Yehle, 2001; Becker & Neuwirth, 2002; Sprengel & Job, 2004). The transition to a new clinical course can be facilitated by having students currently enrolled in the course accept responsibility for assisting the upcoming students for a day, modeling the care delivered and allowing the less experienced students to carry out some of the skills they have already learned. In any situation where students supervise others (peers or agency personnel), it must be done within the parameters of the agency policies and the state Nurse Practice Act.

When students are ready to make the supervision of others the focus of their learning, prior experience in junior/senior-paired assignments can be a valuable foundation. Senior students may then assume the role of team leader, supervising a team composed exclusively of junior students or one in which junior students are incorporated with other agency personnel (Bradshaw, Rule, & Hooper, 2002).

As a part of a given course, students may take on a peer mentoring role in which they are not assigned to a single patient or student, but instead serve as the resource person for a small number of their colleagues in the clinical site (Duchscher, 2001). In this peer-coaching role application, students collaborate in matters of patient care, provide emotional support, assist with the integration of theory and patient data, observe technical and communication skills, and step in to help their peers with patient care as needed. This approach was born from the realities of endeavoring to facilitate student learning given the high acuity and student-faculty ratios and is illustrative of the creative potential of nurse educators.

The final component of facilitating learning through clinical patient assignments deals with student placement. In some clinical courses, students may be rotated to different areas within an agency or go between several different agencies (multiple placements) rather than remaining in a single patient care area during a term (consistent placement). Multiple placements may be necessary to meet the course objectives (e.g., postpartum, labor and delivery, and neonatal nursery), or simply with the rationale of providing more diverse student experiences than would be obtained by remaining on one unit. In the case of a medical-surgical course, consistent placement would require the students to remain on one unit, such as an orthopedic unit, and multiple placements would result in rotations to several different units, such as orthopedics, medical cardiac, and a general surgery unit, or time spent in the operating room or a critical care unit. In a psychiatric/mental health–nursing course, students may remain in one area for the term or rotate between geriatric and adolescent units, outpatient clinics, or acute and chronic inpatient settings. The only recent study exploring the effect of these two approaches on learning outcomes found no quantitative differences with the instruments used (Adams, 2002).

Qualitatively, agency staff indicated a preference for consistent assignments for the same reasons students see them as beneficial: Consistency was perceived as building student proficiency and the relationships between staff and students. With consistent placements, students were mentored to a greater extent, receiving more assistance transitioning into the professional role. Students' comfort levels with and desire for diversity varies; some students not only prefer but also thrive with multiple placements. Adams (2002) suggests that for these students, alternative means outside of the clinical course time could be designed to provide exposure to various nursing roles and specialties. For beginning students, consistent placement is likely to be less stressful and more beneficial in developing student confidence. But as the students progress through the curriculum, experiencing a broader variety of placements provides new challenges, allows students to experience a range of practice options, and may provide increased skill and depth in the habits of the mind and skills of critical thinking.

Clinical Queries

As nurses are taught to use themselves as therapeutic tools in their interactions with patients, so too do clinical coaches use themselves as educational instruments in their interactions with students. Research has substantiated that oral questions are more effective in facilitating learning than those that are written (Cotton, 2001). By asking students meaningful questions, clinical faculty help students develop the cognitive skills needed to understand the theoretical foundations of their nursing practice, use the habits of the mind and skills of critical thinking, and develop clinical nursing judgment (see Chapter 11). Articulation also serves to extend students' engagement in learning (Murphy, 2005). As novices to nursing, students' anxiety often evokes tunnel vision; clinical queries can help them see the "big picture" in patient care situations. As a facilitative coaching activity, clinical queries only begin by assessing the student's theoretical understanding; the true value of questioning rests in the guidance it provides the student and the cognitive growth it encourages (Grealish, 2000). Clinical questioning is a teaching skill that requires practice and continuous self-assessment.

This technique is often given the misnomer of "the Socratic method" in both the literature and popular educator parlance. The questions used by Socrates as presented in Plato's dialogues were actually designed to lead and persuade (Bevis, 1989). They read like philosophic syllogisms; the classic Socratic method moves the student in a lockstep fashion along a progressive line of reasoning to a specific and predetermined endpoint. The questions that are truly educationally meaningful are those that compel students to *think* rather than merely *find* an answer (Ironside, 2003). As used in nursing education, questioning is a well-recognized technique for developing heuristic and other higher-order thinking skills needed for a practice discipline where problems are multifaceted and complex (Oermann, Truesdell, & Ziolkowski, 2000).

It is important for clinical faculty to explain to students how the questioning technique will be done and its usefulness in helping them develop thinking skills before it is initiated (Twibell, Ryan, & Hermiz, 2005). This can be done in the initial meeting with students at the beginning of the term. As course expectations and evaluation are reviewed, teaching methods also should be presented. An obvious advantage to this is that all students are given the same information at the same time. Perhaps less obvious is that clinical queries can be demonstrated with a nonnursing, even humorous, example such as the process of deciding what to wear to school or which route to drive. Orientation to clinical questioning is synopsized in Box 13-8.

The challenge in being an effective interlocutor is in posing questions that stimulate, even necessitate, higher-order thinking on the part of the student. These skills of application, synthesis, analysis, and evaluation are the focus of the majority of questions students will be presented with when they sit for their licensing examination. Lower-order questions are much easier to formulate and do have their place, albeit a limited place. These are factual or descriptive questions that are often prefaced by the words *who, what, when,* or *where* (Cotton, 2001; McKeachie, 2002; Bastable, 2003). This type of question taps into the student's recall of previously acquired information. Answers to factual questions are straightforward and usually brief. These questions draw their value

---

BOX 13-8
Preparing Students for the Technique of Clinical Queries

What it is
Clinical questioning is a teaching tool that helps develop thinking skills and enhance learning.

What it is not
Questions are not designed to diminish you or make you feel badly about yourself. You are not expected to have all the answers (or you wouldn't need to be taking the course!).

Faculty role
Ask questions that are clear. Ask questions to move student thinking to higher levels of meaning.

Student role
Listen to the question; take time to think; don't be afraid to say, "I don't know" or "I don't understand the question."

BOX 13-9
Types and Examples of Lower-Order Clinical Queries

Factual
What is the normal serum potassium level?
When does lente insulin exert its peak effect?
Who is eligible for Medicaid?

Descriptive
What does Maslow mean by a *hierarchy of needs*?
Where should intramuscular injections be administered when a child is not yet walking?
What is the immunization schedule for the first 2 years of a child's life?

---

from their ability to act as building blocks for concepts, generalizations, and higher-order questions. Both factual and descriptive questions deal with facts, but descriptive questions require students to logically organize their thoughts and deliver a longer response (see Box 13-9).

When faculty emphasize lower-order questions and reward only "right" answers, students will respond rapidly by memorizing information and will not become the critical thinkers or develop the clinical judgment needed for nursing practice today and in the future. Higher-order questions cannot be answered from memory; they require students to think beyond the facts; to establish relationships and make inferences; to compare and contrast; and to find cause and effect (Cotton, 2001; McKeachie, 2002; Bastable, 2003). Here is the level of application and analysis, of critical thinking. The starting point for higher-order questions is often, but not always, *why*. The question, "Why does exercise increase heart rate?" is a lower-order question that can be answered with a factual physiologic, rote textbook response. The clinical coach also must bear in mind that, depending on the student's knowledge and experience, what is a lower-order question for one student may be higher-order for another.

Higher-order questions serve specific functions: evaluating, making inferences, comparisons, and predictions (McKeachie, 2002; Bastable, 2003) (Box 13-10). Questions designed to explore evaluation may have rather concrete answers, as in evaluating the effect of a drug, or may lack a right or wrong answer, as in evaluating matters of judgment, value, and choice. In both cases, the higher-order thinking demanded requires the student to establish criteria and then measure the subject against them (McKeachie, 2002; Bastable, 2003). Another type of higher-order question calls for the student to make inferences. When a student takes a premise or a group of facts drawn from recall (lower-order) and then comes to a conclusion based on that information, an inference is drawn. This is a valuable tool for calling the student's attention to how something recently learned relates to prior learning or for helping the student see reason, motive, or

---

BOX 13-10
Types and Examples of Higher-Order Clinical Queries

Evaluative
How will you know that your patient has tolerated ambulating in the hallway?
How did you know your intervention was effective?

Inferential/Interpretive
Why should the nurse assure that the patient has signed the consent for surgery before preoperative medications are administered?
The manifestations of pain differ considerably from person to person. How have your patients today shown they were in pain?
What else might happen if you did that?

Comparative
What is the relationship between mental illness and homelessness?
Is there a connection between the level of education attained and the incidence of abuse?
What is the relationship between the pathophysiology of emphysema and the manifestations your patient presents with?

Heuristic/Divergent/Creative
What would be the effect of a health care system in which nurse practitioners were the dominant health care providers?
How will this hospital going from not-for-profit to a for-profit status affect how this unit is managed?
In what ways would closure of this community center affect the community it serves?

---

cause and effect that can be drawn from the given circumstances (McKeachie, 2002). Responding to these questions involves using deductive or inductive reasoning skills. The student uses deductive reasoning when thinking through from a principle or generalization to the current situation. An otherwise factual question can be moved to a higher-order level that requires deductive reasoning simply by the addition of context. For example, rather than ask a student what a patient should be taught about taking beta-blockers, a clinical coach might say, "Your patient, Mr. Smith, will be taking the beta-blocker metoprolol (Lopressor) when he leaves the hospital. What will you need to teach him related to this medication before he is discharged?" The other approach to inferential questions requires inductive reasoning. Inductive reasoning is used when the student analyzes the current situation and extracts the generalization from the specific situation at hand. Comparative questioning is an especially valuable learning tool and the next type of higher-order question. By helping students relate ideas to one another, look for commonalities and dissimilarities between concepts, and determine whether theories are contradictory, faculty assist students in making linkages that enable long-term memory acquisition (see Chapter 2). This type of question typically employs the words *compare/contrast, connection between,* or *relationship between* (McKeachie, 2002). The final type of higher-order question compels the student to apply analytical and problem solving skills. Generally questions without known answers, those divergent or heuristic questions, are most often predictive in nature and serve to pique student curiosity (Cashin, 1995).

When using clinical queries, additional questions are often required to guide the student beyond the superficial or otherwise help propel thinking forward. These clarifying questions fall between lower- and higher-order questions and so are transitional in nature. Novice faculty will recognize clarifying questions from working with patients in their clinical practice. These questions elicit further information, ask for justification, direct attention to related concepts or examples, or prompt the student's thinking with hints (McKeachie, 2002; Bastable, 2003) (Box 13-11). Sometimes a student's response to a clinical query is unclear to faculty. An effective clinical coach will ask the student to explain an answer in order to identify the accuracy of the thinking process or the point where the student's thinking moved off-track. It is possible that the student may have a good answer that is just different from what faculty had in mind! Student responses to transition questions are then used to loop back to further higher-order questions.

Higher-order clinical queries can promote the development of the habits of the mind and skills of critical thinking discussed in Chapter 11. In some cases the student's cognitive growth is related to the type of question posed, whereas in other circumstances, growth occurs as a result of the querying process as

---

BOX 13-11
Clarifying Questions to Guide Students' Thinking

Seeking information
What do you mean by ___ ?
Can you tell me more about that?

Seeking justification
What data are you using to substantiate that?
What are the assumptions you are making?

Seeking refocus
How does this relate to that?
What else might be responsible for that?

Seeking progression
What other problems would this produce?
What other information about the patient do you need to obtain?

a whole. Some aspects of critical thinking are associated with more than one element of questioning, and their placement in Box 13-12 reflects this. The connection of this pedagogy to critical thinking is substantial.

Clinical queries are a teaching strategy that requires focused thinking on the part of faculty and lots of practice! Students benefit the most when their clinical coaches build a question set, a sequence of questions to propel students' thinking to a higher-order (Prince George's County Public Schools). The power of this pedagogy does not rest in a single question, but in the faculty's ability to combine questions of differing types into a pattern that requires the student to use varied critical thinking skills. Beginning with a lower-level question (facts or descriptions), then moving on to higher-order questions is one approach, but is not always a necessary approach. A higher-order question can

---

BOX 13-12

Relationship of the Habits of the Mind and Skills of Critical Thinking to Clinical Queries

Evaluative questions
Analyzing
Applying standards
Intellectual integrity

Comparative questions
Analyzing
Discriminating

Inferential/Interpretive questions
Intuition
Predicting
Logical reasoning
Inquisitiveness

Heuristic/Divergent/Creative questions
Creativity
Transforming knowledge
Inquisitiveness
Predicting

Questioning process
Confidence
Contextual perspective
Flexibility
Open-mindedness
Perseverance
Reflection
Information seeking

serve as the starting point, or the clinical coach can move smoothly between question types. Setting the focus with the student at the beginning helps avoid tangential thinking, for example, "Let's talk about Joe's behavior in group today." Depending on the desired result, questions can be open-ended to permit the student's exploration of alternative answers, or they may be closed in order to limit the responses. If the student is asked what the daily requirement for calcium is during pregnancy, one right answer is the result. However, by asking for ways that a lactose-intolerant person can meet the daily calcium requirements, the student is required to access a wider knowledge base.

Questioning as a pedagogical approach in nursing education is truly an art that has not been universally mastered by clinical faculty. There are pitfalls lurking along the query pathway (Box 13-13). Besides asking too many lower-order questions, novice faculty are most prone to make the error of telling rather than asking. Anxious to be seen by their students as clinically knowledgeable and competent, new faculty may dole out information to students on request, actually depriving them of significant learning opportunities. Once a question is posed, faculty may commit another common error by providing students with insufficient time to think about the question and construct a response (Cotton, 2001; McKeachie, 2002). As clinicians, new faculty are familiar with the need to allow patients time to assemble their thoughts after being asked a question, and they are comfortable with silence. But with the stress of a new role as a faculty member, tolerance for that quiet moment following a question may be lessened. In those situations, inexperienced faculty either provide the answer outright for a student, or they operate from the assumption that the student does not know "the answer" and too rapidly fire off another question volley. "It is better to be an open-minded, curious questioner than the font of all knowledge" (McKeachie, 2002, p. 35). Student anxiety climbs as it does for faculty, and the overall value of the teaching technique is then lost.

Those who are new to constructing clinical queries may make the mistake of framing questions in such a fashion that the student needs to read the faculty's mind in order to be able to respond. The question and the expected reply may seem logical to the faculty, but from the student's perspective, any response is doomed to failure. It is also important for faculty to listen attentively

---

BOX 13-13

Common Errors in the Technique of Clinical Queries

- Asking excessive numbers of factual questions
- Telling; providing the answers
- Allowing insufficient time for processing the question
- Asking questions with arbitrary answers
- Inadequate listening to student responses
- Poor clarifying and redirecting skills

and thoughtfully to student's answers in order to accurately determine the level of student understanding. As student nurses may follow circuitous roads of thought, or struggle to find a word or phrase, inexperienced faculty can "bulldoze" the discussion, pushing it forward in a direction the student did not intend. If a student seems stuck and presents with the classic "deer in the headlights" expression after a question is presented and sufficient thinking time has been allowed, faculty must decide how best to proceed. Usually, if the question is rephrased, the student becomes "unstuck" and can begin to think through a response. Another approach some faculty are quite skilled with is the use of an analogy, in a nursing context or an everyday one. This method is especially valuable for beginning students. For instance, a coach might say, "Drugs bind to cellular receptors much as Legos® attach to one another, so what happens to the patient if I lay a stick across the Lego receptor?" Or, faculty might suggest an answer (right or wrong) and ask the student to identify the supportive evidence. It may be necessary to redirect the student's thinking by stepping back to some prior question or knowledge that is foundational to the current question. Asking several factual or descriptive questions before moving back to one requiring higher-order thinking skills can sometimes decrease student anxiety during clinical queries.

Clinical faculty may assume they are doing a fine job of teaching because they ask their students lots of questions. But when this assumption is explored, it is often the case that although questions are being asked in quantity, they have limited value beyond basic knowledge assessment. Skills are lacking in building question sets, providing sufficient wait time, and guiding student responses. Even when provided in open-ended format, factual questions do little to move the learner to higher cognitive ground unless they are part of a greater pattern. When clinical faculty coach through the skilled application of clinical queries, both faculty and students experience new enthusiasm for active, collaborative learning. A pinnacle experience for faculty often follows: students begin to query themselves and one another! Students achieve a major benchmark in their educational experience when they learn how to learn.

Technical/Psychomotor Skills

The psychomotor skills associated with the discipline of nursing are primarily embedded within the students' earliest clinical educational experiences. Many sound rationales support this curricular approach, but the primary one is that action supersedes communication and higher-level thinking. Experienced clinical faculty will tell their novice colleagues that when a student is able to safely perform a technical skill while carrying on a conversation with the patient, advanced beginner competency has been attained. When students reach their final clinical courses, the procedural aspects of most technical skills have been adequately mastered and are now being refined. The onus of facilitating students' learning of psychomotor skills falls most heavily on faculty teaching foundational and medical-surgical clinical courses and those who work with students in learning resource centers (LRCs).

Still routinely referred to as *psychomotor skills*, the revised taxonomy of educational objectives (Anderson et al., 2001) redefines the knowledge of how to do something that is specific to a subject or discipline as *procedural knowledge* (see Chapter 2). As one of the four dimensions of knowledge (factual, conceptual, procedural, and metacognitive), procedural knowledge encompasses the skills and algorithms, techniques and methods of a discipline, and also the knowledge of when and where to use them (Anderson et al., 2001). The nursing student learning how to insert an intravenous (IV) cannula must also learn the indications for IV therapy, how to select the appropriate site and needle size, and the criteria for determining successful access. In addition to procedural knowledge, complete skill mastery at the advanced beginner level requires factual knowledge (i.e., terminology) and conceptual knowledge (i.e., principles).

The acquisition of procedural knowledge is heavily grounded in behavioral learning theories (see Chapter 2). Technical skills are learned and carried out in a sequential pattern. Students learn to test the balloon on a retention catheter prior to insertion but after they have donned sterile gloves. New skills are learned by building on prior knowledge. Surgical asepsis is learned as a situational extension of medical aseptic technique. Simple skills are learned before progressing to more complex ones. Students first learn to put on sterile gloves and then learn the process of changing a dressing. The quantity and order of steps comprising each psychomotor skill form an "executive subroutine" (Gagné & Driscoll, 1988) that is established and triggered in the learner's mind by verbal and nonverbal cues provided by the clinical coach. For instance, clinical faculty might remind a student of the executive subroutine of a dressing change by pointing to the Telfa pad or saying, "Put on the Telfa pad before the gauze." Feedback that is immediate and precise guides the learning process and serves as a reward for successful performance. Without being excessively wordy, faculty must communicate the proximity of the performance to the desired standard. Vague feedback fails to support the learning of psychomotor skills (e.g., "That's good."). "The expectancy [of success] that is activated must be confirmed in order to complete the act of learning" (Gagné & Driscoll, 1988, p. 99). Indicating to the student that the injection site has been correctly identified allows progression to the next step and tells the student that site identification was accurately done. Repeated practice of a psychomotor skill facilitates the feedback of the musculoskeletal system, enabling the student to attain both accuracy and smoothness of performance over time (Miracle, 1999).

Behavioral learning theories do not provide the only guidance for facilitating skill acquisition; cognitive learning theories play a role as well (see Chapter 2). Skills are learned within the context of the teacher-student relationship, and as previously discussed, the characteristics and quality of that relationship impact the student's learning, positively or negatively. All of a student's previous learning experiences and the feelings that were engendered by them are brought to bear in learning new psychomotor skills. Individual learning preferences and styles can be capitalized on in the process of skill acquisition. Students who are primarily visual learners benefit the most from observing a skill being performed before attempting to do it themselves. Kinesthetic learners are helped by being encouraged to think about how a skill "feels" and the position of their hands in relation to one another and to the patient. Adult learning theory guides the approach to teaching and learning skills in nursing. Students actively participate in the learning experiences and collaborate with faculty in monitoring their progress. Mental rehearsal is another helpful tool for students learning psychomotor skills. Mentally rehearsing skills provides a mental image of the desired process (Miracle, 1999), and the technique "teaches" muscles how to behave when the skill is performed. The use of mental practice to assist in the learning of complex psychomotor skills has been documented for more than 60 years (Gagné & Driscoll, 1988). The use of imagery for the development and improvement of skill performance is common in sports, and although there is limited nursing research proffering support beyond empirical evidence, what is available is quite encouraging (Miracle, 1999).

Learning theories provide the basis for the tactics and techniques faculty use, whether teaching skills in the LRC or following up practice in the LRC with performance in the clinical setting (Box 13-14). Students must learn that carrying out psychomotor skills is only one aspect of what it is to be a nurse. Technical skill performance, procedural knowledge, is but one knowledge realm tapped in the total process of caring for patients. Competency in all the dimensions of knowledge is required in nursing practice. Once a student has attained some familiarity with manual skills, faculty must incorporate skills into a patient care context and move the student's thinking to a higher level. Students should be expected to introduce themselves to their patients, prepare them for

---

BOX 13-14

Tactics and Techniques for Facilitating Psychomotor Skill Acquisition

- Foster a positive student-faculty relationship
- Capitalize on individual learning preferences and styles
- Encourage a collaborative approach to skill acquisition
- Ascertain student readiness for learning
- Build on prior knowledge when introducing new skills
- Assure the student has the necessary factual and conceptual knowledge
- Break complex skills into smaller units for initial learning
- Facilitate procedural knowledge by emphasizing sequential patterns
- Establish the boundaries of safety; allow controlled mistakes
- Use mental rehearsal/imagery
- Consider skill demonstration
- Use triggers to cue the executive subroutine
- Provide immediate and precise feedback
- Encourage/provide opportunities for practice
- Place the skill within a patient context
- Use clinical queries to exercise higher-level thinking skills

the skill, and respect their privacy. This also can be done in the LRC through the use of mannequins or simulators within a case scenario format (Tarnow, 2005). In both the LRC and the clinical setting, judicious clinical queries are the best tool for facilitating the habits of the mind and skills of critical thinking while integrating procedural knowledge into the student's armamentarium of knowledge and skills.

One of the most difficult teaching skills for novice faculty to master is determining when and how to intercede when students are performing skills. Permitting students to make controlled mistakes within the parameters of patient safety in the clinical setting in order to see the results can be a valuable learning experience (Lichtman et al., 2003), but must be limited in application with novice practitioners. In the LRC, students must learn the boundaries of safety, but can be permitted to overstep them without consequences to an actual patient. In the clinical setting, inexperienced faculty may step in too early and even take the skill over from the student. Reviewing the procedural aspects with the student and discussing the factual and conceptual knowledge associated with the skill prior to approaching the patient can provide faculty with some assurance that the student is adequately prepared. A second valuable technique is to establish with the student in advance certain verbal or nonverbal cues to be given by faculty during skill performance indicative of correct/incorrect procedural steps. Glancing at faculty intermittently while carrying out the skill, the student knows to proceed when faculty give a slight nod of the head. If the student does get off track, try to make the correction as unobtrusively as possible to avoid dispelling the patient's trust in the student. Telling the student "A little higher" or offering a guiding hand is far superior to completely taking over the skill. With adequate direction, usurping a skill from a student should rarely be necessary, other than during an emergency situation.

Facilitating students' acquisition of psychomotor skills can be carried out first in the LRC or in the clinical setting. Primarily for the benefit of increasing patient safety, reducing student stress, and efficient time utilization in the clinical area, the initial practice of skills in the LRC is most common (see Chapter 12). Faculty can most effectively demonstrate skills in the LRC, and demonstration is known to be a valuable tool to facilitate learning (Miracle, 1999). When demonstrating skills, encourage active student participation in learning by asking questions that tap into the students' factual and theoretical knowledge as well as encourage procedural knowledge development. Questions such as, "What is this called/used for?" "What do I do next?" and "Why am I doing this?" are all examples of this technique. Remember to place the skill within a patient context, however general that may be, by way of checking identification, providing introductions and explanations, showing respect for privacy, ensuring comfort, and of course, handwashing! In the LRC, clinical variables are controlled and students can repeatedly practice skills to correct errors and attain at least a minimal level of proficiency before carrying them out with patients.

Opportunities to perform skills that students have not prepared for in advance do present themselves in the clinical setting. Faculty should consider how they might address such circumstances well before they occur. Basically, there are three options: (1) the student may be a nonparticipant observer as the skill is performed, (2) the student may assist with the skill, or (3) the student may carry out the skill with adequate direction and supervision. It may be that the skill is far too advanced for the student; in that situation, it is best that the student observe the skill being carried out by a nurse—faculty or staff member. If a skill is otherwise appropriate, faculty must carefully select the student who is to carry it out. Judgment is required to identify the students who have excelled in skill mastery, actively seek out additional learning experiences, and have the time at the moment to invest in an unscripted activity. If the student is to participate in carrying out the skill, the procedure should be methodically "walked through" with the student, supplies and equipment examined, and triggers for cueing established in advance. Under these circumstances, the feedback provided must take into consideration the student's inexperience with the skill and, perhaps, also provide direction for practice in the LRC after the fact.

Learning technical skills assumes an inordinate amount of student excitement and attention early in the educational experience. It often seems that students must "do nursey things" before they are open to learning the full meaning of what it is to be a nurse. Part of the role of the coach in facilitating skill acquisition is helping students learn to place the technical aspects of nursing in the proper perspective and open their eyes, minds, and hearts to the full scope of what it means to be a nurse.

Affective Skill Development

From the highly tangible aspects of learning to perform technical skills, the transition to the ephemeral affective aspects of nursing practice can feel rather abrupt. However, this is the nucleus of nursing. Affective knowledge is most often perceived of as feelings and emotions, attitudes and values, and the actions derived from them (Krathwohl, Bloom, & Masia, 1956). As previously described, the affective domain is reflected in the nursing student's degree of self-awareness and behaviors associated with professionalism. Self-awareness can be seen in a student's written and verbal communication and professional behaviors identified in the fulfillment of expectations for behaviors such as punctuality and appropriate attire. In both of these areas, faculty guide the student's growth through the feedback provided. But in nursing practice, the internalized affective domain components are externally exemplified primarily through caring behaviors. Caring is the art of nursing, guided by the science of nursing. The development of values, therapeutic communication skills, the knowledge and ability to apply moral and ethical principles, and the entire holistic approach to patient care are all encompassed in the affective domain and are all made tangible in caring nursing practice.

Human caring is the moral context for nursing education (Watson, 1988). In addition to experiences that help students learn to think like a nurse and act like a nurse, they must have experiences that help them learn to *care* like a nurse (Tanner, 2002). "While students must gain knowledge of the human body, mind, and spirit, this knowledge alone is insufficient without the essential component of caring" (Sappington, 2004, p. 223). Benner and Wrubel (1989) take the position that "…caring is primary. Caring is a basic way of being in the world…" (p. xi). "Caring as a focus of study must be made fundamental to nursing education and practice" (Tarnow & Butcher, 2005, p. 375). Refocusing clinical nursing education on helping students learn the process of caring was a part of the curriculum revolution instigated in the late 1980s (Woolley & Costello, 1988). In 1998, the American Association of Colleges of Nursing identified caring, with all its component behaviors, attitudes, and beliefs, to be a primary aspect of baccalaureate nursing education, and its role in practice was affirmed in the 2003 revision of the American Nurses' Association Social Policy Statement. If the attainment of caring competencies is to be an expected outcome of nursing education, students should not be graduated who cannot demonstrate them. "If our goal is to ensure that the student assimilates the process of caring for patients by integrating the necessary knowledge and skills, then a greater portion of clinical time should be spent teaching…the process of caring…" (Woolley & Costello, 1988, p. 91).

Nurse researchers have struggled for decades to describe, define, and measure the concept of caring, but a science of caring may simply never be entirely known (Giguere, 2002). The body of work regarding caring is substantial, and an in-depth examination of it is inappropriate for this venue. Perusing a metasynthesis of caring from the perspective of the patient (Sherwood, 1997), and a more recent one from the vantage point of nursing education (Beck, 2001), certain commonalities emerge. Caring is by nature interpersonal; it is manifested in the reciprocal connection of faculty with student and nurse with patient. Within this relationship, caring requires self-awareness, openness to the other person, and an offering of self. Empathy, support, being present in the moment, and attentiveness are facets of this caring relationship. Caring requires competence. Clinical competency is an important aspect of caring, whether provided by nurses to patients in clinical practice or imparted by faculty to students in educational settings. In nursing education, competency also includes the maintenance of professional standards and fairness in the evaluation of students. Caring in nurses' clinical practice generates therapeutic outcomes for patients and a sense of inspiration and fulfillment for nurses. In nursing education, care is contagious; students learn to care when faculty model caring and provide opportunities to develop the skills of caring practice.

Nurse scholars emphasize that the modeling of caring practices by faculty within the context of the student-teacher relationship is essential in the development of students' caring behaviors (Evans, 2000; Zimmerman & Phillips, 2000; Beck, 2001; Scotto, 2003; Duffy, 2005). "The commitment to care about students is central to concepts of good teaching" (Scotto, 2003, p. 289). Role-modeling caring by clinical coaches is clearly one means of facilitating the learning of caring behaviors by students. Faculty exemplify their caring for students in innumerable ways and Box 13-15 illustrates a few of these. Students witness the openness of caring when faculty share aspects of who they are. Raising children,

BOX 13-15
Some Caring Behaviors Modeled By Faculty

- Allowing students to see them as human beings
- Listening attentively
- Making eye contact
- Using a calm tone and conveying warmth
- Responding to questions
- Allowing and encouraging students to ask questions
- Being kind
- Being patient
- Providing encouragement and support
- Being respectful
- Acknowledging and responding to students' emotions
- Respecting individuality
- Being available
- Being fair and consistent in evaluation

having aging parents, a car that will not start, even having a headache, are all part of the human condition, and emotions are a universal language. Faculty must exercise judgment regarding what and when to share, but the act of sharing is a part of caring. Many of the caring behaviors faculty model are related to communication skills, both verbal and nonverbal, whereas others are indicators of empathy, sincerity, and respect. Caring is reflected when faculty offer students anticipatory guidance before encountering disturbing sensory stimuli such as diarrhea or vomitus; coach while assisting and demonstrating a patient transfer from bed to chair; and help students identify the ethical issues in patient care situations. Reason alone tells us that when faculty are caring toward students, the behaviors are likely to be reciprocated and mirrored in the students' practice.

As early as the mid-1950s, psychologists reviewing educational research concluded that there was more than sufficient evidence that, like cognitive and psychomotor behaviors, when the appropriate learning experiences are provided, affective behaviors are developed over time (Krathwohl et al., 1956). Nonetheless, the complexity of the concept of caring makes it especially challenging to create pedagogical approaches to help nursing students develop caring behaviors (Duffy, 2005; Lee-Hsieh, Kuo, & Tseng, 2005). "Teaching students to recognize caring behaviors and to conceptualize caring as the foundation of expert nursing practice remains challenging" (Sappington, 2004, p. 223). Caring practice is the visible outcome of nurses' feelings and emotions, attitudes and values. "Understanding caring as a practice, rather than as pure sentiment or attitudes apart from the practice, reveals the knowledge and skill that excellent caring requires" (Benner, 2001, p. x). The pedagogical approaches

BOX 13-16
Pedagogical Approaches to Teaching Caring

Reflective journaling
Self-awareness development
Identification of caring behaviors in others
Values clarification
Developing a personal philosophy of caring nursing practice

Clinical conferences
Caring narratives
Role-play
Exploration of value-laden issues and ethical conundrums in practice

Written assignments
Caring narratives
Analyses of books, film, art, or poetry from a caring perspective
Creative writing

Clinical practice
Caring within therapeutic relationships
Caring in verbal and nonverbal communication
Caring practices within patient context

to teaching caring must include helping students develop this internal affective foundation and recognize and develop caring behaviors (Box 13-16).

The most common and effective approach described in the literature for helping students explore and enhance their self-awareness is reflective journaling (Duffy, 2005) (see Chapter 11). The process of reflecting on their care endeavors teaches students about caring and provides insight as their caring practices evolve (Schaefer, 2002). Students can be artfully guided to examine the feelings and emotions within their care experiences through teacher-posed questions. These feelings and emotions serve as windows to students' attitudes and values. Self-awareness also can be developed through the observations of others. Sappington (2004) had students keep a "caring journal" to record and examine examples of caring displayed by themselves and others during a clinical practicum. Caring observations might be incorporated into students' reflective journaling, becoming the focus for a period of time, or one part of each weekly or daily entry. Using journaling as one strategy for teaching students about caring, Zimmerman and Phillips (2000) found their students initially had difficulty focusing on feelings, finding it much easier to "talk" about patients. In this case, faculty feedback provided the necessary redirection. Values clarification exercises also can be included in journals to help students examine their feelings about health, illness, and diversity and how these feelings affect the care they provide. The development of a personal philosophy of nursing is a common assignment in programs of nursing. Recasting this to focus on the caring practice of nursing and placing it in a reflection journal allows individualized feedback of a more intimate nature.

Clinical conferences or seminars, when students gather together as a group, offer another avenue to learning about caring. These venues provide a sanctuary for the safe and open exploration of clinical situations imbued with conflicting values—circumstances in which the ethical principles from the classroom become complicated by real human faces. In the company of their colleagues and with the assistance of clinical coaches, students grapple with the actualities of patients who are unlikable, barriers to communication, and practice challenges with no clear answers. In these situations, the teacher must avoid proselytizing and violating the student's right to explore ideas and values and make choices. Critical thinking simply cannot be fostered if faculty even subtly convey an expectation that students conform to their thinking. "The teacher's task is often directed not so much toward attitude change as toward increased sensitivity to other points of view and increased understanding of the phenomena to which the attitude applies" (McKeachie, 2002, p. 41).

In clinical conferences, students can be introduced to narrative pedagogy as they listen to the caring stories of their peers and faculty (Eifried, 2003). Narrative pedagogy serves to "engage students and teachers in collectively interpreting narrative accounts of their experiences in practice education" (Ironside, Diekelmann, & Hirschmann, 2005, p. 154). Here, narrative pedagogy makes caring more visible. With an understanding of cultural and contextual norms, students can receive help from one another in accessing and verbalizing their feelings, and in reflecting on their practices. Faculty can use this opportunity to assist students in identifying themes of caring within the stories. As they explore one another's narratives, students can identify commonalities in caring behaviors. What it means to know and connect with patients emerges (Ironside et al., 2005).

Role-play during clinical conferences can be another valuable means of allowing students to explore caring behaviors within a therapeutic relationship. Caring can be placed within context by creating miniscenarios dealing with common experiences such as admitting a patient, preparing someone for surgery, working with a dying patient, or those in physical or emotional pain. The group can identify and discuss caring behaviors within the given context, and the student "patient" can describe how it felt when the student "nurse" did or said certain things.

In addition to journaling, students can write caring narratives in more depth and detail as written assignments. As a part of the assignment, students could be asked to apply some of the relevant literature related to caring. This allows students to explore the extensive theoretical foundations of caring and move from the level of theory to that of application. Other approaches to written assignments might include the incorporation of analyses of poetry, books, films, or art in light of caring. Students could explore caring through metaphoric creative writing or the creation of poetry or art.

Students' clinical practice experiences offer many opportunities to focus their attention on caring practices. From their first experience with a patient, students begin to learn the reality of a therapeutic relationship. They learn the role of authenticity and the antecedent role of self-awareness. "Authenticity in therapeutic relationship [sic] is important because healing relationships depend on the nurse's genuine presence and caring. Authenticity requires self-awareness as well as confidence in relationship skills" (Lennerts, 2003, p. 160). Students need to experience the impact of their own personalities, the strengths and limitations of their interpersonal skills, on their relationships with patients (Lennerts, 2003). As they learn to use themselves as therapeutic tools, students begin to learn caring communication. Not surprisingly, students report faculty are less likely to assist them in developing communication skills than in learning technical skills in the clinical setting (Kotecki, 2002). As with all aspects of practice acumen, experiences over time will refine nurses' communication repertoire as they progress through the stages of their professional development (Benner, 2001). Thankfully, the nearly paralyzing fear of saying the wrong thing to a patient that is ubiquitous in the neophyte nursing student population passes with time and experience. From their perspective as students, they know that mistakes are a part of the learning process, but as novice nurses they are aware of the impact mistakes can have on their patients' welfare (Kotecki, 2002).

To help students learn caring behaviors, including those related to verbal and nonverbal communication, Lee-Hsieh, Kuo, and Tseng (2005) used patient interviews to identify specific behaviors by nurses that were seen as reflective of caring. Analyzed and thematically organized, then succinctly worded from the perspective of a patient, these interviews evolved into the "Caring Code" found in the "Clinical Toolbox" (see Chapter 20, p. 343). Students were introduced to the code by their clinical faculty, who reviewed its components and intent with them. Printed on laminated cards that they carried in their pockets, students referred to this "Caring Code" before approaching their patients. Such a teaching tool provides a ready resource "crutch" for student learning. Students reported the "Caring Code" offered guidance in meeting the holistic needs of their patients, helped with the development of empathy and positive relationships with patients, afforded affirmative feedback regarding the care they gave, and encouraged attitudinal and behavioral changes. Faculty offered much the same insights in their evaluation of the teaching strategy. When the efficacy of the strategy was tested using an experimental longitudinal design, the researchers found significantly higher scores in caring behavior in the experimental student group. Designed for use with adult, hospitalized patients, the tool can easily be modified for any setting or patient population, with credit to the original source provided. Content that is not applicable can be removed, and examples can be changed to reflect the clinical context from inpatient pediatrics to community-based settings.

The exploration of caring practices can be focused on patient context in a variety of creative fashions. A patient population (e.g., pediatrics), a concept (e.g., comfort), a setting (e.g., emergency department), or a health/illness topic (e.g., chronic illness; diabetes) can all become the contextual focal point for the study of caring in clinical practice. Zimmerman and Phillips (2000) describe a number of affective teaching strategies used in a rehabilitation nursing course with both theoretical and clinical components. Classroom experiential learning activities such as conceptual drawings and presentations were augmented in the clinical setting by reflective journaling. Schaefer (2002) applied a theoretical framework of knowing derived from the literature as the basis for reflecting on patient suffering through caring narratives in a graduate course, but the approach could be transposed for use with beginning students.

If caring is indeed primary, synonymous with the work of nursing, clinical nursing faculty are obligated to provide opportunities for students in which affective skills can be learned. The historical emphasis of nursing education on the acquisition of technical skills and tools to "do *things* to, for, and with people" must continue to be reconceptualized (Bevis, 1989, p. 354). The affective aspects of nursing practice are not learned spontaneously in some magical vacuum; caring does not become an inextricable part of students' nursing practice by oblivious osmotic absorption. By intentionally attending to the expressions of caring in nursing practice, faculty can help students become more self-aware, recognize caring behaviors, and fulfill the fundamental purpose of nursing.

Access To Resources

Students' knowledge and utilization of resources significantly impacts their ability to be successful in a clinical course, their entire program of learning, and eventually as advanced beginners in practice. The scope of resources is much more than the *Physician Desk Reference* and diagnostic/laboratory test books. Today's students use more than library and agency materials and personnel as resources in planning, providing, supervising, and evaluating patient care. They also make substantial use of online and computer-based resources.

Mobile technologies, such as personal digital assistants (PDAs), previously limited to advance practice, are beginning to be employed in clinical practice and nursing education (Huffstutler, Wyatt, & Wright, 2002; Miller et al., 2005). PDAs have been found to save personnel time, diminish mistakes, and make it easier and more suitable to seek information at the patient's bedside (Miller et al., 2005). Software programs are available as companions for textbooks, for purchase, or as online freeware. Programs include drug references, medical dictionaries and abbreviations, laboratory references, and medical terminology in other languages, and more programs continue to evolve. The availability of downloadable drug databases such as the ePocrates Rx™ system from www.ePocrates.com eliminate the need for students (or faculty) to tote drug reference texts to the clinical site (Lehman, 2003). In addition to providing ready access to informational references, PDAs also have calendars and memo pads to help organize information, as well as the ability to connect to desktop computers to facilitate backups and transfers of data (Huffstutler et al., 2002). In a study by Miller et al. (2005), nursing students made considerable use of their PDAs and agency personnel while significantly reducing their dependency on their textbooks and clinical faculty.

Increasingly aware of the diminishing half-life of knowledge, clinical coaches are acutely aware that they cannot be the only resource available to their students. They must be knowledgeable regarding the types of resources available and the means to access them, and then serve as a sort of relay station between students and the applicable resources for their needs. All clinical faculty should thoroughly explore services, personnel, and materials available in their clinical agency and educational institution. Then, depending on the focus of the course, other informational avenues may be incorporated into the clinical faculty's repertoire. This might include local branches of national organizations and services such as the American Heart Association, local agencies offering specialized services for the medically indigent or respite care, and valid and reliable online resources for patient teaching materials. As students become resource explorers, they will help supplement their faculty's inventory of resources as well.

It is sometimes difficult for novice faculty to accept that they serve their students far better as information coaches, directing learners to resources rather than simply providing answers themselves. Besides, it is just not possible for any faculty to have all the answers; the stress of that self-expectation can place a monumental weight on a faculty member's shoulders. Realizing the importance of access to tools is itself an eminent teaching tool. Whatever the discipline, a vital goal of postsecondary education is helping students learn where and how to access information.

Teaching/Learning Moments

Carpe momentum—seize the moment, and then make the most of it. Experienced faculty can describe innumerable teaching moments they have had with their students—times when theory was so well integrated into the situation at hand that students' faces glowed with understanding and the pleasure of learning. These instants of incredible joy in the synchronicity of teaching and learning are characterized by a mental receptivity of both faculty and student. Minds merge, insights are discovered, and the empowerment of understanding makes a profound impact on the student. It is in these moments that faculty experience the essence of what it is to be a teacher.

Learning moments cannot be scripted, constructed, or predicted; they arise spontaneously and are by their very nature short-lived and transitory (Reinsmith, 2003). To make the most of these opportunities, faculty must watch for them and be prepared to take advantage of them when they present themselves. Reinsmith (2003) has said that teachers must "learn to live on the balls of their feet, expecting the unexpected" (p. 7). As novice faculty, it is especially challenging to recognize and respond to teaching moments because simply learning to function within the routine parameters of a clinical course consumes so much time and attention. When unexpected occurrences develop in the clinical setting, neophyte faculty often see them as situations to simply survive, to get through, rather than as potential learning moments for students. Until their comfort range on site expands, new faculty can begin by applying some tools

---

BOX 13-17

Tools for Teaching/Learning Moments

- Know and build on students' theoretical and experiential backgrounds
- Change the perspective
- Use everyday analogies
- Draw from reflective journals and critical incidents
- Look, listen, jot down ideas

---

for identifying and seizing teaching moments in seminars and from within students' reflection journals. As they become more attuned to the teaching-learning process in the clinical agencies, and more relaxed and skilled in their teaching, these tools will become even more helpful to clinical coaches (Box 13-17).

Teaching moments depend a great deal on the faculty's knowledge of what students have learned in their theory classes and experienced in clinical practicum. But more than this, faculty teaching clinical courses come to know their students as individuals, including many of the life experiences and cultural foundations that make each one unique. In a teaching moment, learning is stimulated by the student's personal reality intersecting with an experience or piece of information to ignite an explosion of comprehension. A student's clinical time spent with a dying patient, a woman in labor, a schizophrenic adolescent, or a child with cystic fibrosis can result in the most meaningful learning when faculty are aware of what the student brings to the experience. Issues are embedded in each of these situations, and extracting them for discussion individually or within the clinical group can lead to a wonderful synergism of teaching and learning.

Looking at clinical situations from unexpected perspectives often can make students sit up, take notice, and engage. Encourage students to step into the shoes of other family members or health care professionals in a given situation. Transpose a scenario from a large medical center to a small rural hospital or change a key variable like socioeconomic status. Analogies can be very useful as a pedagogical approach in the clinical setting. Using analogies between clinical situations and routine life experiences can help provide clarity to complicated concepts. This approach is especially useful when the experience used for the analogy is personalized for the individual student.

Teaching/learning moments are more often lost than captured. This happens simply because they are not identified or there is insufficient time to make adequate use of them. Take advantage of students' reflective journal entries and their identification of critical incidents as potential sources. Jot down occurrences and thoughts during or following the time students are in their clinical settings that might be returned to and used later on.

The student response to a teaching/learning moment serves as its own reward for faculty effort. An "aha" space in time has occurred, and both teacher and learner are electrified by the experience. Students will say things such as, "I've read and heard about this over and over, but never really understood before. I get it now!" Teaching/learning moments provide additional richness and meaning to the faculty experience.

When Things Go Wrong

There is something to be learned even in the less than desirable circumstances that may arise in students' clinical practice. For most students, anxiety levels are higher in the clinical practicum than the classroom, and so is the sense of vulnerability (Keith & Schmeiser, 2003). Clinical settings are inherently unpredictable. As students practice applying their fledgling knowledge and skills, they are constantly reminded that they are novices. Others seem so efficient, so capable and skilled; their own inexperience and uncertainty seems that much more obvious to students. When they make an error, or personnel or patients say something hurtful or act in what students perceive as a hurtful way, they can be crushed. In these situations it is the role of the clinical coach to support students emotionally while helping them learn from the experience.

It is a rational and logical statement to say that making mistakes is part of the learning process. It is also rational and logical to say that students are just learning to be nurses; they are not there yet. Intellectually students understand that. But they often impose high expectations on themselves in the clinical setting and can become very distressed when they make a mistake. Probably the most common error that students make in the clinical arena is related to medication administration. Faculty must guide the student through the process of notifying the appropriate people, documenting the occurrence, and taking whatever corrective action is indicated. The next step is to explore with the student how a similar error might be avoided in the future. The coach's goal is both remedial, in terms of the error itself, and educative to help the student learn from the experience. The process requires a gentle hand. Disparagement from clinical faculty has no real place here; students castigate themselves for mistakes they make far more thoroughly than faculty ever could or would. The learning that occurs from such an experience requires some further thought and reflection when the student is away from the clinical site, as in writing a reflective journal entry, having a subsequent conversation with faculty, or both. Whenever faculty consider sharing a mistake a student has made with the rest of the group for educational purposes, it should always be discussed with the student in advance and never disclosed if the student seems uncomfortable or objects. This is a part of the student's rights for privacy and confidentiality (see Chapter 6).

Racism, sexism, and harassment are societal realities that students may experience in the microcosm of a clinical agency. Often presenting as a patient who refuses to be cared for by a student because of gender or ethnicity, or a staff member who seems to be constantly badgering students, such conduct is unfortunately not uncommon. Behaviors that reflect prejudice are hurtful to others wherever they occur, but for vulnerable students the experience can be overwhelming. Students often personalize the attack, perceiving its origin to be in who and what they are rather than in the attitudes, beliefs, or personality of others. Patients have the right to refuse the care of a nurse or a student based on any rationale they choose, regardless of its validity. This is not meant to legitimize patients' prejudices but rather to protect them from additional stress when they are less able to protect themselves. Faculty can use these experiences to help students understand this while beginning to learn to step outside of their own needs and into the role of patient advocate. Prejudice or harassment from agency personnel, however, is not appropriate and should be addressed. How these situations are managed may be partially determined by the policies and procedures of the agency. Depending on the student, staff, and situation faculty may intercede for the student with the staff member or manager or guide the student in addressing the matter directly. Rehearsal through role-playing may be helpful in the latter case. Ignoring the behavior is truly not an option; it does not model professionalism for the student nor does it resolve the problem. Again, student-faculty dialogue should provide the opportunity for the student to express feelings as well as to explore how to deal with such situations when they occur in the future... because they will!

Contingency Plans

As life is unpredictable for students, so it also is for faculty. Faculty get the flu, are called to jury duty, and are otherwise impacted by life's inevitable chance occurrences. For more lengthy periods of faculty absence, such as those required for major illness or surgery, the administrators of the nursing program are typically forced to devise longer-term alternatives such as restructuring faculty assignments or hiring clinicians to provide the needed course coverage. Unfortunately, there are usually no faculty to spare who have the time and ability to step into one or more unfamiliar clinical agencies and provide coverage for short-term faculty absences. It is to each clinical faculty member's advantage to build in some contingency learning experiences for these brief unforeseen absences. Box 13-18 provides some suggestions for consideration.

Faculty need to consider strategies that will develop students' critical thinking skills and are applicable to the individual clinical course while not involving the provision of direct, unsupervised patient care. The value of clinical learning is diminished if faculty simply give students the 1 or 2 days off or consider the time to be "payback" for the time required for completion of course assignments. Contingency plans are most effective and challenging for students if one is prepared for use early and another for later in the term when students are more knowledgeable and experienced in the course content. The assignments and any supportive materials should be centrally located and easily accessible by the students when faculty are unavailable. A file in the library is one option, or materials could be posted online, or e-mailed directly to the students in the clinical group.

BOX 13-18
Techniques for Making Contingency Plans

■ Make contingency learning experiences that enhance critical thinking skills
■ Design plans for both early and later in the term
■ Make assignments accessible without faculty assistance
■ Suggested approaches:
  ■ Learning resource center activities
  ■ Written case studies
  ■ Field trips
  ■ WebQuest activities
■ Consider additional faculty work required to evaluate learning

---

Many of the suggestions in Chapters 12, 14, and 15 could be adapted to meet faculty needs for contingency plans. If the learning resource center at your school can provide the necessary support, faculty can arrange for selected computer-based learning activities, or they may prepare case studies for use in role-playing or to be used with mannequins or simulators (Chapter 12). If this is not feasible, written case studies (Chapter 15) can be prepared for students to work on separately or in small groups from home or in the library. Some of the outside experiences and projects discussed in Chapter 14 also might be appropriate. Field trips to pharmacies, grocery stores, food banks, or toy stores are an enjoyable change of pace, and learning goals can be prepared to address foci for different courses and leveled for differing points in the term.

Unforeseen circumstances might present an opportunity to help students integrate the humanities into their nursing practice. Smith et al. (2004) describe a variety of pedagogical approaches for incorporating the arts into graduate nursing education, and some of these could be very effective for beginning nursing students. For example, students could take a field trip to an art gallery, or view preselected pieces of art exemplifying caring, illness, family, or other relevant topics. This experience then forms the basis for students' guided reflection in a paper or journal.

WebQuest activities have the potential to be exciting and entertaining inquiry-based learning experiences for today's computer savvy students. Directed by the faculty-created design, students use the resources of the Internet to gather information and solve problems. In the case of short-term faculty absence, students can obtain the assignment and then work from home. Billings and Kowalski (2004) provide a summary of the application of WebQuests to nursing education and a number of relevant resources. Other helpful online sites include the following:

WebQuest Resources: http://wneo.org/WebQuests/WebquestResources.htm
  (additional links provided)

WebQuest News: http://webquest.org/ (news views about the WebQuest model)

The WebQuest Page: http://webquest.sdsu.edu/webquest.html (supported by San Diego State University).

Contingency plans can generate presentations prepared in advance for the clinical group or even guidelines for assignment of group or individual papers. If faculty choose these options, they need to be prepared to adjust other preestablished assignments or seminar plans. Grading criteria cannot be changed once the syllabus has been given to the students (see Chapter 10). It is more efficient, for both faculty and students, if the products of contingency assignments can be incorporated into some preexisting format such as reflective journal entries. The additional work faculty put into the preparation of emergency learning activities should not result in additional work when they return to their courses.

SUMMARY

A good coach shows enthusiasm and joy for the game. The excitement and pleasure of accomplishment in clinical teaching is primarily derived from the coaching aspect of the faculty role. The feelings engendered when the look in a student's eyes says, "I got it!" are beyond description by all but a poet. And when coaching is well done, faculty know it intuitively, much as they know when they have done well in their clinical practice. Here is the elation that counter-balances the physical and emotional expenditures of teaching. And for the student, having clinical experiences guided by good coaches provides the knowledge and skills essential to the launching of a successful professional life.

REFLECTION EXERCISE 13

Thinking About Clinical Coaching

◆ Conduct a motivational assessment (Box 13-2) on yourself in relation to your own motivation to improve your abilities as a clinical coach.

◆ Conduct a self-assessment using the characteristics of an effective clinical coach listed in Box 13-1. Where are your strengths? Your limitations? Create a plan for your growth. Write several learning goals related to enhancing your coaching skills using the information in Box 13-3 as a guide.

◆ Consider your experiences in providing feedback to patients and colleagues in your clinical practice. How is providing feedback to students the same? How does it differ?

◆ In the clinical course you currently teach or will most likely teach, what approaches to making student assignments would facilitate student learning?

◆ Reflect on your current or on a previous clinical practice setting. Choose a single practice day and assess dangerousness in your own clinical practice (see Box 13-6). How can you use this experience to help students assess dangerousness in their clinical practice?

◆ Return to the definitions of the habits of the mind and skills of critical thinking presented in Chapter 11 and examine them in light of the higher-order clinical queries presented in Box 13-12. Does their placement make sense? Are others reasonable? Imagine a nursing student is with you in a recent clinical practice scenario. Create some question sets, using this situation as the foundation, that would be appropriate for a beginning student and others for a student who has nearly completed a nursing program.

◆ Consider any psychomotor skill that is performed in your area of clinical practice. Imagine you are teaching this skill to students in an LRC and describe how this would be carried out.

◆ Record and reflect on a caring narrative from your clinical practice that would be useful in helping students develop their affective skills.

◆ Reflect on the caring behaviors modeled by faculty in Box 13-15. Are there areas you need to work on? How might you do this?

◆ Consider the academic, clinical agency, and community informational resources that would be beneficial to nursing students in the course you currently teach or will most likely teach.

◆ Consider a learning moment you remember from your own clinical experiences. What were the circumstances? How was that learning facilitated?

◆ Think back to a mistake you made or some especially discomforting experience that happened to you when you were a student. What was done to help you through it? Were things done or said that were counterproductive, made you feel worse? When you make a mistake, how do you want to be treated?

◆ What contingency plans might you create for the course you are currently teaching or anticipate you will be teaching?

References

Adams, V.J. (2002). Consistent clinical assignment for nursing students compared to multiple placements. *Journal of Nursing Education, 41*(2), 80-82.

American Association of Colleges of Nursing (AACN). (1998). *The essentials of baccalaureate education for professional nursing practice.* Washington, DC: Author.

American Nurses' Association. (2003). *The social policy statement for nurses.* Washington, DC: Author.

Anderson, L.W., Krathwohl, D.R., Airasian, P.W., Cruikshank, K.A., Mayer, R.E., Pintrich, P.R., et al. (Eds.). (2001). *A taxonomy of learning, teaching, and assessment: A revision of Bloom's taxonomy of educational objectives.* New York: Longman.

Bastable, S. B. (2003). *Nurse as educator: Principles of teaching and learning for nursing practice* (2nd ed.). Sudbury, MA: Jones and Bartlett.

Beck, C.T. (2001). Caring within nursing education: A metasynthesis. *Journal of Nursing Education, 40*(3), 101-109.

Becker, M.K., & Neuwirth, J.M. (2002). Teaching strategy to maximize clinical experience with beginning nursing students. *Journal of Nursing Education, 41*(2), 89-91.

Benner, P. (2001). *From novice to expert: Excellence and power in clinical nursing practice* (Commemorative edition). Upper Saddle River, NJ: Prentice-Hall.

Benner, P., & Wrubel, J. (1989). *The primacy of caring: Stress and coping in health and illness.* Menlo Park, CA: Addison-Wesley.

Bevis, E.O. (1988). New directions for a new age. In National League for Nursing, *Curriculum revolution: Mandate for change.* (pp. 27-52). New York: National League for Nursing.

Bevis, E.O. (1989). Making a difference. In E.O. Bevis, & J. Watson, (Eds.), *Toward a caring curriculum: A new pedagogy for nursing.* (pp. 345-367). New York: National League for Nursing.

Billings, D., & Kowalski, K. (2004). Using WebQuests to promote active learning. *Journal of Continuing Education in Nursing, 35*(5), 200-201.

Blythe, H., & Sweet, C. (2003). Five more ways sports coaches model good instruction. *The teaching professor, 17*(9), 5.

Bradshaw, M.J., Rule, R., & Hooper, V. (2002). A joint junior-senior clinical experience. *Nurse Educator, 27*(2), 56-57.

Broscious, S.K., & Saunders, D.J. (2001). Clinical strategies: Peer coaching. *Nurse Educator, 26*(5), 212-214.

Burst, H.V. (2000). The circle of safety: A tool for clinical preceptors. *Journal of Midwifery and Women's Health, 45*(5), 408-410.

Cashin, W.E. (1995). Asking and answering questions. Prince Georges Community College, Reasoning Across the Curriculum Newsletter, 1(4). Retrieved May 11, 2005, from http://academic.pg.cc.md.us/~wpeirce/MCCCTR/cashin~1.html.

Cotton, K. (2001). Classroom questioning. NW Regional Educational Library. Retrieved May 11, 2005, from http://www.nwrel.org/scpd/sirs/3/cu5.html.

Diekelmann, N., & Scheckel, M. (2004). Leaving the safe harbor of competency-based and outcomes education: Re-thinking practice education. *Journal of Nursing Education, 43*(9), 385-388.

Duchscher, J.E. (2001). Peer learning: A clinical teaching strategy to promote active learning. *Nurse Educator, 26*(2), 59-60.

Duffy, J.R. (2005). Want to graduate nurses who care? Assessing nursing students' caring competencies. *Annual Review of Nursing Education, 3*, 59-76.

Eifried, S. (2003). Bearing witness to suffering: The lived experience of nursing students. *Journal of Nursing Education, 42*(2), 59-67.

Evans, B. (2000). Clinical teaching strategies for a caring curriculum. *Nursing and Health Care Perspectives, 21*(3), 133-138.

Gagné, R.M., & Driscoll, M.P. (1988). *Essentials of learning for instruction.* (2nd ed.). Englewood Cliffs, NJ: Prentice Hall.

Giguere, B. (2002). *Assessing and measuring caring in nursing and health science.* New York: Springer Publishing.

Grealish, L. (2000). The skills of coach are an essential element in clinical learning. *Journal of Nursing Education, 39*(5), 231-233.

Hayden-Miles, M. (2002). Humor in clinical nursing education. *Journal of Nursing Education, 41*(9), 420-424.

Huffstutler, S., Wyatt, T.H., & Wright, C.P. (2002). The use of handheld technology in nursing education. *Nurse Educator, 27*(6), 271-275.

Ironside, P.M. (2003). New pedagogies for teaching thinking: The lived experiences of students and teachers enacting narrative pedagogy. *Journal of Nursing Education, 42*(11), 509-516.

Ironside, P., Diekelmann, N., & Hirschmann, M. (2005). Learning the practices of knowing and connecting: The voices of students. *Journal of Nursing Education, 44*(4), 153-155.

Keith, C.L.B. & Schmeiser, D.N. (2003). Student issues: Anxiety—What's in a word? *Nurse Educator, 28*(5), 202-203.

Kotecki, C.N. (2002). Baccalaureate nursing students' communication process in the clinical setting. *Journal of Nursing Education, 41*(2), 61-68.

Krathwohl, D.R., Bloom, B.S., & Masia, B.B. (1956). *Taxonomy of educational objectives: The classification of educational goal—Handbook II: Affective domain.* New York: David McKay.

Lee-Hsieh, J., Kuo, C.L., & Tseng, H.F. (2005). Application and evaluation of a caring code in clinical nursing education. *Journal of Nursing Education, 44*(4), 177-184.

Lehman, K. (2003). Clinical nursing instructors' use of handheld computers for student recordkeeping and evaluation. *Journal of Nursing Education, 42*(1), 41-42.

Lennerts, M.H. (2003). Teaching personal knowledge as a way of knowing self in therapeutic relationship. *Nursing Outlook, 51*(4), 158-164.

Lichtman, R., Burst, H.V., Campau, N., Carrington, B., Diegmann, E.K., Hsia, L., et al. (2003). Pearls of wisdom for clinical teaching: Expert educators reflect. *Journal of Midwifery and Women's Health, 48*(6), 455-463.

Luparell, S. (2005). Why and how we should address student incivility in nursing programs. *Annual Review of Nursing Education, 3*, 23-36.

McKeachie, W.J. (Ed.). (2002). *McKeachie's teaching tips: Strategies, research, and theory for college and university teachers.* (11th ed.). Boston: Houghton Mifflin.

Merriam-Webster's Collegiate Dictionary (11th ed.). (2004). Springfield, MA: Merriam-Webster.

Miller, J., Shaw-Kokot, J.R., Arnold, M.S., Boggin, T., Crowell, K.E., Allegri, F., Blue, J.H., & Berrier, S.B. (2005). A study of personal disgital assistants to enhance undergraduate clinical nursing education. *Journal of Nursing Education, 44*(1) 19-26.

Miracle, D.J. (1999). Teaching psychomotor nursing skills in simulated learning labs: A critical review of the literature. In K.R. Stevens & V.R. Cassidy (Eds.). *Evidence-based teaching: Current research in nursing education* (pp.71-103). Sudbury, MA: Jones and Bartlett.

Murphy, J.I. (2005). How to learn, not what to learn: three strategies that foster lifelong learning in clinical settings. *Annual Review of Nursing Education, 3*, 37-55.

Oermann, M., Truesdell, S., & Ziolkowski, L. (2000). Strategy to assess, develop, and evaluate critical thinking. *Journal of Continuing Education in Nursing, 31*(4), 155-160.

Prince George's County Public Schools. Questioning to promote higher-order thinking. Retrieved May 15, 2005, from http://www.pgcps.pg.k12.md.us/~elc/isquestiontopromote.html

Redman, B.K. (2001). *The practice of patient education* (9th ed.). St. Louis: Mosby.

Reinsmith, W.A. (2003). Make the most of the learning moment. *The Teaching Professor, 17*(10), 1, 7.

Sappington, J.Y. (2004). Caring in action. *Nurse Educator, 29*(6), 223.

Scotto, C.J. (2003). A new view of caring. *Journal of Nursing Education, 42*(7), 289-291.

Schaefer, K.M. (2002). Reflections on caring narratives: Enhancing patterns of knowing. *Nursing Education Perspectives, 23*(6), 286-293.

Schmeiser, D.N., & Yehle, K.T. (2001). Decreasing anxiety for the nursing student entering the acute-care clinical setting. *Nurse Educator, 26*(4), 169, 174.

Sherwood, G. (1997). Meta-synthesis of qualitative analyses of caring: Defining a therapeutic model of nursing. *Advances in the Practice of Nursing Quarterly, 3*, 32-42.

Smith, R.L., Bailey, M., Hydo, S.K., Lepp, M., Mews, S., Timm, S., & Zorn, C. (2004). Integrating humanities in nursing education. *Nursing Education Perspectives, 25*(6), 278-283.

Sprengel, A.D., & Job, L. (2004). Reducing student anxiety by using clinical peer mentoring with beginning nursing students. *Nurse Educator, 29*(6), 246-250.

Stokes, L., & Kost, G. (2005). Teaching in the clinical setting. In D.M. Billings and J.A. Halstead (Eds.), *Teaching in nursing: A guide for faculty* (2nd ed.) (pp. 325-346). Philadelphia: Saunders.

Tanner, C.A. (2002). Clinical education, circa 2010. *Journal of Nursing Education, 41*(2), 51-52.

Tarnow, K.G. (2005). Humanizing the learning laboratory. *Journal of Nursing Education, 44*(1), 43-44.

Tarnow, K.G., & Butcher, H.K. (2005). Teaching the art of professional nursing in the learning laboratory. *Review of Nursing Education, 3,* 375-392.

Tsai, M.T., & Tsai, L.L. (2004). Critical success factors of transferring nursing knowledge in hospital's clinical practice. *Journal of the American Academy of Business, 5*(1/2), 193-197.

Twibell, R., Ryan, M., & Hermiz, M. (2005). Faculty perceptions of critical thinking in student clinical experiences. *Journal of Nursing Education, 44*(2), 71-79.

Watson, J. (1988). A case study: curriculum in transition. In National League for Nursing, *Curriculum revolution: Mandate for change.* (pp. 1-8). New York: National League for Nursing.

Weimer, M. (2003). 10 characteristics of effective feedback. *The Teaching Professor, 17*(10), 5.

Westberg, J., & Jason, H. (2001). Fostering reflection and providing feedback: Helping others learn from experience. New York: Springer.

Woolley, A.S., & Costello, S.E. (1988). Innovations in clinical teaching. In National League for Nursing (Ed). *Curriculum revolution: Mandate for change,* (pp. 89-105). New York: National League for Nursing.

Youngblood, N., & Beitz, J.M. (2001). Developing critical thinking skills with active learning strategies. *Nurse Educator, 26*(1), 39-42.

Zimmerman, B.J., & Phillips, C.Y. (2000). Affective learning: Stimulus to critical thinking and caring practice. *Journal of Nursing Education, 39*(9), 422-425.

CHAPTER 14

Group Learning Experiences: Seminars and Conferences

A portion of the total number of hours allocated for a clinical course is characteristically designated for seminar or conference use. This is time set aside for clinically based group learning experiences that is generally separate from that spent in the clinical setting. Commonly, these meeting times are orchestrated in one of several patterns depending on the course. Each clinical day may be preceded and/or followed by a clinical conference, or the conference time may occur following one or more clinical experiences on a weekly or on an even more frequent intermittent basis over the term. Occasionally, again depending on the clinical course, all or part of this time is used for psychomotor skill instruction or perhaps evaluation in the learning resources center. But in most cases, this time is an opportunity for all of the students in one or more sections of a clinical course to meet together, virtually by some technologic method or in physical proximity, for other types of group learning experiences.

Clinical conferences are seen by faculty as one of the primary approaches for promoting critical thinking in clinical nursing education (Twibell, Ryan, & Hermiz, 2005). But the success of this approach is highly dependent on how faculty use the time. Little learning occurs during most conferences held just prior to a clinical day; these preconferences serve the purpose of briefly addressing individual students' questions and/or allowing faculty to gather information to facilitate organizing their own day. Learning is rarely optimized during "post" clinical conferences either. Having been educated during the realm of conventional pedagogies (i.e., outcomes or competency-based nursing education) in which knowledge acquisition and its application ruled and being driven by an overfull curriculum and the perceived need to "cover the content," clinical faculty often use this time to present material in teacher-focused didactic lessons. Tossing out an occasional question during the presentation is not enough to qualify it as an active learning experience! Alternatively, thinking they are making the most of the students' clinical learning, faculty begin with a summary or question about what has happened that day and then endeavor to "go with the flow" as students share some of their experiences. Any learning that occurs with this method is usually serendipitous, and even when guided by the most skilled facilitator, the resulting learning experience can prove wan and boring.

Reconceptualizing clinical conferences using the new pedagogies requires faculty to identify and challenge their assumptions of teaching and learning and cast content in an equal relationship with thinking (Diekelmann & Smythe, 2004). These small group environments are ideal for active learning experiences, and in this more intimate setting, each student's insights can be valued and teacher-student relationships can be strengthened to a degree not possible in the larger classroom of 50 or more students. Dialogue is opened as teachers and students engage in thinking together, and the true complexity of clinical practice emerges. "Content [is] the necessary, but not sufficient, background for thinking" (Diekelmann & Smythe, 2004, p. 344).

The type of clinical course (e.g., foundations, community health), the level of the students (e.g., first term, final term), and the type of educational program (e.g., baccalaureate, associate degree) primarily affect the content of learning experiences in these clinical seminars, but most formats are broadly applicable. Some approaches lend themselves more to having students together physically in the same room, while others can be adapted for interactive activities via the Internet when students are geographically dispersed.

During clinical conferences, classroom theory can be artfully integrated into practice, analyzed and critiqued. Faculty do need to put some advance thought into their clinical conferences and consider the pedagogical method most suitable to the circumstances. Variety maintains vigor in learning, and given the numerous options to choose from, there is no need to use the same approach week after week. Faculty do take the lead in the clinical conference learning experience, but only to a certain point. They may select, design, and initiate the activity, and then become an observer or a participant as the students become more involved, as in group concept mapping or case studies. Or they may provide guidance in advance, such as making the structure available for case presentations or debate topics, and then allow the seminar to be student lead. Students are quite perceptive of the needs of their colleagues after a long day in the clinical setting, so when they are responsible for leading an activity, they usually endeavor to make the experience both edifying and enjoyable (Herrman, 2002). Students also should be involved in providing feedback to one another. Faculty often underestimate the impact of "peer power;" positive and constructive feedback from other students can significantly impact learning (Ridley, 2004) both for the initiator and the recipient. The potential for facilitating learning and stimulating thinking during clinical conferences is often untapped.

■ CREATING THE ENVIRONMENT

Faculty assume primary responsibility in establishing an environment that will be conducive to learning. This includes setting the general tone of this learning time. Clinical practice is a stressful time for students, as they strive to build their competency within the context of various settings and personalities. Students often carry this stress into clinical conferences, so faculty will find learning is enhanced when student stress is reduced. Relaxation techniques can be used to help decrease stress, but when dealing with the time constraints of a clinical conference, this may not be ideal. As effective as it is when the faculty member is coaching in the clinical setting (see Chapter 13), humor is a wonderful stress reducer and enhances the learning environment in clinical conferences. Hayden-Miles (2002), in her study of humor in clinical nursing education, noted numerous earlier studies demonstrating the role of humor in increasing the cohesiveness and morale in groups. Laughing together, individuals form bonds, and an environment is created where opinions can be expressed and criticisms addressed without damaging students' self-concepts (Hayden-Miles, 2002). It is certainly possible to teach and interact with students using humor, while still maintaining one's position as a faculty member.

Much of the discussion in Chapter 10 regarding the first meeting with the students is also applicable to clinical conferences. Remember to consider whether providing food for the group is appropriate and financially feasible. If the seminar is at the end of a long day of classes or a clinical day, feeding the masses will nourish the brain (Mann, 2004). The brain needs the equivalent of 250 M&Ms® to provide for its daily glucose needs! Remember all of the potential sources of glucose, and strive for nutritionally sound snacks. Consider any special dietary needs of the students, such as food allergies or metabolic disorders. Bringing snacks could be a responsibility rotated among the students. Food could also be a focal point of a seminar exploring the other cultures in the population served by the clinical agency.

Consider the dynamics of the group members, and use clinical conference time as an opportunity to use strengths and build on limitations in how each student interacts within the group. If the location of the seminar is to be in the clinical setting, privacy from patients and personnel is essential. Students should be reminded of the confidential nature of any discussion of their patients that may occur during these seminars.

Use the skills of "creating the set" to begin the seminar and provide a closure that will not only verify it is the end of the conference but also kindle ongoing curiosity and even advocate further action (Gustafson, 2003). Remember the power of provocative questions! These can be excellent both for opening and closing a clinical conference and can be applied during the conference itself. Students love to hear stories about their faculty's experiences as students or in clinical practice, and one of these might make a good opening for a clinical conference if it is applicable—especially if the story is a funny one!

▩ SHARING EXPERIENCES WITH A PURPOSE IN MIND

Obviously, faculty teaching clinical courses want their students to learn from their practice experiences, and within a conference setting, the students in the group can learn a great deal from one another and gain additional insights into themselves. The errors that some faculty make are (1) allowing this sharing of experiences to be haphazard instead of focused in nature and (2) repeatedly using this approach as the only or dominant learning approach used in clinical conferences. When a random approach is used, there may not be adequate time to fully process or effect closure of the topic being addressed, and therefore, student learning is not optimized.

Focus on What is Important

Starting from the perspective of the student, rather than that of the faculty, what is important to the students is what most merits discussion. Rather than move around the group with a general question about what happened to them today, faculty can employ an activity the students do quietly and independently to help them reflect on the day and determine their most meaningful moments. Taking a few minutes at the beginning of the conference period, students might use Herrman's (2002) "quick writes" strategy to jot down brief situational reactions, dilemmas, or even notes to their patients. Herrman suggests quick notes can be shared or kept private, but if the activity is introduced as something to guide group discussion, students will understand the purpose and select their subject matter accordingly. If reflective journaling is being used in the course, quick writes that were not addressed in seminar can be incorporated there; in that way faculty will still have an opportunity to dialogue with the students about their most significant issues. One or two quick thoughts can generate meaningful discussion, yet not consume the entire seminar period.

Make Stimulating Critical Thinking a Priority

Review the habits of the mind and skills of critical thinking presented in Chapter 11. Consider how, within the context of the discussion, they might be fostered in the students. Positive feedback and encouragement, combined with questioning are the best tools faculty have available to accomplish this (see Chapter 13). When a student recounts the experience of doggedly pursuing information to respond to a patient's request, identify and commend the perseverance demonstrated. Ask students to predict what might happen next in a situation, or what the results of a particular therapeutic intervention might be. Encourage inquisitiveness and creativity; guide logical reasoning.

Postulate "what if" questions to help the students develop flexibility. And model intellectual integrity in the pursuit of truth as assumptions are identified and challenged.

Practice the Pedagogy of Relational Inquiry

Often, wrapped up in their focus on performing skills and doing the right thing at the right time, students may overlook what it truly is to be a nurse. At the heart of every clinical experience that students have is their interaction with patients. Exploring this relationship during clinical conferences, students learn to relate in a profound and genuine manner (Doane, 2002). In the process of listening to the call of the patients, how they are living through their experiences, students find ways to understand and bond with them at a deeply intense level (Ironside, Diekelmann, & Hirschmann, 2005). Historically, formalized methodologies addressing the nurse-patient interaction have emphasized rigid behaviors and constraining rules, communicating to students that there are certain right and wrong behaviors in every patient situation. Reconceptualizing relational practice as a spontaneous, unself-conscious interface creates a flow experience that Doane (2002) sees as having a transcendental nature.

As one becomes skillful in conscious participation, the automaticity of known patterns that seek to still the flux of human life and relationships is diminished. The spontaneous compassion that arises when one is not caught in habitual patterns is released. The heart awakens (Doane, 2002, p. 402).

Students can be encouraged to role-play, discuss, and reflect on their interactions with patients as a means to learn and expand their relational practice (Doane, 2002). Faculty can open discussions by telling a story of a practice experience of their own, where listening to the patient, simply being present, was especially powerful. Another method could be to have each student conduct an interview of a patient with a general common experience, such as feelings about pregnancy or living with a chronic disease. This could be done during or outside of their clinical experience. The interview results can be brought to clinical conference and used to stimulate reflection when commonalities and differences are shared within the group (Staib, 2003). Seeking patients' stories in order to better understand the health care experience from their perspective and endeavoring to participate in relationships with them with authenticity and presence permits the enactment of the caring essence of nursing practice.

▪ STUDENT CASE OR TOPICAL PRESENTATIONS

Having students prepare presentations for the group that are related to a specific case from their clinical experiences or a topic applicable to the content of the course is a common approach to clinical conferences. This active group learning experience develops oral communication and teaching skills. Students may be provided with structural guidelines in advance, especially if the presentations are to be graded. Or they may be encouraged to use their creativity in selecting a method of sharing information with their peers. In these cases, students often generate games or other active learning experiences around the subject matter. Case presentations tend to generate a greater likelihood of boredom within the group, even with the most animated presentation. One way to make the learning experience more enjoyable and active is to combine the presentation with nursing rounds. In any case, faculty may have to assist the student presenter in making the entire experience more enjoyable and stimulating critical thinking by the group through posing questions and facilitating discussion of possible application. Learning is enhanced through the provision of faculty and/or peer critiques.

This learning activity can consume an inordinate amount of time if every student in the clinical group is required to do a case or topical presentation, leaving little time over the course of the term for other activities. If, for instance, there are 10 students in the group and each student is given 30 minutes for a presentation, at least 5 hours would be required, and time for set-up and breaks has to be included as well. Faculty can address some of these problems by further restricting the time allocated for presentations (e.g., 15-20 minutes), interspersing them between other activities over the term, or making them one option among a selection of learning activities from which students may choose.

▦ NURSING ROUNDS

Nursing rounds are a pedagogical approach in which the actual patient is incorporated into the learning experience. Evolving from the bedside teaching practice of medical students and physicians-in-training, the patients are the focus of demonstrations of assessment techniques, illustrations of key findings, interviews, and discussions among those in attendance. In some cases, students prepare and present their own patients; in others, faculty design the entire experience. Students should be given guidance in the preparation for rounds under both circumstances in order to maximize learning. Permission must be obtained in advance from the patient, or from family members in the case of children or those unable to provide permission themselves. The purpose of the rounds should be explained, and patients should be told in advance if there is to be any physical exposure. Privacy and respect must be maintained during the rounds, and most of the case discussion should be held in another room following the interaction with the patient. After the portion requiring the patients' participation, appreciation should be extended for their contribution to the students' learning. In a separate setting, the students can work through complicated patient issues as a group (Herrman, 2002). Within the context of the interaction with the patient, with supplemental data provided as needed, faculty can address relevant questions to the students to stimulate their thinking and develop clinical judgment.

Although traditionally carried out at the bedside of hospitalized patients with acute health problems, nursing rounds can take place anywhere patients are located. They can be used with beginning students in extended care facilities and with more experienced students in community health settings. Properly done, conducting nursing rounds is an excellent approach for encouraging critical thinking skill development. Identifying relevant data and interpreting it as part of the process of assigning meaning is a key component in synthesizing diverse components into an integrated whole—what faculty and students alike often call "putting it all together" (Twibell et al., 2005). Many of the habits of the mind and skills of critical thinking can be incorporated into this pedagogical strategy.

GROUP CONCEPT MAPPING

Concept mapping is discussed in detail in Chapter 15 as one approach to clinical preparation, but it also can be used in a number of ways as a group learning experience (Baugh & Mellott, 1998; Brock & Butts, 1998; Herrman, 2002; King & Shell, 2002). The process itself can be initially taught in a clinical conference, as faculty provide the disparate data and then guide the students to identify the conceptual nodes and create linkages (King & Shell, 2002). Once the skill has been developed, it can be used as a group activity, or students can form teams to address highly complex topics (Herrman, 2002). Alternatively, students can present the concept maps they have previously constructed and now use during their clinical time, obtaining feedback from their peers and learning to appreciate the variance in patient presentations (Baugh & Mellott, 1998), examining cause and effect relationships (Brock & Butts, 1998). Creating concept maps for prototypical conditions currently being discussed in accompanying theory courses allows all students in the group to actively participate in the transfer of theory to practice.

By virtue of the dynamic nature of concept mapping, actual clinical practice is more accurately reflected, and students find the activity entertaining and engaging (King & Shell, 2002). Time in clinical conference can be allocated for the revision of individual concept maps based on the day's experiences, encouraging reflection and further dialogue as clues in the maps are identified that could have been used to predict occurrences. Faculty provide guidance in the process, using questioning techniques and helping students gain new insights and seek additional data (Baugh & Mellott, 1998). Group concept mapping is an intellectually active learning experience that can facilitate growth of the habits of the mind and skills of critical thinking. Examples of concept maps are found in the "Clinical Toolbox" (see Chapter 20, pp. 366-367).

CASE STUDIES

The examination of case studies provided by faculty, as a mode of stimulating critical thinking within a clinical group, is a common pedagogical approach. Since cases can be designed for students from the first to the last clinical course, be drawn from virtually every clinical setting, and leveled to meet expectations for students in every type of academic program, they are one of the most flexible teaching methods available.

Case studies can be explored in writing as formal assignments (Chapter 15) or as part of contingency plans for faculty absence (Chapter 13). Here, as group learning experiences, they can be used with online discussion boards (discussed later) or as a face-to-face activity. Their design and presentation is discussed here in detail. The "Clinical Toolbox" (see Chapter 20, pp. 346-348) provides several examples.

Theory presented in the classroom is applied to actual practice situations in an active learning experience as students respond to faculty prompts in the form of discussion questions. Cases may reflect situations similar to ones students have experienced, or they may provide the opportunity to examine a number of patient problems before they are encountered in the clinical setting. In some cases, this may be the only exposure students have to some clinical experiences that are not attainable in the practice environment.

Case studies can be quite simple, brief, and straightforward or highly detailed and complex. Some authors call the shorter format *case method*, rather than case studies (Gaberson & Oermann, 1999), but the term *case study* is sufficiently generic as to incorporate the full range of extent and difficulty. Usually the cases are presented in written form, but case studies in video format give faculty the added advantage, when used during clinical conference, of pausing the dialog as needed for questions or discussion. The case may be presented as a scenario in which the students are asked to *make* decisions or to *analyze* a decision made by a nurse depicted in the case (Oermann, Truesdell, & Ziolkowski, 2000). Critical thinking is encouraged as students employ reflection to scrutinize their assumptions, explore problems from multiple perspectives, and choose and prioritize interventions (Staib, 2003). Many of the habits of the mind and skills of critical thinking are galvanized through the skillful implementation of case studies. Used in a group format, students' thinking is stimulated by their peers, new insights are achieved, and the dynamic of the group adds a significantly different flavor to the learning experience.

For a discussion in a clinical conference to flow smoothly, students should have learned the necessary knowledge beforehand and should have resources readily available; this will help the conference proceed on schedule and within the allotted time. Typically, the case study incorporates questions posed at the beginning, within the text, or at the conclusion. The case study and planned discussion questions can be provided in advance, and the students can be required to come prepared to address them in the seminar. Another approach is to give the students the general topic in advance, encouraging them to find relevant research or clinical articles to incorporate into the discussion. Alternatively, the case can be presented verbally or in writing at the time of discussion, and the group facilitator (student or teacher) can have some general questions in mind, deviating from them as needed based on the discussion that evolves.

The faculty role as facilitator of the group and the advancement of the learning activity is a key aspect in the use of case studies. Whenever possible, the case analysis is guided through the thoughtful presentation of open-ended questions. The discussion may be initiated by having the group identify the major issues in the case, the problem or problems. Then a variety of questioning approaches direct the progression of the activity. Probing and analytical questions move the students to dig deeper; predictive questions assist in projecting consequences; linking questions draw the application of theory; summary questions facilitate closure and identification of what was learned (Tomey, 2003). Working together, the students accomplish collaborative problem solving. Evaluation of group process can be a terminal activity, conducted after students have completed the assignment and the results have been summarized by the faculty (Tomey, 2003). Faculty may need to intercede by acting as arbitrators during disagreements, encouraging full participation of all members of the group, and redirecting thinking (Tomey, 2003).

Group discussions are ideal for exploration of legal and ethical topics. Responding to diversity necessitates that students identify their own beliefs and attitudes and how these affect the care they provide. Immediacy is often the most effective timing for these issues; face-to-face discussion encourages students' most accurate insights, so it might be best to avoid providing the case in advance. Again, general questions should be prepared in advance, but the facilitator needs to take cues that arise in the discussion and move with the flow accordingly.

Tomey (2003) provides an in-depth review of the history, design, and use of case studies. Written case studies are commercially available, but faculty often find that when they create and tailor the cases themselves, they are more valuable. Drawn from actual practice experiences or current events or created from one's knowledge base and applicable references, case studies can incorporate issues of public policy, leadership and management, ethical problems, and an endless number of other topics. In discussing design, Tomey (2003) suggests that the content within the case be sequenced, from simple to more complex, building upon itself so that students' thinking is continuously being advanced. She recommends faculty set aside a case they have written after completing it, allow a sort of incubation period, and then reevaluate it for clarity and adequacy. Every effort should be expended to anchor case studies contextually. Supportive documents applicable to the scenario should accompany the case (e.g., graphics, photos, cardiac rhythm strips) (Oermann et al., 2000; Tomey, 2003). These could be displayed with overhead projectors, fastened to the wall, or drawn on a whiteboard. For case studies presented by a group, it is not necessary for every participant to have their own copies of supplemental materials.

The literature is replete with suggested approaches and topics for case studies. Cases may be designed to address emergency situations in a given clinical setting (Tong & Henry, 2005). These are a common focus of the National Board Examination, and a competency expectation for graduate nurses, yet many students are not exposed to them beyond the theoretical level during their programs of study. Welk (2002) placed these emergency situations within the context of pattern recognition and had students identify relevant and irrelevant data pertaining to risk factors and signs and symptoms within a case study of a patient experiencing a myocardial infarction. Minicases are the basis of Ridley's (2004) "sticky situations." She prepared problem-solving situations on Post-It© notes and stuck them to the wall of the conference room. As students entered the room for their clinical conference, each one randomly selected a sticky note, determined the appropriate interventions, prioritized them, and then the results were shared within the group. Every clinical course has emergency situations that could be approached through case studies.

Others may actually be brought into case study discussion. If appropriate, patients or family members may be included. Staff may be involved, presenting an actual scenario and guiding the discussion, while a faculty member contributes as a participant and facilitates discussion as necessary (Staib, 2003). Members of other health care disciplines, or students in those areas, can participate along with nursing students in interdisciplinary case studies (Youngblood & Beitz, 2001). This would be a wonderful opportunity for students to learn the roles of other health care providers and the value of collaborative care models.

Case studies also have been used to establish the context for student role-playing experiences (Van Eerden, 2001). This approach could be used for a variety of clinical experiences. Cornelius (2004) described it as one aspect of an HIV/AIDS experiential learning module. Students can be asked to match the assessment findings within a case study to applicable interventions, with a focus on patient outcomes (Youngblood & Beitz, 2001). Or, using another approach to this connection tactic, students can link the major mechanisms of prototypical drugs or clinical conditions within case studies (Youngblood & Beitz, 2001). Innovative strategies for case study approaches that are especially conducive to group work appear regularly in the literature and are generally adaptable to any clinical focus.

■ SHARING OUTSIDE EXPERIENCES AND PROJECTS

Students may be assigned a variety of projects and independent learning experiences (Chapter 3) over the course of the term, and clinical conferences are ideal for spreading the wealth of the learning. Students may prepare topical poster presentations such as they might use in a nursing in-service program or for group client teaching projects. They may share the results of field trips to pharmacies to compare label instructions or to grocery stores to examine the sodium content of foods. They may return to the full group to discuss the results of small group/team tasks such as community assessment projects, or the development of clinical orientation manuals for student use in community agencies where they are lacking (Lehman & Brighton, 2005). The point is, learning is expanded and strengthened when students share within the group, and faculty have the opportunity to enrich the experience by fostering further critical thinking.

■ INTEGRATING RESEARCH/EVIDENCE-BASED PRACTICE

The prominence of research within a nursing curriculum primarily depends on the terminal degree awarded. Baccalaureate students receive more theory and a greater emphasis is placed on research in their programs of study. However, all novice nurses should enter the profession with an understanding of the importance of evidence-based practice and a spirit of inquiry. This can be fostered at the appropriate level in a variety of ways in clinical courses and carried into clinical conferences. All levels of nursing students should develop some degree of sensitivity to research-related issues within the clinical environment during their education. Baccalaureate students may generate research questions (Callister, Matsumura, Lookinland, Mangum, & Loucks, 2005) during a clinical conference in which discussion revolves around the identification of practices that are not research-based. Or, these questions can serve as the foundation for poster presentations in clinical conferences or the larger college community (Callister et al., 2005). Research findings can be incorporated into a wide variety of clinical conference approaches (e.g., debates, student case or topical presentations, and group project seminars). Agency personnel, from nursing and other health care disciplines, can be invited to speak about aspects of ongoing research projects, leveled based on the student audience. Group critiques of published research can be especially valuable to beginning students who are just learning the language of research.

▦ DEBATES

Debates allow participants to actively develop their thinking, verbal, and listening skills to a remarkable degree and can add a unique flavor to the clinical conference mix of learning experiences. Debates have been used to inform and sway points of view throughout history (Candela, Michael, & Mitchell, 2003). When arguments are based on evidence rather than simply opinion, the habits of the mind and skills of critical thinking are brought to bear. Confidence in verbal expression and reasoning abilities is enhanced; proficiency in researching, analyzing, and validating information is gained; dexterity in establishing inferences and seeking justification in the evidence is increased; and open-mindedness is fostered as divergent positions are presented and biases exposed.

A wide variety of real-world topics applied to nursing can be the subject of debates (Herrman, 2002), topics that may not be as effectively addressed through any other venue. This format encourages student participation in issues of public policy as they relate to nursing, and the examination of nursing's role within the health care system (Herrman, 2002). Many clinical and ethical scenarios can be used as the basis for debates between faculty and students, or between students within a clinical group (Youngblood & Beitz, 2001). Ethical debates are especially useful in aiding in the development of positions corroborated in the scientific literature and examination of the conflicts that develop in nursing practice (Candela et al., 2003). Students have the opportunity to apply ethical principles such as autonomy and beneficence presented in the classroom to the conundrums of clinical practice.

Adequate preparation for debating will require time to explore and evaluate the topic, identify positions, and then seek evidence to substantiate them. Students on each team will need the opportunity to distribute their research to other members and then assemble it into a coherent and credible argument (Candela et al., 2003). Classical debate format should be followed, with strict time allocations for the presentation of positions and rebuttal. Under most circumstances, faculty will assume the moderator role, monitoring time limits, and perhaps providing an overall summary at the conclusion. With clear direction, debates lend themselves well to grading.

GAMES

In addition to games students and faculty may have designed in previous terms and the wide variety and availability of commercially prepared ones, new games can be created that are contextually appropriate to any clinical course. Faculty may create games or students may do so as a means of presenting relevant topics.

One of the most popular formats is that of the television game show Jeopardy®. Students are divided into teams, and the faculty member or a student assumes the role of game host, providing the "answer" and awarding points for the quickest accurate question provided. The content of the answer/question combinations varies with the course, but any topic can probably be used (i.e., terminology, drugs and nursing considerations, developmental milestones, signs and symptoms, nutrition content).

Glendon and Ulrich (2005) followed the *Family Feud®* format for a game they called "What's the Intervention?" as two teams of students were given a scenario, with the interventions hidden. Members of each team compete in the identification of interventions, earning points or striking out with each turn. The classic game show of the 1950's, *Name That Tune®* became "Name That Drug" as teams endeavored to identify the drug first, as clues ranging from general to specific were presented.

Other television game show formats can be the source of clinical nursing games. The advantage of these formats is that most of the students are familiar with them. A Price is Right® format could be used to help students grasp the cost of supplies such as bags of intravenous fluid, dressing materials, and urinary catheterization trays. The formats of *Wheel of Fortune®, Pyramid®,* or *Password®* could all be adapted for a clinical course at minimal cost.

Some creative educators have published information about original games they have designed (Youseffi, Caldwell, Hadnot, & Blake, 2000; Ridley, 2004). Youseffi et al. (2000) developed a card game to be used for skills testing. Each of the designated skills was broken down into an equal number of steps, which were written on cards (index cards would work). Duplicate cards were prepared anytime the same step was required in more than one skill (such as hand washing or documentation). The result was the same number of cards for each skill (e.g., 7-10). All the cards were combined to form a deck, shuffled, and dealt out to the group so that each person had the number of cards equal to the total number of procedural steps plus one. The remaining deck was placed face down, and one card turned face-up beginning the discard pile. Dubbed "Recall Rummy," the game proceeded as a rummy game, with the goal to be the first player to put together a complete procedural skill sequence (plus discard). For her "Contraceptive Grab Bag," Ridley (2004) indicated that any container can be used, although she uses a commercially prepared knitted uterus that she prefilled with a variety of contraceptive devices for a game with her maternity nursing students. Taking turns in drawing out a device, students then led the discussion and answered questions within the group. Clearly, the potential of gaming as a teaching strategy in clinical conferences is enormous and the only limitation is imagination.

ACTIVE AFFECTIVE LEARNING

In their revised *Taxonomy for Learning, Teaching, and Assessing*, Anderson et al. (2001) critique previous efforts to differentiate knowledge into three discrete domains for the isolating effect it produced, since "…nearly every cognitive objective has an affective component" (p. 258). Yet in common educational parlance, the cognitive, affective, and psychomotor knowledge domains are routinely addressed separately in an effort to emphasize the given topic. Nurse educators likewise know that in every psychomotor skill there are cognitive and affective components, yet still refer to this entirety as teaching psychomotor skill performance. So, although affective components are key features of many of the clinical conference approaches previously presented, there are some strategies in which affective learning is foremost.

The development of communication skills is a foundational part of nursing education. Students are often concerned that they might "say the wrong thing" to a patient in a particularly stressful situation. One approach to reducing this anxiety is role-playing, and in a group setting this can be followed by discussion. Ridley (2004) suggested this approach with skits in a maternity setting for students to practice assisting a grieving mother following a stillbirth, but it could be broadly applied to any number of contexts. Students can learn how to deal with angry and belligerent patients, as well as those who are demanding, depressed, fearful, or have any other anxiety-provoking emotion. This approach can be used for emotionally charged exchanges between the student as nurse and physicians or other health care providers. Done within the clinical conference, the experience and subsequent discussion can be beneficial to all of the students.

Many different experiential approaches can be used to explore topics in clinical conferences. Students can be urged to imagine themselves in a myriad of situations, and then discuss their responses as a group. Interpretive dance can be used to simulate fetal monitoring strips (Ridley, 2004) or cardiac rhythms. Marshall (2003) wrote about having students in a psych/mental health clinical course create mandalas as a means of developing interpersonal skills and self-awareness, while learning about Buddhism, Jung, and Peplau. Poetry, art, and music all can be used to help students get in touch with universal experiences of humanity such as childbirth, aging, pain, suffering, and dying.

ONLINE DISCUSSION BOARDS

The role of the internet in education is growing exponentially. At the postsecondary level, online students can take not just isolated classes, but complete entire degree programs. For the Net-Gen students especially, computer technology is second nature. In clinical courses for students in their initial programs of nursing study, the Internet is a dominant source of information, especially for planning care and patient teaching.

Faculty may also explore the use of the Internet for communication with individuals or groups through e-mail, online office hours, and discussion boards with threaded dialogues through software support programs such as Blackboard©. These discussion boards provide a group experience of sorts, so could be used for one or more clinical conferences. This methodology could be especially useful for students in geographically dispersed clinical sites in rural nursing courses or for capstone experiences.

Some of the conference approaches, such as student presentations, could be modified for online use, but it is important to realize and make allowances for the effect of this medium on group dynamics. Faculty feedback and facilitation are especially important for online discussion boards (Halstead & Billings, 2005). Case studies might lend themselves to this medium especially well. Each discussion question could be posted as a separate discussion board topic. Each student would then be required to post an answer and also to build on previous student postings with additional ideas or critiques. Web links to additional resources could be easily embedded within the case study. Faculty may consult with the information technology support personnel if they are interested in initiating online discussion boards for their clinical courses.

SUMMARY

Clinical conferences can be stimulating and enjoyable teaching and learning experiences if faculty put the necessary effort into their format and the creation of an environment conducive to active group learning. It is in these seminars that faculty teaching clinical courses can be the most inventive and daring in their implementation of some of the newest pedagogical strategies. Not everything works every time in every setting for every student, but part of the educator's role is to model the habits of the mind and skills of critical thinking and take some risks to facilitate growth.

REFLECTION EXERCISE 14

Thinking About Group Learning Experiences

Clinical conferences and seminars are a platform on which clinical faculty can apply the new pedagogical approaches in inventive and exciting ways to create truly memorable learning experiences for their students. Using the suggestions provided in this chapter as a starting point, consider your own unique gifts and perspectives and the clinical course you are teaching, or will be likely to teach.

◆ How have your previous assumptions about how clinical conferences "should" be conducted blocked your current exploration of alternatives?

◆ How might you create the learning environment for group learning experiences? What changes might be necessitated by the various approaches you might use?

◆ How might you determine what is important to the students as initial discussion items?

◆ Reflect on how you might practice the pedagogy of relational inquiry within the context of your clinical course/setting.

◆ Consider how two or three of the strategies discussed in this chapter could be applied or adapted to your clinical course.

◆ What criteria would you use to determine whether a clinical conference was "successful"?

References

Anderson, L.W., Krathwohl, D.R., Airasian, P.W., Cruikshank, K.A., Mayer, R.E., Pintrich, P.R., et al. (Eds.). (2001). *A taxonomy for learning, teaching, and assessing: A revision of Bloom's taxonomy of educational objectives.* New York: Addison Wesley Longman.

Baugh, N.G., & Mellott, K.G. (1998). Clinical concept mapping as preparation for student nurses' clinical experiences. *Journal of Nursing Education, 37*(6), 253-256.

Brock, A., & Butts, J.B. (1998). On target: A model to teach baccalaureate nursing students to apply critical thinking. *Nursing Forum, 33*(3), 5-10.

Callister, L.C., Matsumura, G., Lookinland, S., Mangum, S., & Loucks, C. (2005). Inquiry in baccalaureate nursing education: Fostering evidence-based practice. *Journal of Nursing Education, 44*(2), 59-64.

Candela, L., Michael, S.R., & Mitchell, S. (2003). Ethical debates: Enhancing critical thinking in nursing students. *Nurse Educator, 28*(1), 37-39.

Cornelius, J.B. (2004). To be touched by AIDS: An HIV-experiential teaching method. *Journal of Nursing Education, 43*(12), 576.

Diekelmann, N., & Smythe, E. (2004). Covering content and the additive curriculum: How can I use my time with students to best help them learn what they need to know? *Journal of Nursing Education, 43*(8), 341-344.

Doane, G.A. (2002). Beyond behavioral skills to human-involved processes: Relational nursing practice and interpretive pedagogy. *Journal of Nursing Education, 41*(9), 400-404.

Gaberson, K.B., & Oermann, M.H. (1999). *Clinical teaching strategies in nursing.* New York: Springer.

Glendon, K., & Ulrich, D. (2005). Using games as a teaching strategy. *Journal of Nursing Education, 44*(7), 338-339.

Gustafson, M. (2003). Get going! Get done! Introductions and conclusions for your class. *Journal of Continuing Education in Nursing, 34*(4), 149-150.

Halstead, J.A., & Billings, D.M. (2005). Teaching and learning in online learning communities. In D.M. Billings & J.A. Halstead (Eds.), *Teaching in nursing: A guide for faculty* (pp. 423-439). Philadelphia: Saunders.

Hayden-Miles, M. (2002). Humor in clinical nursing education. *Journal of Nursing Education, 41*(9), 420-424.

Herrman, J.W. (2002). The 60-Second Nurse Educator: Creative strategies to inspire learning. *Nursing Education Perspectives, 23*(5), 222-227.

Ironside, P., Diekelmann, N., & Hirschmann, M. (2005). Students' voices: Listening to their experiences in practice education. *Journal of Nursing Education, 44*(2), 49-52.

King, M., & Shell, R. (2002). Teaching and evaluating critical thinking with concept maps. *Nurse Educator, 27*(5), 214-216.

Lehmann, S.P., & Brighton, V.A. (2005). The clinical orientation manual: A student/preceptor educational resource. *Nurse Educator, 30*(2), 47-49.

Mann, A.S. (2004). Eleven tips for the new college teacher. *Journal of Nursing Education, 43(9)*, 389-390.

Marshall, M.C. (2003). Creative learning: The mandala as teaching exercise. *Journal of Nursing Education, 42*(11), 517-519.

Oermann, M., Truesdell, S., & Ziolkowski, L. (2000). Strategy to assess, develop, and evaluate critical thinking. *Journal of Continuing Education in Nursing, 31*(4), 155-160.

Ridley, R.T. (2004). Teaching tools: Creative collaborative clinical quickies. *Nurse Educator, 29*(4), 135-136.

Scheffer, B.K., & Rubenfeld, M.F. (2000). A consensus statement on critical thinking in nursing. *Journal of Nursing Education, 39*(8), 352-359.

Staib, S. (2003). Teaching and measuring critical thinking. *Journal of Nursing Education, 42*(11), 498-508.

Tomey, A.M. (2003). Learning with cases. *Journal of Continuing Education in Nursing, 34*(1), 34-38.

Tong, V., & Henry, D. (2005). Performance-based development system for nursing students. *Journal of Nursing Education, 44*(2), 95-96.

Twibell, R., Ryan, M., & Hermiz, M. (2005). Faculty perceptions of critical thinking in student clinical experiences. *Journal of Nursing Education, 44*(2), 71-79.

Van Eerden, K. (2001). Using critical thinking vignettes to evaluate student learning. *Nursing and Health Care Perspectives, 22*(5), 231-234.

Youngblood, N., & Beitz, J.M. (2001). Developing critical thinking with active learning strategies. *Nurse Educator, 26*(1), 39-42.

Youseffi, F., Caldwell, R., Hadnot, P., & Blake, B.J. (2000). Recall rummy: Learning can be fun. *Journal of Continuing Education in Nursing, 31*(4), 161-162.

Welk, D.S. (2002). Designing clinical examples to promote pattern recognition: Nursing education-based research and practical applications. *Journal of Nursing Education, 41*(2), 53-60.

Written Assignments

Written assignments in clinical courses include those done by students prior to a clinical experience, self-evaluation assignments, and those chosen to meet other course goals. The inclusion of written assignments beyond those required for preparation for clinical experiences must be very carefully considered. The process of preparing for a clinical experience can be very time consuming. Students may spend hours preparing to go to the clinical site: practicing psychomotor skills, investigating medications, and researching pathology, diagnostic assessments, and interventions, then prioritizing the day's care and creating an effective organizational plan. Additional student time may be required for other course expectations, such as the development of teaching or discharge plans, and group learning activities related to nursing rounds or clinical conferences/seminars (see Chapter 14). And always bear in mind that students are enrolled in courses other than their clinical ones! Time is a valuable and often scarce resource for both students and faculty. Students' lives encompass more than school, and caring faculty recognize this and respect students' time for learning. A considerable amount of faculty time should be devoted to the design of assignments and to the provision of prompt and meaningful feedback to students. The addition of other writing expectations must meet specific educational goals appropriate to the course that cannot be addressed as effectively in any other fashion.

■ CLARITY OF PURPOSE

It should be possible for faculty to explain the purpose of every learning activity, including written assignments, that they require. Students will complain about requirements they perceive as meaningless or unbeneficial to their learning. Ideally, the purpose should be provided in writing along with the assignment directions in such a way as to plainly describe the intent from the perspective of the students. Redundancy of assignments should be avoided at all costs. Students have been known to submit the same paper to faculty in more than one course; if the assignment is appropriately constructed, this should not be possible (or someone should eliminate an assignment!). Clinical courses also have multiple sections, taught by several different faculty, and students will compare the amount of work required by their faculty with that of other course groups. Complaints of too little work do not seem to occur, but complaints that a faculty member requires too much work are common.

This should not be construed to mean that there is no place for written assignments in clinical courses. The development of effective communication skills is an integral part of nursing education. Interpersonal communication is practiced and refined in accordance with the goal that novice graduates will become capable of interacting with their colleagues and patients meaningfully. Additionally, there is an expectation that as an educated person, the beginning nurse should demonstrate a degree of scholarly writing expertise beyond the level of simple documentation in patient records. Assignments that allow students to practice and refine their writing skills and enhance the habits of the mind and skills of critical thinking can be very valuable within the context of clinical practice courses. Since both writing and critical thinking skills can be addressed in other, nonclinical courses, the context of the current clinical setting is the key differentiating factor.

■ DEVELOPMENT OF WRITTEN COMMUNICATION SKILLS

As an educational tool, writing is essential. In the late 1970s and early 1980s, a pedagogical reform movement called Writing Across the Curriculum (WAC) gained momentum in the United States (University of Missouri, 1996; Purdue University Online Writing Lab, 2004; Questia Media America, Inc., 2004). In response to a perceived decline in literacy rates among college students, WAC programs were introduced beginning in elementary schools and continued through collegiate education. Curricular innovations evolved grounded in educational theories regarding the diverse and creative ways learning occurs beyond the rote and lecture formulaic approaches. Connections between writing, learning, and thinking are encouraged early in the educational process and facilitated with informal assignments such as journals and response papers. Then, in postsecondary programs, writing focuses on differences between disciplines.

Recognizing that each discipline has its own unique conventions of language use and style, discipline-specific assignments such as research papers and article reviews are added to the writing repertoire.

Colleges and universities may establish global expectations as part of initiating WAC programs, accompanying expectations with new or expanded resources for faculty and students. Programs of study may be required to have a specified number of "writing intensive" courses, mandating that students be enrolled in one of these each term of the curriculum. Online Writing Laboratories sponsored by the institution are commonplace, providing student services including writing and researching assistance. Faculty development programs and resource centers are often provided to assist faculty in meeting institutional expectations for students' quality and quantity of writing.

Nursing faculty routinely use writing assignments for evaluation; the role of writing as a learning tool for students is far too often overlooked and under appreciated. Increasingly, the results of educational research suggest that writing can make possible more creative and active learning of course content, and help students learn more about negotiating the contextual aspects of discipline-specific situations (University of Missouri, 1996). But writing also facilitates learning at an intensely personal level. As articulated by Bevis (1989), nurse educator, scholar, and poet:

> To write is to make commentary on oneself, on lived as well as imagined life; to battle with cause, effect, and correlation; to defend, determine, make assessments, and find meanings. And in the end, it is to attempt to balance merit, compassion, justice, and need. To write is also both to mask and reveal ourselves in layers of meanings that are often unanticipated, building on steps of assumptions and illusions, sometimes unidentified, often unilluminated. This is what enables writing to be a great tool for unraveling mystery and seeking feeling tones that hide in logic's shadow. Writing stretches the inner resources as does nothing else. (p. 237).

Judiciously used, writing assignments in clinical nursing courses support the development of both the professional and the person.

■ PROVISION OF WRITING STANDARDS

Students need to be provided with guidance in their writing, and the first aspect of that guidance lies in the directions and resources provided for the assignment. Instructions to the students should be clear, while encouraging creative thought and critical thinking. But, if something specific is expected to be included, it should be incorporated into the directions. Provision of a model, representative of the quality of the work expected, may be appropriate. Differing approaches to the same assignment in Box 15-1 illustrate the movement of assignment instructions from simple but highly structured to complex but less structured. Complexity is increased by more involved intellectual activity, and stimulates more of the habits of the mind and skills of critical thinking.

Although the structure of the assignment may vary significantly between a journal and a scholarly paper, there are universal expectations regarding

---

BOX 15-1
Sample Writing Assignments Differing in Complexity and Structure

Simple and high structure
Write a four-page paper addressing the etiology, significance, and interventions for one common surgical complication. Cite two research studies. Use correct grammar and APA format. Follow the attached outline.

Complex and less structure
Submit a scholarly paper exploring a common surgical complication. Incorporate the nurses' role in interdisciplinary collaborative care, both preventative and therapeutic.

---

grammar and professional writing that should not have to be reiterated with each assignment. Students should come to their secondary educational program with elementary grammatical skills, but reality often deviates from this expectation! With grammar check routinely available with word processing programs, it seems unnecessary to tell students to use them, but it *is* necessary. The mastery of the appropriate use of the semicolon, use of active voice, even the structure of sentences is an art that is not inherent. Syntax may be quite different among various types of assignments. Professional writing in a journal entry does not necessitate complete sentences, but correct spelling and the avoidance of sexist language should be an expectation. Students should have access to a good collegiate dictionary, in addition to a medical dictionary. A thesaurus is a useful tool that may be included with word processing programs or available for purchase in book format. Grammar and syntax references such as the classic *Elements of Style* by Strunk and White (2000) and *The Gregg Reference Manual* (2004) are very helpful. Scholarly papers typically require an established format, usually selected at a programmatic level. The reference manuals for the two most commonly used formats, APA (American Psychological Association, 2001) and MLA (Gibaldi, 2003), also provide writing guidance in addition to format styles for the papers and citations. A review of the issue of plagiarism may be very appropriate (see Chapter 8). Reference materials should be available in the school library, and many are also accessible online.

▇ PROVISION OF QUALITY FEEDBACK ON WRITING ASSIGNMENTS

The second aspect of faculty guidance for student writing is the written feedback provided. Offering feedback that is constructive, opportune, and enhances critical thinking is one of the two key ways to help our students learn (the other being fostering reflection) (Westburg & Jason, 2001). Clinical faculty do this verbally in the clinical setting in their role as coach (Chapter 13) and with many group teaching activities (Chapter 14), and they do it in writing with students' written assignments and written evaluations (Unit V). The importance of providing feedback cannot possibly be overstated; it is vital to learning. Students do not inherently know how to analyze, synthesize, or critique, any more than they innately know the rules of grammar!

Learning in educational settings is enabled by a variety of scholarly modalities (Bevis, 1989), some of which are as follows:

- Analysis
- Critiquing
- Recognizing insights
- Identifying and evaluating assumptions
- Inquiring into the nature of things
- Projecting, futuring, anticipating, predicting, or hypothesizing
- Searching for structural or organizational motifs (patterns) or building them
- Engaging in praxis (the enabling of theory and practice to inform and shape one another)
- Evaluating (assessing merit using criteria and expert judgment)
- Viewing wholes, not just parts in relation to each other
- Acknowledging paradigm experiences and cases in ways that enable them to be useful in practice and theorizing
- Finding meanings in ideas and experiences (pp. 235-236)

Students use these modes with varying degrees of proficiency depending on their individual expertise and the standard imposed by the educational level (i.e., associate degree, baccalaureate, graduate students). "Furthermore, it is the types of conclusions, ideas, and insights that are derived from these modes and the quality of abstractions that can be elicited from them by the student that distinguishes the educated mind" (Bevis, 1989, p. 236). The role of the teacher is to guide the student in the development of these scholarly modes, so that optimal results are obtained. Feedback is essential to this process and requires a thoughtful and often delicate hand.

Many of the feedback considerations for written work are the same as those for verbal responses for clinical performance, but the alteration in the medium of communication necessitates some substantive changes. As with verbal feedback, written feedback possesses distinctive qualitative, even emotional aspects. Without inflection or nonverbal behavioral cues, written feedback can be misinterpreted, so faculty need to consider the feeling tone they are communicating as well as the content of the feedback. Always tell students to speak to you directly if they do not understand or have concerns about the feedback they receive (Westburg & Jason, 2001). Even avoiding the use of red ink (or red highlighting when tracking changes and comments electronically) improves the emotional tenor of feedback (Mann, 2004). Purple is becoming popular; some educators find it packs the power of red with the tranquility of blue, calling the eye's attention without being hostile (Aoki, 2004). Pick a favorite blue, green, or purple pen; rotate or alternate the colors used on student papers to avoid evoking the Bloody Mary (or Marvin) moniker.

As with verbal feedback, positive observations in writing are very important. But be concrete and descriptive in positive remarks as well as constructive criticisms (Westburg & Jason, 2001). Rather than a margin note of "Good" or "Well done," tell the student specifically what was done well and what it was that made it good work. This input provides students with criteria they can use later to judge their intellectual work themselves. The positive feedback may provide a bridge of sorts to suggestions for further consideration or areas of weakness (Westburg & Jason, 2001) (e.g., "You are so right in your identification of this assumption. Now, consider how this assumption influenced your decision. What would be different in the future, without the bias this assumption imposed?") Own up to any subjectivity in your feedback, by accepting personal accountability (e.g., "I think...", "It seems to me..."). Such an approach implies that this is opinion and opens the door to further dialogue and exploration with the student (Westburg & Jason, 2001).

Avoid jumping to conclusions and making judgments (Westburg & Jason, 2001); pose questions to help clarify interpretations (e.g., "I'm not sure I understand your point about family relationships. Did you mean...?"). Also, as with verbal feedback, avoid feedback overload and recognize the student's level of receptivity (Westburg & Jason, 2001). Clinical faculty get to know their students quite well and are capable of accurate determinations regarding whether the feedback is too complicated for the neophyte to interpret and integrate, or whether the individual student's current emotional and intellectual status or recent clinical or life experiences may negatively affect receptivity. Excessive, inadequate, vague, or nonspecific feedback will not provide the impetus for growth that students want or need.

WRITING ASSIGNMENTS FOR CLINICAL PREPARATION

It is essential that any assignment relating to any patient or client in any setting be devoid of individually identifiable health information in order to meet legal requirements for patient privacy (see Unit II).

Clinical "Prep Sheets"

Not necessarily used in all clinical settings, faculty-designed clinical "prep sheets" are used primarily to meet the need for assuring patient safety at an elemental level and providing organizational structure for faculty and students. Some faculty attempt to combine clinical preparation formats with some form of self-evaluation through guided questions and reflection; the database used at the Decker School of Nursing is an example of this approach (Smith & Johnston, 2002). Clinical preparatory forms alone are typically inadequate to meet overall faculty needs for assessing students' knowledge, understanding, and thinking processes. In response to these deficits, faculty using these forms often add supplemental written requirements and/or rely on verbal dialogue with students in the clinical setting. It might be wiser for faculty to use some other approach to written clinical preparation that would more effectively and efficiently meet their needs.

Clinical preparatory sheets are most often used in acute care settings, especially in medical-surgical clinical courses. A sample form used for this type of course is provided in the "Clinical Toolbox" (see Chapter 20, p. 372). Faculty teaching these courses also often require that students prepare some sort of a time-management tool, especially for when they are caring for multiple patients or are involved in some leadership experience in which they are supervising other personnel. This may be a separate tool or included as part of other forms.

Nursing Process and Nursing Care Plans

The formulaic, rule-driven problem-solving format dubbed "nursing process" is a direct outgrowth of the behavioral learning theories and educational framework, and the traditional pedagogies of outcome-based education (Bevis, 1989) (see Chapter 2). The dedication of many nurse educators to nursing process, nursing diagnoses, and nursing care plans remains unswerving. "…Nursing faculty throughout the western world have both reified and deified the nursing process" (Tanner, 2000, p. 338). It can indeed be a useful tool in helping students think through many aspects of their care, but the insufficiency of nursing process as the customary modality used in the education of professional nurses is increasingly apparent. Tanner (2000) notes that even one of the forbearers of modern nursing, Virginia Henderson, remarked that what is termed the *nursing process* is not the only process used by nurses, nor is it a process exclusive to nurses.

Problem solving in health care cannot be approached linearly and in disciplinary isolation; it is a multidimensional, interrelational, often interdisciplinary, process of inquiry. In one qualitative study of 12 nurse educators in New Zealand, Walthew (2004) found that "…a number of the participants…considered the nursing process to actually inhibit critical thinking by stifling creativity, which they considered to be an essential component of critical thinking" (p. 410). Creativity is but one of the habits of the mind and skills of critical thinking that fails to be supported by either the nursing process or the construction of nursing care plans. A significant body of research substantiates that the nursing process is inadequate in capturing the thought processes used in clinical practice by either the novice or the expert nurse (Tanner, 2000; Mueller, Johnston, & Bligh, 2001). There is no question that the nursing process and nursing diagnosis model is inconsistent with the reality of today's managed care health care system. It is a model that generates work; managed care limits it (Barnum, 1999).

Standardized nursing care plans (NCPs) are available in numerous textbooks, and students have been known to resort to copying them verbatim, effecting little if any true learning (Mueller et al., 2001). Or students are required to spend hours prior to their clinical experiences meticulously endeavoring to create their own, provide rationales for every potential intervention, and address every actual and potential nursing diagnosis. Students then find nursing care plans to be of variable value in the clinical setting and expend hours more of their time working on them after their clinical day is over with, and an uncertain amount of learning occurs as a result (Welk, 2001). The North America Nursing Diagnosis Association (NANDA), Nursing Outcomes Classification (NOC), and Nursing Intervention Classification (NIC) rigorously dictate the structure and language to be used in the nursing care plan, and interventions often regress to the level of minutia. In the reality of clinical practice, nursing diagnoses impede the ability of nurses to effectively communicate with other disciplines at a time when interdisciplinary collaboration is increasingly essential. In this age of cost containment through managed care, our focus is more appropriately on what the health care professionals have in common, on collaboration and even joint educational experiences (Barnum, 1999). Indeed, as Barnum succinctly puts it:

> This pattern is in distinct contrast with a faculty's focus on discrete nursing theories and unique nursing terminology—for example, making nursing diagnoses that were different from medical diagnoses. Nursing faculties now have to question this kind of insularity and seek ways to participate in greater intimacy with professional peers. (p. 23).

Who else understands the student's discharge concerns for a patient when they are couched as Ineffective Therapeutic Regimen Management? Would a clinical pharmacist appreciate the differences in drug therapy for a patient with Decreased Cardiac Output when the etiology is heart failure versus hypovolemic shock? Nursing care plans are uncommon in the clinical arena today. More often clinical (critical) pathways delineate the care to be provided to patients with common health problems by the members of the health care team.

The furor engendered by the dogmatic acceptance of traditional nursing care plans by some faculty in a nursing program, and their rejection by others, can generate considerable confusion among the students. Ideally faculty in nursing programs will initiate a dialogue and attain some reasonable consensus in how nursing process will be taught and care plans will be used within their curricula. Such discussion will be universally beneficial and provide a consistent message to students.

It is certainly accurate to say that the nursing process concepts of organization (assessment, planning, interventions, evaluation) continue to be one useful tool for beginning nursing students, and there are some creative interpretations and applications of nursing care plans in the recent literature (e.g., Welk, 2001). However, there are other strategies available that are reflective of cognitive learning theories and more progressive educational frameworks and pedagogies, while simultaneously being more applicable to today's nursing practice. Clearly, the one currently receiving the greatest amount of attention by faculty, and being prolifically addressed in the literature, is concept or mind mapping.

Concept/Mind Maps

The traditional nursing care plan emphasizes format over content; the wording and structure is rigidly stylized (Koehler, 2001; Mueller et al., 2001). A major criticism of NCPs is that students expend precious hours endeavoring to locate references for known activities and an insufficient amount of time thinking. The process of creating concept maps emphasizes thinking, helps students establish priorities, find relationships, and build on their prior knowledge (Koehler, 2001). It assists students to progress beyond their predilection for memorization of facts, to the level of identifying and operationalizing concepts (All, Huycke, & Fisher, 2003). The nonlinear approach of concept mapping enables the generation of connections of one patient problem to another that is essential for effective nursing practice (Mueller et al., 2001). Concept mapping encourages the development of all of the habits of the mind and skills of critical thinking.

The theoretical foundations of concept mapping are found in the educational literature (Schuster, 2000), reaching back to the field of cognitive learning theory that addresses information processing, specifically the assimilation of information into long-term memory (All et al., 2003; Staib, 2003). Information is processed in short-term memory by reordering it into "chunks," which move into long-term memory to be stored as a result of linkages to preexisting knowledge. Concept mapping expedites this process by visually connecting, or linking, concepts to related concepts within geometric figures (nodes) (All et al., 2003). Information is organized and represented by concept maps in the same fashion as it is in human memory (Harpaz, Balik, & Ehrenfeld, 2004). Students can literally "see" the relationships, depict directionality through the lines forming the links, and the strength of the correlations by using solid and dotted lines. Colored pens may be employed as an additional organizational tool (Mueller et al, 2001). Risk factors, etiologies, diagnostic test results, adverse effects of drugs, and much more can be incorporated.

As a teaching strategy, concept mapping exemplifies the existential belief in individual reality, and many of the educational frameworks and pedagogies it spawned. Through inquiry learning, meaning is individually created, learning is active, insights are attained, and contextual perspective is achieved. An investment in learning is promoted and a holistic view of the patient is facilitated through the process of concept mapping (Baugh & Mellott, 1998; Harpaz, Balik, & Ehrenfeld, 2004).

The use of concept maps as a means to both teach and evaluate critical thinking in the clinical setting has been widely supported (Schuster, 2000; Mueller et al., 2001; King & Shell, 2002; Staib, 2003; Harpaz et al., 2004). Theory and practice are linked in concept maps (King & Shell, 2002; Harpaz et al., 2004). Creativity is encouraged as the students select and organize concepts, and contextual perspective becomes apparent as relationships emerge (Staib, 2003). The level of student understanding is increased through the use of concept maps (Schuster, 2000), and the "big picture" revealed (King & Shell, 2002).

Concept mapping is used broadly in nursing education (All et al., 2003). Nursing faculty may employ them as a teaching strategy in the classroom or for curriculum and organizational planning, and students may use them as a note taking or study tool (All et al., 2003). There are multiple structures used for concept mapping (Schuster, 2000; Mueller et al., 2001; King & Shell, 2002;

All, Huycke, & Fisher, 2003; Harpaz, Balik, & Ehrenfeld, 2004). Concept mapping can be used by all levels of students and in a variety of clinical settings. It is a tool that is very responsive to situations in which patients have multiple health problems (King & Shell, 2002). Legal and ethical issues, as well as those pertaining to leadership and management, may be analyzed and synthesized via concept mapping (King & Shell, 2002). A medical diagnosis or the reason for seeking care can be used as the initial starting point (King & Shell, 2002; Harpaz et al., 2004), as can a nursing diagnosis (Schuster, 2000), or a psychosocial concept such as pain or coping mechanisms (Baugh & Mellott, 1998). The components of the nursing process may be used as organizational features (Mueller et al., 2001).

Used for clinical nursing education, concept maps are usually prepared by students prior to their clinical experience, drawn from relevant assessment data and applicable literature (All et al., 2003). Students bring their maps to the clinical setting, where they may be shared with faculty, and revise them over the course of the experience. Concept maps may provide fodder for clinical questioning (Schuster, 2000; Mueller et al., 2001; King & Shell, 2002), as described in Chapter 13. They are then typically submitted to faculty, who are able to provide further feedback on the students' grasp of concepts and their relationships. Knowledge gaps and misinterpretations can be identified and explored (King & Shell, 2002; All et al., 2003). It has been reported that the time involved in preparation and revision by students and that expended in faculty evaluation declines over the course of the term (Schuster, 2000). This is most likely a reflection of the development of expertise by both students and faculty.

If this approach to clinical preparation is to be successful, students must be taught what concept mapping is, how to create them, and their potential value to them in learning. This may be integrated into the curriculum as part of a class for broad usage by students (Mueller et al., 2001) or presented by faculty in the context of a clinical course during a seminar or clinical conference at the beginning of the course. Computer programs are available to facilitate learning mapping techniques for both faculty and students (All et al., 2003). *Mosby's Nursing Concept Map Creator* (Giddens & Kennedy, 2005) is one such tool. It could be required for students in their first clinical course, and then used throughout the program. As with the use of nursing care plans, it would probably be ideal if all faculty teaching a given clinical course used concept mapping, but this is certainly not a requirement. One approach to teaching concept mapping is to create a generic one with student participation to introduce the process and terminology, using a nonnursing scenario such as a vacation trip (Mueller et al., 2001). Following this, a case study can be used with the group to demonstrate the application to a nursing context. For example, with beginning students, a concept such as infection could be used. The related assessment data, physiologic effects, dependent and independent nursing interventions, and evaluation would form the conceptual relationships. Next, students could be provided with a case study, working alone or in pairs, to design a concept map. Group discussion would follow this, allowing further refinement of the method.

From a faculty perspective, there are some concerns regarding the use of concept mapping that must be considered prior to initiating their use in a clinical course. Faculty feedback on students' clinical concept maps is essential to facilitate maximal learning. Initially, this process will be time consuming, so faculty should incorporate this as part of their time management plan for the term. Feedback also can be complicated by the fact that students will differ in the organization of their concept maps. Connections can be made in a variety of ways (Mueller et al., 2001), reflecting the uniqueness of students' thinking processes. Individuals are believed to attain their distinctive mental structure of conceptual organization over the course of many years; an atmosphere that recognizes and values varied ways of ordering and grouping concepts is essential (All et al., 2003). Such an approach moves both faculty and students away from the trap of the "one right answer" mentality, but may require increased faculty efforts to attain clarity of students' intent. Concept mapping uses a visual spatial methodology to guide students' attainment, association, and display of information (All, Huycke, & Fisher, 2003), and for students whose preferred learning style is not visual or who are linear thinkers, this strategy may be difficult to master (Mueller, Johnston, & Bligh, 2001). It might be best to provide students with options for their clinical preparation (Emerson & Groth, 1996), making concept mapping one of the potential choices, while accepting different styles of concept mapping. Nurse educators have yet to create an ideal learning tool for students in the clinical setting. Tools are only as valuable and effective as they are presented and used in the clinical area by faculty and students, and as such possess unique strengths and limitations. Sample concept maps are provided in the "Clinical Toolbox" (see Chapter 20, pp. 366-367).

WRITTEN ASSIGNMENTS FOR STUDENT SELF-EVALUATION

The active role students play in their own learning and the role of faculty facilitation in the learning process are key aspects of cognitive learning theories, and all of the educational frameworks and pedagogies that evolved from existential philosophy. In order for these functions to be fulfilled, dialogue between faculty and students is essential. In addition to the interactions occurring during the clinical experience itself (Chapter 13), some sort of communication regarding overall progress should occur on a routine, usually weekly, basis. Formative and summative student evaluation are addressed in more detail in Unit V; here, the formats alone are mentioned briefly as a part of the total writing expectations for students in clinical courses.

Student Self-Evaluation Forms

Completed by students on a routine basis, usually weekly, and submitted to faculty for feedback, self-evaluation forms add another expectation for student writing. Faculty use this approach primarily to help both students and faculty "stay on the same page" in their interpretation of how students are progressing in the course. Faculty also often find such a tool to be beneficial in identifying what students have accomplished that may otherwise have been overlooked during busy clinical days or when students are not under direct faculty observation.

A variety of formats are used, depending on the course and faculty preference. Often, using the course objectives as a guide, students address how they felt when they met expectations, identify their strengths and limitations, and establish learning goals for the next clinical experience. Faculty then provide their interpretations, and the form is returned to the students.

Open dialogue between students and faculty regarding progress in clinical courses is essential, and such a tool can meet this need, but faculty may find other venues more effective. Brief weekly face-to-face exchanges may be better, or self-evaluation may be a component of student reflective journaling.

Journaling for Reflection

As previously discussed (Chapter 11), journaling is an extremely effective heuristic for the development of critical thinking skills and clinical judgment. Self-evaluation is integral to this process. Through the journaling medium, students can dialogue with faculty regarding their clinical performance, addressing how goals were met, identifying strengths and limitations, and exploring future learning goals. Self-evaluations can become rote; journaling helps students develop maturity in their self-analyses and in the analysis of their environments (Diekelmann, 2003). The mentoring role faculty play in the journaling dialogue with students enhances the individualized guidance that is unique to the clinical practica. Reflective journaling has an important role in helping students find the meaning of their experiences while growing as critical thinkers (Bilinski, 2002; Blake, 2005). As always, the method by which journaling is implemented by the faculty is vital to its ultimate success (Yonge & Myrick, 2005). The self-evaluative function of reflective journaling is an important aspect in the development of critical thinking. Chapter 11 provides detailed guidance in this process.

■ WRITTEN ASSIGNMENTS TO MEET OTHER LEARNING GOALS

Once needs are met for students' written clinical preparation and self-evaluation, faculty must carefully consider whether additional writing assignments should be incorporated into their clinical courses. It may be that verbal communication skills can be developed while these learning goals are being met, and student presentations, debates and discussions, nursing rounds, and other activities presented in Chapter 14 would be more appropriate than papers. Or, alternatively, reflective journaling assignments could incorporate these topics more efficiently and effectively. The decision to add a formal paper as a writing assignment in a clinical course must be cautiously and judiciously appraised in light of other written assignments and course expectations.

Integration of Research

Clinical courses often have objectives related to the incorporation of research at some level, depending on the anticipated degree. This focus on evidence-based nursing practice is yet another reflection of the philosophic and intellectual shift away from behaviorism. Helping beginning nursing students see and understand the role of research in clinical nursing practice is an important educational outcome (Brock & Butts, 1998). In the clinical arena, the prominence of evidence-based practice is escalating; the educational obligation then is to graduate novice nurses who are, at minimum, capable of appreciating its importance (Callister, Matsumura, Lookinland, Mangum, & Loucks, 2005).

Incorporation of research occurs most often in some form of written assignment or in discussions and presentations during clinical conferences. As a written assignment, research may be integrated as part of a formal paper addressing the application of theory (see below), or less formally submitted as a weekly research article critique, or the identification and exploration of a clinical problem in a brief paper or in the student's reflective journal. This is an important topic, and clinical practice courses are the best location for the identification of nursing's "sacred cows" and to demonstrate the value and application of research-based practice (Callister et al., 2005). But both faculty and student time much be considered; a scholarly paper required in a clinical course may not be the most efficient method of exploring the role of research in clinical practice. Whatever methods are chosen, faculty must select strategies that are appropriate to the educational level of the students.

Critical Incidents/Challenging Exemplars

Examining critical incidents is an excellent method for the facilitation of critical thinking, and one that students seem to especially enjoy. In addition to helping students cope with the stresses of intense practice situations and build their critical thinking skills, discussing critical incidents in writing can assist in the development of abilities that will enhance future practice and coping skills (Craft, 2005). Challenging exemplars provide an opportunity for students to critically examine their decision-making processes and explore their learning in terms of their future practice (Tanner, 1998). Such an approach is active, contextual, and all about the evolution of individual meaning. This can be done in reflective journaling or as a formal paper allowing the evaluation of scholarly writing skills and the incorporation of relevant theory. Basic elements to the exploration of critical incidents are the setting, time, persons involved, descriptions of physical and emotional responses, themes and meaning, and actions taken (Craft, 2005). As the student shifts from the point of view of participant to that of narrator, new insights and meanings evolve (Craft, 2005). The "Clinical Toolbox" (see Chapter 20, p. 354) provides Gordon and Benner's (1984) guidelines for recording critical incidents that could be used as the basis for both approaches, as well as a sample formal paper format. Critical incidents are intensely personal and subjective experiences, and the decision to treat their examination as graded assignments may put students in the position of writing for the faculty rather than for their own enrichment and enlightenment. For this reason, dealing with critical incidents through reflective journaling, or as one potential writing topic among a selection of others, may be most beneficial (Craft, 2005).

Theory Application

Writing assignments can be used as a means for incorporating a wide variety of relevant theories into clinical practice. Ethical conundrums, leadership and management topics such as conflict and power, exploration of diseases and treatments, topics such as pain management and the effects of immobility are all appropriate for theoretical application in a formal written assignment. Students can identify "microthemes" or schemas from their clinical practice (e.g., physiologic patterns, social situations, psychologic commonalities) and explore relevant theory (Youngblood & Beitz, 2001). Since these are all quite general topics, and therefore potentially interchangeable between students and even courses, every effort should be made to contextually ground the subject matter in specific student experiences associated with the given clinical course. After observing peers or practicing nurses, students might write brief reaction papers, critiquing what they observed (Youngblood & Beitz, 2001). Or students in a community health clinical course might attend a town meeting or city council meeting, then write a paper about the experience incorporating relevant theory. Something similar could be done by students in a pediatric rotation following a day spent in an outpatient clinic or observing developmental testing or by students enrolled in a psychiatric nursing clinical course after observing group meetings. The key factor is the incorporation of relevant theory at an analytical level within the actual clinical context.

Creative Writing

There are many options for assignments that allow students to develop their abilities to express themselves in writing that are less conventional, tapping into ways of knowing that are highly individual. Perhaps as alternatives among other options, students might write letters to the editor or editorials, compose poetry, even create crossword and anagram puzzles. Like all other written assignments, the decision to add creative writing assignments must be weighed against other course demands on the students.

▉ STUDENT WRITING PORTFOLIOS

Many disciplines are now using student portfolios as a means of presenting the body of work generated during the educational experience. These portfolios may be used to provide a longitudinal assessment of academic growth or be viewed as a reflection of the skills and abilities of the individual graduate for employment or educational advancement (Billings & Kowalski, 2005). In nursing education, such portfolios typically include a compilation or representation of written work generated by a student, documentation of skills evaluated during the program, documentation of special honors or certifications (e.g., Advanced Cardiac Life Support), letters of support and reference, and a resume, all organized in a dossier either in written form or electronically. Since such portfolios are increasingly being used in clinical practice as a resourceful and valuable method for recording learning experiences and outcomes reflecting competency attainment (Billings & Kowalski, 2005), beginning the process while in school seems a logical initiation to professional development.

SUMMARY

Written assignments in clinical courses vary considerably based on the setting and population served, the goals of the course, the specific point in the program, and the overall curriculum. Faculty should carefully evaluate the need and potential value of any written assignment within the comprehensive course expectations. At all costs, busy work should be shunned; the purpose of the assignments should be clear to students and faculty alike. And any written work students prepare deserves meaningful faculty feedback to achieve full educational value.

REFLECTION EXERCISE 15

Thinking About Written Assignments

Consider Bevis's "scholarly modalities" listed on p. 220 and the potential sources of written assignments discussed in this chapter in light of the clinical course you are teaching, or will be likely to teach.

◆ As appropriate to the course expectations/outcomes/objectives, what applicable assignments could be used to assist students in their utilization and development of these modes?

◆ Within the confines of the course, are written assignments the best method of addressing them? Would some group activity (Chapter 14) or some clinical experience (Chapter 13) be better?

◆ What assumptions underlie your determination of "best" and "better" in the previous question? Does this reflection provide you with new insights or clarify how you view your role as a clinical faculty member?

References

All, A.C., Huycke, L.I., & Fisher, M.J. (2003). Instructional tools for nursing education: Concept maps. *Nursing Education Perspectives, 24*(6), 311-317.

American Psychological Association (APA). (2001). *Publication manual of the American Psychological Association* (5th ed.). Washington, DC: APA.

Aoki, N. (2004). Harshness of red marks has students seeing purple. Retrieved September 2, 2004, from http://www.Boston.com/News/Education/K-12/articles/2004/08/23/harshness_of_red_marks.

Barnum, B.S. (1999). *Teaching nursing in the era of managed care.* New York: Springer.

Baugh, N.G., & Mellott, K.F. (1998). Clinical concept mapping as preparation for student nurses' clinical experiences. *Journal of Nursing Education, 37*(6), 253-256.

Bevis, E.M. (1989). Teaching and learning: A practical commentary. In E.M. Bevis & J. Watson (Eds.). *Toward a caring curriculum: A new pedagogy for nursing* (pp. 217-259). New York: National League for Nursing.

Bilinski, H. (2002). The mentored journal. *Nurse Educator, 27*(1), 37-41.

Billings, D., & Kowalski, K. (2005). Teaching tips: Learning portfolios. *The Journal of Continuing Education in Nursing, 36*(4), 149-150.

Blake, T.K. (2005). Journaling: An active learning technique. *International Journal of Nursing Education Scholarship*. Retrieved September 12, 2005, from http://www.bepress.com/ijnes/vol2/iss1/art7.

Brock, A., & Butts, J.B. (1998). On target: A model to teach baccalaureate nursing students to apply critical thinking. *Nursing Forum, 33*(3), 5-10.

Callister, L.C., Matsumura, G., Lookinland, S., Mangum, S., & Loucks, C. (2005). Inquiry in baccalaureate nursing education: Fostering evidence-based practice. *Journal of Nursing Education, 44*(2), 59-64.

Craft, M. (2005). Reflective writing and nursing education. *Journal of Nursing Education, 44*(2), 53-57.

Diekelmann, N. (2003). Thing-in-action journals: From self-evaluation to multiperspectival thinking. *Journal of Nursing Education, 42*(11), 482-484.

Emerson, R.J. & Groth, K. (1996). The verbal connection: Effective clinical teaching maximizing student communication skills. *The Journal of Nursing Education, 35*(6), 275-277.

Gibaldi, J. (2003). *MLA handbook for writers of research papers* (6th ed.). New York: Modern Language Association.

Giddens J.F., & Kennedy, E. (2005). *Mosby's nursing concept map creator*. St. Louis: Mosby.

Gordon, D.R., & Benner, P. (1984). Guideline for recording critical incidents. In P. Benner, *From novice to expert* (pp. 300-302). Menlo Park, CA: Addison-Wesley.

Harpaz, I., Balik, C., & Ehrenfeld, M. (2004). Concept mapping: An educational strategy for advancing nursing education. *Nursing Forum, 39*(2), 27-30, 36.

King, M., & Shell, R. (2002). Teaching and evaluating critical thinking with concept maps. *Nurse Educator, 27*(5), 214-216.

Koehler, C.J. (2001). Nursing process mapping replaces nursing care plans. In A.J. Lowenstein & M.J. Bradshaw (Eds.), *Fuzzard's innovative teaching strategies in nursing* (3rd ed.) (pp. 303-313.). Gaithersburg, MD: Aspen.

Mann, A.S. (2004). Eleven tips for the new college teacher. *Journal of Nursing Education, 43*(9), 389-390.

Mueller, A., Johnston, M., & Bligh, D. (2001). Mind-mapped care plans: A remarkable alternative to traditional nursing care plans. *Nurse Educator, 26*(2), 75-80.

Purdue University Online Writing Lab (2004). Writing across the curriculum and writing in the disciplines. Retrieved February 9, 2005, from http://owl.english.purdue.edu/handouts/WAC/.

Questia Media America, Inc. (2004). Writing across the curriculum. Retrieved February 9, 2005, from http://www.questia.com/popularSearches/writing_across_the_curriculum.jsp.

Sabin, WA (2004). *The Gregg Reference Manual*, (10th ed.). Columbus, OH: McGraw-Hill.

Schuster, P.M. (2000). Concept mapping: Reducing clinical care plan paperwork and increasing learning. *Nurse Educator, 25*(2), 76-81.

Smith, B., & Johnston, Y. (2002). Using structured clinical preparation to stimulate reflection and foster critical thinking. *Journal of Nursing Education, 41*(4), 182-185.

Staib, S. (2003). Teaching and measuring critical thinking. *Journal of Nursing Education, 42*(11), 498-508.

Strunk, W., & White, E.B. (2000). *The elements of style*, (4th ed.). New York: Longman.

Tanner, C.A. (1998). Lessons on learning. *Journal of Nursing Education, 37*(5), 195-196.

Tanner, C.A. (2000). Critical thinking: Beyond nursing process. *Journal of Nursing Education, 39*(8), 338-339.

University of Missouri. (1996). Writing Across the Curriculum. Retrieved February 9, 2005, from http://www.umsl.edu/~klein/WAC_links.html.

Walthew, P.J. (2004). Conceptions of critical thinking held by nurse educators. *Journal of Nursing Education, 43*(9), 408-411.

Welk, D.E. (2001). Teaching students a pattern of reversals eases the care plan process. *Nurse Educator, 26*(1), 43-45.

Westburg, J., & Jason, H. (2001). Fostering reflection and providing feedback: Helping others learn from experience. New York: Springer.

Yonge, O., & Myrick, F. (2005). Shadows and corners: The other side of journaling. *Annual Review of Nursing Education, 3*, 331-341.

Youngblood, N., & Beitz, J.M. (2001). Developing critical thinking with active learning strategies. *Nurse Educator, 26*(1), 39-42.

CHAPTER 16

Challenging Student Situations

- EMOTIONAL OUTBURSTS: ANGER AND TEARS
- UNPREPARED STUDENTS
- RETURNING STUDENTS
- WHEN ENGLISH IS A SECOND LANGUAGE
- STUDENTS WITH A DISABILITY
- UNSATISFACTORY CLINICAL PERFORMANCE
- SUMMARY
- *REFLECTION EXERCISE 16: EXPLORING SOME ASSUMPTIONS ABOUT CHALLENGING SITUATIONS*

As a novice faculty member teaching a clinical course, new and challenging situations initially seem to arise on a daily basis. Some are more trying than others, but most can be addressed relatively easily. The tardy student, the one with bad breath, the one who ducks learning opportunities, or the one who clings like a limpet can be managed with tact and consistency. Some difficulties are related to the clinical site and require variable amounts of time and finesse to resolve them. Many of the suggestions made in Chapter 9, if continued throughout the term, will act as prophylactic interventions for agency problems. But the situations faculty find the most challenging usually involve the students themselves. Knowing the policies and procedures of the agency and academic institution and the norms for clinical courses in advance of the first day will provide a degree of security in the actions taken. But the more emotionally charged or protracted circumstances exact a toll from even the most experienced faculty. In these instances, collegial support is invaluable. Colleagues can offer additional insights and perspectives, proffer suggestions for approaches, and provide comfort subsequent to emotionally draining or time-consuming decisions and interventions. These are the types of challenging situations presented in this chapter—those that require time and energy and are often affectively highly charged.

EMOTIONAL OUTBURSTS: ANGER AND TEARS

At some point or another, every faculty member experiences a situation in which a student displays inappropriate anger behaviors or bursts into tears. In both cases, faculty may be caught unaware, but may see warning indicators in retrospect. There are reasons for these losses of composure. Certain faculty interventions will decrease the likelihood they will occur; others will help faculty deal with them when they do.

People respond differently to stressful situations, and students that are angry may cry (Mezeske, 2003); act out with verbal abuse, threats, or other disrespectful and inappropriate behavior; demonstrate covert passive-aggressive behaviors; or internalize and deliberate on their anger without demonstrable behavior (Lashley & deMeneses, 2001). The five most common reasons for students' anger are (1) feelings of faculty partiality, stringency, or discrimination, (2) expectations that are perceived as out of proportion, (3) feeling their faculty are being excessively critical, (4) unanticipated changes in course assignments or deadlines or in administrative matters such as scheduling or fees, and (5) unsettled family matters (Thomas, 2003).

Clearly, there are actions faculty and administrators can take to address these etiological factors. From the faculty perspective, this includes identifying course expectations and policies at the start of the term. Feedback and evaluation problems are reduced by being consistent and fair in evaluation, providing students with clear feedback in terms of areas of strength and how they can improve, and being cognizant of any possible partiality. Being alert to students' behaviors that might indicate rising levels of frustration or dramatic changes in demeanor is also important. Administrators should endeavor to provide notification well in advance of changes that impact students and present reasonable options if at all possible. Nursing programs also should provide access to counseling services for students and have clear expectations for student conduct that are supported by the administration, which will dissipate concerns of legal reprisals when enforcement of rules of conduct is necessary (Thomas, 2003).

If at all possible, when an angry outburst occurs in the clinical setting, discussion between the student and faculty member should be conducted privately and should be postponed until a later time if possible (Thomas, 2003). If the situation is so explosive and involves so much enmity that a discussion cannot be deferred, then a private space needs to be located and adequate time allocated to deal with it. This is very hard to do during a busy day in a clinical agency, and it is perfectly appropriate to share with students that you want to give the time and attention their concerns merit, and so would prefer to wait at least until the end of the day. Ask if this is acceptable, being sure to convey that this situation is seen as a priority. If the student agrees, determine a time and place, then suggest a break to allow the student an opportunity to establish equanimity before returning to patient care. If this is not acceptable or possible, faculty should create the time to address the situation immediately; giving the student what could be perceived as a brush off could have serious ramifications.

When meeting with the student, it is most important to listen assiduously without interrupting or trying to justify or defend the faculty or administrative actions or positions (Thomas, 2003). Endeavor to gain the student's perspective and then validate what was heard by paraphrasing. Remain calm, use a soft tone of voice, and empathize with the frustration that is so often at the heart of anger. Maintaining the focus on the problem at hand, acknowledge the validity of complaints when it exists, and offer options if possible to address the feeling of powerlessness students often find contributes to their anger (Thomas, 2003).

It is entirely possible that this experience may prove to be a meaningful learning moment for the student (Mezeske, 2003).

Verbal abuse is unacceptable, so establish the ground rule of mutual respect from the outset; if the student is unable to regain control, the meeting should be terminated and another appointment arranged (Thomas, 2003). Under these circumstances, inform a faculty supervisor or administrator of the situation, and consider bringing in another person to mediate and assist with the subsequent discussion. It is important to be familiar with the nursing program's policies; rather than initiating a mediation session, some other intervention such as counseling or even suspension may be required.

Belying the pastoral outward appearance, academia is a societal microcosm and the potential for violence in academic settings is real (Facts and Figures, 2000; Langford, 2004). Cultural misconceptions of anger as an inherent proclivity, an uncontrollable response, or a cathartic release of pent-up emotional pressure have lead to a societal desensitization to aggressive behaviors (Thomas, 2003). As nursing faculty, we care deeply about our students. At the same time, we have not only the right but also the obligation to protect ourselves, our colleagues, and other students from violent behavior. And, in anticipation of students' entry into the profession, we are obliged to take action to ultimately protect the public.

Although students' tears may be an angry response to something faculty may have done or said, other potential reasons for crying are common (Mezeske, 2003). For many students, attending college is their first significant move toward independence from their family support systems. Adjustments are profound under these circumstances, and students may easily feel overwhelmed. Many students work long hours outside of school to fund their education and/or support families. Some are single parents or are trying to cope with aging parents, disabled family members, or spouses who are unemployed. Even when students are immersed only in the demands of school, life goes on. Cars break down, family members become ill or die, separation and divorce occur, and the content of nursing courses can unearth in students emotional histories related to abuse or other violent episodes. The demanding requirements of nursing programs may be unanticipated, and students' unrealistic expectations for their own performance may crash head on with their less than stellar outcomes. Grades are a major source of anxiety, especially as students try to cope with financial aid requirements and define career goals for further education. Student life is notorious for evoking poor sleeping, eating, and exercise patterns. Identifying the cause for a student's loss of composure is an essential aspect of faculty intervention (Mezeske, 2003).

It is important that the student has a private place in which to regain self-control and talk out the problem. Next, faculty should again listen in such a way that attention and concern for the student are tangible, paraphrasing and endeavoring to clarify the problem as needed (Mezeske, 2003). It may be that the student's perception of the problem is based on inaccurate information, so rectifying that may resolve the issue. Helping the student see the matter from a more realistic and accurate perspective can be helpful, but it is always best to guide students' thinking rather than offer solutions, thereby "fixing" the situation for them. The student may not be aware of pertinent resources that are available, such as an emergency fund available through the school, counseling services, mentoring programs, or student organizations.

After regaining composure, the student is likely to feel embarrassment. The student may be visibly uncomfortable, so it is important for faculty to make an effort to reequilibrate the relationship. Acknowledge the discomfort at the moment and offer the student the opportunity to follow-up on the discussion later. At the time of the next interaction, treat the student no differently in public, but find a private moment to inquire if things are better (Mezeske, 2003).

Faculty teaching clinical courses are often closer to their students on an emotional level than are their classroom counterparts. If students sense this connection with faculty, it is easier for them to lower their emotional guards, even knowing they are exposing their vulnerability. By modeling the caring practices of nursing, being genuine and facilitative, we can encourage effective problem solving and assist our students through these challenging experiences.

UNPREPARED STUDENTS

From the first meeting with the students, when faculty discuss the course expectations, the students' ethical and legal obligations to come to the clinical site prepared for the reasonably expected activities should be established. Within this expectation, there are two addendums: (1) unanticipated incidents will occur and (2) there are consequences for not being prepared for the anticipated ones.

Learning opportunities spontaneously arise during the students' clinical time, and the students' role in these learning moments will vary, as discussed in detail in Chapter 13. In some cases, faculty will determine it is best for the student to be a passive observer, whereas in others it may be acceptable for the student to assist in some way. It may be possible for the student to do some preparation at the time and then be guided through the experience by faculty, preceptors, or staff. It is important to bear in mind that in most cases, the more actively involved the student can safely and appropriately be, the more actual learning will occur. Whether to allow this involvement is a judgment call that is affected by innumerable variables. Ultimately, faculty must determine how best to manage each learning moment individually.

The consequences for lack of preparation for anticipated patient care also must be appropriate to the situation. For instance, if a student does not know about a prn medication that has been previously ordered, the student may be given the time to look up the drug and then give it, or the administration responsibility may have to be directed to agency personnel. How the faculty member then addresses this illustrative incident is affected by many variables such as the level of the student, the point in the term, the urgency for administering the drug, whether lack of preparation has occurred previously, or whether a pattern of unsafe performance is emerging.

The student may have to leave the clinical setting for a time to prepare or even be sent home or to the learning resources center for part or all of the day. Totally removing the student from the clinical site for the day is certainly an option, but one that should be rarely exercised. It is definitely perceived by the student as punitive, and little real learning will occur if the student is not present in the agency and meaningful alternatives are not available. The seriousness of the situation can be communicated in other ways. The day's assignment may need to be modified, or the student may be partnered with a peer or staff member. Faculty may have to explore the specific circumstances at a later time. The student may be given a formal notification of unsatisfactory performance for the day, which may put the successful passing of the course in jeopardy.

Faculty should take the time to thoroughly assess any occasion on which a student is unprepared for the clinical experience and endeavor to identify the underlying problem. The issue may be a blatant disregard of adequate preparation or a lack of knowledge and/or understanding. The student may have been too ill to adequately prepare in advance or had some other family emergency arise. Interactions with the student should be caring and respectful, while clearly communicating the unacceptability of the behavior.

▨ RETURNING STUDENTS

Eventually, all faculty will have a student in their clinical course who previously failed and is repeating the course or is returning after having withdrawn for any number of reasons. The decision to permit students to repeat a course or reenroll in a nursing program is usually made following a strict organizational protocol involving both administrative and faculty oversight. Much of this process is legally mandated and designed to protect the rights of the student as well as those of the academic institution (see Unit II). The point here is that the circumstances have been carefully considered, and the decision has been made to allow the student to retake the course; clinical faculty must operate from this stance, doing everything possible to facilitate a successful outcome.

Many times, faculty do not know that a particular student is returning to the program or repeating a course, so they are unaware of any of the circumstances. Sometimes this information can be elicited by a broad question included on the information sheet faculty may have students fill out at their first meeting (see Chapter 10), or the student may ask to meet with faculty privately to discuss the particular circumstances. Certainly there is an advantage to this, because the insight faculty gain can be used to assist the student throughout the term. However, the antithesis is also possible; faculty may find their perceptions of the student's performance are colored by knowing the reasons for the failure or withdrawal. Probably no single right answer to this dilemma is right; rather the key lies in the relationship between the faculty member and student.

Faculty assume the primary responsibility for creating a facilitative learning environment and engendering a potential relationship with students characterized by openness and trust. This effort will be successful when students reciprocate and a relationship evolves in which both parties respect one another and participate in the learning experience with mutuality. Consistent with this spirit of communal caring, students are more likely to share significant aspects of their educational history, and faculty are more likely to be able to treat this information appropriately to the benefit of the student.

WHEN ENGLISH IS A SECOND LANGUAGE

In recognition of and response to the increasingly multicultural population in the United States, nursing programs have added cultural content to curricula, sought faculty with advanced preparation in transcultural nursing theories, and admitted applicants from diverse ethnic and cultural groups (Klisch, 2000; Etowa, Foster, Vukic, Wittstock, & Youden, 2005). In today's global society, nursing programs increasingly find their environments enriched by the diversity of students from other countries. Wherever an academic institution is located, having students from other countries facilitates heterogeneity in world perspectives, the arts, and cultural norms. Along with all of these benefits, these students also bring educational challenges to nursing programs, particularly in the areas of language, culture, and academic expectations (Pardue & Haas, 2003).

Generically labeled as students for whom English is a second language (ESL), English may actually be one of several languages these students have mastered at some level. Some evaluation of their English reading, writing, and speaking abilities is done, often voluntarily, prior to or following admission to the academic program. The challenge of learning the language of medicine and nursing, which all students face, is compounded for ESL students by the fact that their written and verbal fluency in English often is not as advanced as their skill level in the language of their country of origin. Obviously, these students embody a wide range of linguistic abilities, often reading more easily than speaking or writing, and in some cases still mentally translating between languages. Additionally, the academic challenges associated with ESL students' communication difficulties may be compounded by the expectation of conformity with very different cultural norms. These students often find things such as the differences in their relationships with faculty, that is, being encouraged to assertively ask questions and seek clarification and forcefully challenge information and assumptions, to be troublesome. In the clinical setting, asking intimate questions of patients and attending to their personal care, being exposed to family dynamics that are different from their own home culture, and encountering different beliefs about role obligations, illness, and death can all pose difficulties for ESL students.

Implications for the recruitment and retention of ESL students and for curricular and pedagogical alterations in nursing programs' classrooms are being explored increasingly in the literature (Klisch, 2000; Pardue & Haas, 2003; Richardson, 2005). The availability of international faculty and/or student role models and support services for language and cultural immersion will benefit nursing students in their clinical courses. But the clinical setting is unique, and what is lacking in the literature is sufficient discussion related to facilitating ESL students' success in their clinical courses.

BOX 16-1

Suggestions for Working with ESL Students in Clinical Courses

- Allow time during group orientation for ESL students to share their backgrounds.
- Keep clinical groups smaller when composition includes ESL students.
- Consider placing two ESL students in a clinical group to provide mutual support.
- Be aware of institutional supports available (tutors, library and writing assistance, etc.).
- Solicit life experience and nursing practice objectives from them.
- Assess individual needs related to language and cultural adjustment.
- Have all students in the group initially prepare clinical documentation for faculty review, providing assistance to any who may require it.
- Assess cultural biases regarding touch, eye contact, intimate personal care, interactions with the opposite gender and authority figures (teachers, doctors).
- Ask questions ("What questions do you have about ...?") or request students provide explanations to assess comprehension.
- Encourage the use of reflective journaling as an interaction modality with faculty and means of increasing self-awareness.

Each situation will be a bit different, but some general suggestions for faculty who are teaching clinical courses with ESL students are provided in Box 16-1. Having ESL students in a clinical group adds a richness and complexity. If possible there should be only one or two ESL students in each clinical group, and depending on their overall skill level, the total number of students in the group may need to be decreased to allow faculty to devote additional time and attention to the ESL students without depriving the other students in the group. Two ESL students of the same ethnicity in the group can provide an inherent support system for them. All students, regardless of ethnicity, tend to create subgroups; avoid criticizing ESL students for doing so any more than you would any other students for the same behaviors.

Information about organizational resources for both faculty and ESL students is usually available in faculty handbooks. When everyone shares background information during the initial orientation to the course, faculty need to encourage ESL students to participate; this provides experiential information as well as an opportunity for an initial spoken/written language assessment. All faculty should make the effort to learn elements of the cultural circumstances of their ESL students in order to know best how to expedite their learning (Klisch, 2000). Faculty need to know how to appropriately interact with ESL students in recognition of their cultural norms, while helping them learn to interact in accordance with the dominant cultural norms when providing patient care.

To help students improve their English writing skills and conform to the documentation requirements of the clinical setting, faculty often need to continue to review students' notes prior to those notes being entered into records beyond the time when other students have mastered these skills. Due to cultural differences, ESL students are often extremely hesitant to ask questions or request clarification from authority figures such as teachers. Routinely encouraging their questions both assesses their understanding and allows them to see that questioning is expected and encouraged. They also may be uncomfortable with faculty-initiated queries (see Chapter 13). Faculty may choose a variation of this approach, and ask students to explain something in return that has been discussed previously—a sort of verbal return demonstration. As time passes, they usually become increasingly comfortable with clinical queries. Reflective journaling provides ESL students with practice communicating their thoughts in writing, and as with other students, increases self-awareness and dialogue with faculty. It is necessary that faculty plan for the additional time that working with ESL students typically requires, in the clinical setting and often in additional meetings. Although teaching ESL students demands extra faculty time, attention and persistence; the experience is a rewarding one (Klisch, 2000; Pardue & Haas, 2003).

▇ STUDENTS WITH A DISABILITY

Increasing numbers of men and women with a variety of disabilities are choosing to enter programs of nursing. These students are taking advantage of Titles II and III of the Americans with Disabilities Act of 1990, which requires "reasonable accommodations" for students in public and private postsecondary institutions who self-identify as having a disability (Frank & Halstead, 2005; U.S. Equal Employment Opportunity Commission, 1997). These students have diagnosed learning disabilities, physical disabilities (visual, auditory, and mobility issues), chronic illnesses (physical and mental), or chemical dependency problems, and have followed the law by notifying their institutions and requesting accommodations. Accommodations can be designed only if this is done and approval is obtained. At the beginning of the term, faculty need to announce the policy regarding disabilities. In order to obtain reasonable accommodations, students with disabilities must self-identify (Selekman, 2002). The office of disability services at the institution, together with the students and faculty, will then explore what arrangements can be made in both the classroom and clinical settings to provide the reasonable accommodations that will allow the students to pursue their career choice. Clinical faculty are not expected to have expertise in disability accommodations, but rather to understand the accommodations to be made and demonstrate a willingness to work with the students and experts to offer equal, but different, learning and performance opportunities (Sowers & Smith, 2002).

In a study conducted in 2000 and 2001, Sowers and Smith found the attitudes of nursing faculty to be a significant barrier for disabled students (2004). Discrimination still exists in the application processes as well as the openness to the provision of assistance and services that will allow these students to meet the programs' academic goals (Sowers & Smith, 2002; Carroll, 2004). Institutional standards should not be lowered, and technological advances will allow more accommodation options in the future, but only rarely will situations occur that will not be amenable to reasonable adaptations. Under those circumstances, one creative resolution is task trading between disabled and nondisabled students; this team divides the work to be done based on the strengths and limitations of the members (Carroll, 2004). Although a commonly voiced concern, no data suggest that disabled nurses or nursing students pose any greater risk to the safety of their patients than their nondisabled counterparts (Sowers & Smith, 2002; Carroll, 2004; Sowers & Smith, 2004). Practicing nurses and nursing students must be cognizant of their limitations; safety is an issue for all. As is true for those without disabilities, some individuals with disabilities are not qualified to be nurses or the profession is not a good match to their personalities and interests (Carroll, 2004; Sowers & Smith, 2004). In actuality, what is important to the practice of nursing are the characteristics that enable coming to know the patient within the nurse-patient relationship; due to their life experiences, disabled students may have developed de facto these characteristics more abundantly (Carroll, 2004).

In advance of exploring potential accommodations, nursing faculty need to examine their curricula and available educational resources. Faculty should determine the essential knowledge and skills embedded within their curricula and be open to alternative means of attaining them (Frank & Halstead, 2005). It is important to separate this set of knowledge and skills (e.g., clinical problem solving), which are behaviors and role functions related to nursing, from physical attributes such as seeing or hearing (Sowers & Smith, 2002). Once the program and course objectives appropriately address this essential set of knowledge and skills, it becomes the end-point that must be attained in order to graduate. All students are expected to reach this end-point; it is the means by which this requirement is met that is open to reasonable accommodation (Selekman, 2002). Focusing on a process-based technical standards model (essential or core competencies) emphasizes a rigid method as opposed to the end result (Carroll, 2004). In the future, nursing curricula will become more responsive to the multiplicity of roles beyond those of the traditional bedside nurse, relinquishing the narrow perspective of nursing practice as merely a compilation of technical competencies (Sowers & Smith, 2002; Carroll, 2004).

The specific accommodations made depend on the clinical site, course expectations, and the given disability. Much like working with ESL students, assisting students with disabilities is a diversity issue (Sowers & Smith, 2002). Like differences in language and culture, disabilities involve differences in communication, learning, and mobility. Such differences should not be taken to mean an inherent insufficiency or inadequacy. Indeed, like students from other countries, students with disabilities can bring a fresh point of view to patient care (Sowers & Smith, 2002). Students with a history of chemical dependency may be required to submit routine urine tests and be monitored by faculty for behavioral, personality, and physical indicators of being under the influence of drugs or alcohol. Clinical agencies may limit these students' access to controlled substances. Nursing programs should have clearly articulated policies related to the management of situations in which chemical abuse is historical as well as when it is currently suspected (Frank & Halstead, 2005). The treatment plan for chronic mental illness may employ medication and therapy, but in any case, faculty need to remain vigilant for behavioral changes that could signal poor stress management and a potential relapse. Physical and learning disabilities bring the greatest challenges to faculty teaching clinical courses. Auditory limitations may be addressed with amplified stethoscopes and vibrating pagers to communicate in the clinical setting (Frank & Halstead, 2005). Stethoscopes are even available that translate auditory stimuli into a visual readout (Sowers & Smith, 2002). Visual impairments may require alternative learning environments or partnering with a preceptor (Frank & Halstead, 2005) or clinical tutor. Alternative modes of attaining essential clinical course expectations may be found for the student with a prosthetic limb or mobility aids such as a cane or wheelchair. Institutional resources such as those of the learning resource center may prove to be especially valuable in providing alternative learning environments for some students, and multimedia learning approaches for others (Frank & Halstead, 2005).

Learning disabilities are not the province of children only. In postsecondary education, learning disabilities are the most common disability encountered and often are only then diagnosed (Selekman, 2002). Encompassing a collection of diverse neurologic disorders, the diagnosis of a learning disability is made following specific testing criteria. Learning disabilities are present in people of normal intelligence who have problems with the brain's ability to handle or understand sensory information it receives (Selekman, 2002). These individuals may have trouble accurately interpreting data coming from what they see, hear, or touch. They may have speech difficulties or problems with fine motor skills. Or their challenges may arise in how they manage or use the data that has been received (Selekman, 2002).

In nursing education, identification that a student may have an undiagnosed learning disability most often occurs when a dichotomy between clinical and classroom performance is noted (Frank & Halstead, 2005). The student may have no problem in the clinical arena, yet have great difficulty receiving, processing, and interpreting content or passing examinations in the classroom. This is due to the wide variety of ways in which learning disabilities may manifest. The literature abounds with the delineation of specific behaviors in the classroom and suggested interventions in that setting, but little specifically addresses either facet when disabilities are noted in the clinical setting. Much of what follows has been extrapolated to accommodate this environment.

In the clinical setting, students with learning disabilities may have problems with organizing and prioritizing their care and its subsequent documentation, may struggle with nonverbal or the subtler forms of verbal communication with patients and staff, or may demonstrate difficulties with number or word transpositions involving drug calculations or transcribing orders (Selekman, 2002). Achieving a passing score on a mandatory medication calculation examination may seem an insurmountable obstacle, well beyond the more typical level of math anxiety. For some students with learning disabilities, carrying out effective problem solving, from data analysis to the preparation of a comprehensive plan of action, is extraordinarily difficult (Selekman, 2002). Like the neurologic deficits that manifest after a brain attack, some students are verbally fluent but unable to communicate their thoughts clearly or legibly in writing, whereas others have verbal difficulties but can communicate in writing (Frank & Halstead, 2005). The impaired auditory processing and discrimination seen in some individuals with learning disabilities can produce a high degree of distractibility and difficulty with understanding detailed, sequential directions (Selekman, 2002). These problems potentially have a broad impact on practice, which may include the inability to differentiate abnormal from normal auscultatory assessment data, respond appropriately in an emergency situation, and accurately interpret physicians' verbal orders or faculty feedback. As with auditory problems, it is not the equipment of the eye that causes the problems with vision—the etiology is in the brain's interpretive abilities (Selekman, 2002). In the clinical setting, learning disabilities that result in altered visual receptive input may present as errors in copying information from resources or transcribing physician's orders, in the accuracy of the memory of what was read or seen, or in the meaning of symbols. Difficulties with psychomotor skill mastery can occur due to cognitive deficits and present as problems in remembering the fine points of relevant theory, the sequence of actions, or the meaning of concepts (Selekman, 2002; Frank & Halstead, 2005). Manual skill development can be impaired due to motor and expressive disabilities, presenting as poor eye-hand coordination, poor visual memory, and other perceptual deficits (Selekman, 2002). Students with expressive learning disabilities affecting their speech may stutter or have difficulty with articulation (Selekman, 2002). In practice courses, this can affect students' interactions with faculty, staff, peers, and patients. Verbal presentations or contributions in clinical conferences may be challenging for these students. Detailed patient teaching projects, interviews, collaborations with other personnel—these may all be difficult for students affected by expressive learning disabilities.

The manifestations of learning disabilities are varied, and faculty are not usually educationally prepared to properly diagnose them. A complete series of psychologic tests must be performed by qualified professionals in order to specifically define each student's capabilities and limitations (Selekman, 2002). If faculty suspect an undiagnosed learning disability is interfering with a student's education, the first step is to assist the student to recognize the problem and agree to participate in the evaluation process. This must occur before faculty can make a referral for professional evaluation. Denial and resistance are often significant barriers to progress, and it is the responsibility of faculty to act in a caring fashion to help the student see the impact this possible disability has had on day-to-day functioning in academia in a caring fashion. Faculty should refer to their handbooks or inquire directly about how referrals are managed at their institution. Certainly, not all academic difficulties are due to learning disabilities, but an evaluation will also eliminate other potential etiologies (Selekman, 2002).

Nursing faculty are also not provided with the academic preparation needed to determine how best to accommodate the needs of students with learning disabilities, so it is essential they work with the student and the campus disability services personnel to create an accommodation plan. Specific guidance can then be provided through the resultant plan (Frank & Halstead, 2005). This plan is important; it is individualized to meet the unique needs of the student, facilitating the further development of distinctive assets and offsetting limitations, while at the same time providing explicit direction for teaching and learning. Components addressing remediation and accommodation are often included in the plan (Frank & Halstead, 2005).

The details of what is expected of the student and the faculty should be incorporated into the written plan to avoid potential accusations of discrimination in a grievance action (Selekman, 2002). Typically, additional time is required to help students with learning disabilities, during and outside of the clinical course hours, and they are more closely supervised in the clinical setting (Selekman, 2002). Other students may misinterpret the supplementary time and attention as evidence of preferential treatment. The components of the plan vary with each student's assessment and needs. Box 16-2 presents some common interventions that may be appropriate, depending on the circumstances.

Both faculty member and student have an investment in the plan and an obligation to support it. The plan should include arrangements for periodic bilateral review and the potential for updating as needed. There should be a sound rationale for each intervention, grounded in the thorough assessment previously performed. For example, designing and sticking to a plan of care (e.g., time and type of assessments, treatments, teaching) helps some learning disabled students with organization and sequencing and assures thoroughness of care (Selekman, 2002). A record to help monitor and document technical skill development should be used for the entire program or each clinical course. Until a faculty member signs the student off on a technical skill, she may choose to observe every skill performed by the student (Selekman, 2002). Assignment directions should be provided in writing (Selekman, 2002); faculty should make them straightforward, refraining from using sentences that are structurally complex, such as those with double negatives (Frank & Halstead, 2005). Students should prepare written assignments with a word processor whenever possible; this allows them to take advantage of grammar and spelling features, as well as correct for legibility issues. Use of calculators in the clinical areas where medications are to be administered is no longer optional. This is especially beneficial for those students with learning disabilities related to mathematics (Selekman, 2002). Summarizing is known to help many students with learning disabilities discern essential information from that which is supportive or embellishing (Selekman, 2002); adding a closing activity that incorporates a summary at the

---

BOX 16-2
Common Aspects of a Plan for Students With Learning Disabilities

Faculty responsibilities
Plan additional time in clinical or meetings following clinical to guide the student in integrating concepts with practice.
Assist with the student's preparation of detailed, prioritized plan of care; facilitate adherence.
Review and approve documentation in advance of transposition into records.
Directly observe all skill performances until approved and documented.
Provide written directions for all assignments.
Provide a summary closure for group learning activities.
Assist in creation of course(s) schedule of activities and requirements.

Student responsibilities
Anticipate additional time will be spent in discussion and interactions with faculty.
Prepare and follow detailed, prioritized plan of care.
Prepare documentation and initially review with faculty.
Anticipate closer observation and assistance in learning skills.
Use word processor with editorial support for written assignments.
Create course(s) schedule of activities and requirements.

---

end of group learning experiences would likely be a useful intervention. Students whose learning disabilities include difficulties in processing and recovering data have been described as inflexible and having a preference for making and following schedules (Selekman, 2002). Helping them create a master schedule for the course (or all courses being taken) on a calendar can be mutually beneficial.

Selekman (2002) identified multiple benefits of incorporating students with disabilities into the nursing community. For disabled nurses, dealing with a personal disability generates even more caring and empathy in their provision of patient care. Those nurses may have enhanced some sensory skills in compensation because sensory disabilities have robbed them of others, making their assessments keener and more intuitive in some cases. As more disabled students enter nursing practice, the negative attitudes of some of the nondisabled nurses may be dispelled. As the biases of the nursing profession diminish due to experience or exposure, the care provided to the disabled will ultimately improve. There is no question that the attitudes and creativity of clinical nursing faculty will play a significant role in meeting these goals (Selekman, 2002).

■ UNSATISFACTORY CLINICAL PERFORMANCE

Chapter 8 addresses the legal and ethical aspects of the nurse educator's role related to students' unsatisfactory performance in a clinical course, including the need for valid and reliable data and the provision of due process. Here, the discussion focuses on how faculty and students can work together to deal with the deficiencies in order to, if possible, avoid a course failure.

First, consider the meaning of student failure to the academic institution, faculty, and students. With long lists of applicants waiting for acceptance, the current and projected societal need for more practicing nurses, the additional institutional costs associated with students repeating clinical courses, and the litigious nature of the American public, nursing programs may exert overt or covert pressure on faculty to expedite the success of students who are struggling to pass. Failing a course has major personal and financial consequences for students too. Being in danger of failing can bring these anxieties to life. Students worry about the impact having to repeat a course will have on their timely access to the other courses they need to graduate, what will happen to their financial aid, and the embarrassment associated with telling peers and family members of their failure. Knowing they are "not getting it," students worry about the safety of their patients, but feel intense pressure to succeed while faculty hover over them, and they may become angry and defensive or depressed and hopeless. Faculty all too often respond in kind. As physicians often experience the death of a patient as a personal failure, nurse educators report that they feel a student's inability to pass is a reflection of their inability to adequately facilitate learning—their own failure (Diekelmann & McGregor, 2003).

The entire process of nursing education is designed to assist students to learn the basics of nursing art and science prior to entering the profession, where they will continue to learn. We often seem to lose track that learning is the purpose, what with our outcomes-oriented curricula, conventional pedagogies, and competence-based evaluation tools. The fact is that the emphasis on always "doing it correctly" gives students little opportunity to make errors, which are truly a part of the learning process. It is understandable that students may feel there is only time in clinical courses for evaluation, and none for learning, and that they experience evaluation as a series of personal attacks (Diekelmann & McGregor, 2003). The obligation to protect patient safety is important, to be sure, but some mistakes can be safely made in order to further the learning process.

Learning is an incremental process, and the rate at which it occurs is impacted by many variables; individual variation is the norm. Some students progress with little direction or redirection, whereas others require more faculty time and attention. All courses have endpoints, and only a certain number of clinical hours are available. Both knowledge and skills must be attained at a specified "minimal" level prior to progression to a new course, with its own set of knowledge and skills. For some students, due to a variety of internal and external reasons, more time and attention are required to learn. Assisting students to be successful is certainly a shared value between administrators and faculty, but there must be limits to remediation; there is indeed a point in the term beyond which success cannot occur (Diekelmann & McGregor, 2003). Until that time, faculty and students need to work together within their relationship, and using the resources available to them, they must devise and invest in an approach to learning that is mutually respectful and makes the most of the students' strengths.

The student who is unsafe is most definitely failing, but there are other situations that can place a student in jeopardy of failing. Some of these, such as violations of codes of conduct, may have interventions proscribed by the institution. Other "non–safety-based" situations that can result in course failure include excessive absenteeism, not submitting assignments, or interpersonal difficulties with patients or personnel. The key to determining how best to proceed when a student's progress is unsatisfactory is in the early, accurate, and specific mutual identification of the problem. Faculty begin to assess their students from the very first meeting with them (the same can be said of the students!). Faculty watch, listen, and read the students' written work, fulfilling their role of coach by providing feedback and encouraging the students' developing self-awareness of their own thinking and practice. Large and small obstacles to the students' progress are identified and addressed, by both faculty and students.

As the term progresses, faculty may find that the student has missed the maximum number of days of clinical experience possible. Given the rate at which learning has been occurring for the student, further absenteeism raises the risk of failing due to an inability to attain the course knowledge and skills. The faculty member must then meet with the student and describe this observation, listening to the student's view of the problem and thoughts about how best to approach it. When only faculty are involved in the identification of the problem and solutions, they may make significant errors. Faculty efforts to independently fix the situation can unintentionally dishearten the student, leaving behind feelings of impotence and hopelessness (Diekelmann & McGregor, 2003). Such an approach is also clearly antithetical to current educational philosophies, frameworks, and pedagogies. These all support students' personal growth and responsibility for their learning, multiple perspectives of reality, and decreased power inequities with increased collegiality and trust between faculty and students. Conversing with the student, previously unknown information may come to light. The problem of absenteeism may be due to inadequate childcare options for an ill child. The faculty may be able to help the student identify alternatives not previously considered. Excessive absenteeism may be due to unreliable transportation; alternative transportation options such as carpooling or public transportation could then be explored. The clarified problem and plan of approach should, of course, be appropriately documented for the faculty, student, and institution.

The student who is failing due to unsafe behaviors in the clinical setting presents a moral, ethical, and nursing educational conundrum. Maintaining patient safety is a professional obligation, but providing the opportunity for the student to correct deficiencies, learn, and potentially pass a course are also faculty obligations. Institutional policies may provide some guidance, mandating certain courses of action in given situations. The first step is to schedule a meeting with the student, provide an initial description of the issues from a faculty perspective, then listen to the student's view of the problem. The faculty and student can then explore together how best to approach it. As a part of exploring options, ask students if they can think of anyone else, a peer or another faculty member, who might help them in relation to the problem. This opens the door to accessing collective wisdom and expertise of the entire educational community (Diekelmann & McGregor, 2003). Each student's response is affected to a certain degree by the quality and quantity of feedback previously provided and how faculty present the concern. If the student becomes angry, tearful, or defensive, faculty must keep cool while acknowledging feelings and endeavoring to gradually redirect the focus to the problem at hand. Stressing the faculty member's interest in the student's well-being is very important in defusing anxiety and overcoming defense mechanisms.

When student performance is unsafe, interventions depend on the problem and the individual student. Faculty should avoid unilateral and preemptive problems and plan delineation. For example, if preparation for the clinical experience is inadequate, the student may need further guidance in how to sufficiently prepare for clinical (e.g., what information to collect, how to organize and analyze it, or how to put time management skills in order). Often seeing another student going through the process properly provides the needed insight. Assigning a clinical buddy from the group to show the student how to do it or offering a clinical tutor will provide an uncertain student with a peer model. This approach also lessens the direct faculty role and may help reduce some of the student's anxiety. Some problems also can be addressed outside of the clinical setting (e.g., difficulties with medication calculation, weak analytical and synthesis skills, or inaccurate or incomplete documentation). However, the most common areas in which unsafe behaviors are observed involve patients and returning the student to the clinical setting often poses direct challenges to patient safety.

When the student returns to the clinical site with the knowledge that course failure is a possibility, the anxiety levels of both student and faculty rise exponentially, escalating the risk of error (Haskvitz & Koop, 2004). Faculty, preceptors, or staff feel the need to supervise the already anxious student closely, making thinking harder and increasing the odds that mistakes will occur (Diekelmann & McGregor, 2003). In some cases, faculty may choose to request that another colleague observe the student's clinical performance, usually to validate the assessment of unsatisfactory functioning and reduce the possibility that the assigned faculty member can be accused of bias. Increased faculty scrutiny is well intentioned; faculty truly believe they are more available to both protect the patient and assist the student. Nevertheless, from the perspective of the student, this intense scrutiny is the hovering of a bird of prey, and faculty are poised to "catch" them in a misstep and make complete course failure a reality. How much better it is if the student has had the opportunity, in advance of returning to the clinical setting, to attain a satisfactory level of proficiency and increased self-confidence! This is one of the most valuable uses of the learning resource center: remediation for students having difficulty applying their knowledge and skills in the clinical setting. Using the high-fidelity simulators currently available, the desired clinical setting can be reconstructed from both a physiologic and physical perspective (Haskvitz & Koop, 2004). Of course, the use of less sophisticated low-tech, as well as other high-tech resources can be used to create minimilieus and, combined with case scenarios, give the student a safe environment in which to build skills and confidence. Students can stop and correct their errors and repeatedly practice the experience to reach the desired level of proficiency. They become more self-assured that their acquired experience will be available to them when they return to the actual clinical setting (Haskvitz & Koop, 2004).

SUMMARY

Certain student situations can be especially challenging for faculty teaching clinical courses, especially those with limited academic teaching experience. Having some insight into how to approach and respond to some of the most common of these can provide the neophyte with increased confidence.

REFLECTION EXERCISE 16

Exploring Some Assumptions About Challenging Situations

◆ What assumptions do you have that might impact how you work with challenging student situations?

◆ How do you feel when others show emotional extremes, such as crying or angry behaviors? Are you drawn to them, or do you find yourself distancing from them? In those situations, what are your thoughts and feelings *about* the person? What, if any value judgments do you make about them?

◆ Imagine there is a student in your clinical group for whom English is a second language. What information about their cultural norms would you want to know about that would enable you to better help this student learn? If you were a patient being cared for by such a student, what concerns would you have?

People with disabilities are primarily handicapped by others' negative attitudes. Spend some time thinking about your own beliefs regarding disabilities, using the following questions to guide your thinking:

◆ Do you feel differently about people with different types of disabilities? If so, why?

◆ You are introduced to a new faculty member who is clearly blind. What are your immediate thoughts about this person's ability to fulfill the role? Pause now to explore the assumptions behind those thoughts.

◆ You arrive for work in your practice setting and find you are to precept an orientee who is deaf. What thoughts go through your head? Step back and examine your assumptions.

References

Carroll, S.M. (2004). Inclusion of people with physical disabilities in nursing education. *Journal of Nursing Education, 43*(5), 207-212.

Diekelmann, N., & McGregor, A. (2003). Students who fail clinical courses: Keeping open a future of new possibilities. *Journal of Nursing Education, 42*(10), 433-436.

Etowa, J.B., Foster, S., Vukic, A.R., Wittstock, L., & Youden, S. (2005). Recruitment and retention of minority students: Diversity in nursing education. *International Journal of Nursing Education Scholarship, 2*(1); Article 13. Retrieved August 12, 2005, from http://www.bepress.com/ijnes/vol2/iss1/art13.

Facts and figures: Crime on college campuses. (2000). *Chronicle of Higher Education*. Retrieved March 7, 2005, from http://chronicle.com/stats/crime/.

Frank, B., & Halstead, J.A. (2005). Teaching students with disabilities. In D.M. Billings & J.A. Halstead (Eds.), *Teaching in nursing: A guide for faculty* (pp. 67-84). Philadelphia: Saunders.

Haskvitz, L.M., & Koop, E.C. (2004). Students struggling in clinical? A new role for the patient simulator. *Journal of Nursing Education, 43*(4), 181-184.

Klisch, M.L. (2000). Retention strategies for ESL nursing students. *Journal of Multicultural Nursing and Health, 6*(1), 21-28.

Langford, L. (2004). Higher Education Center: Preventing violence and promoting safety in higher education settings: Overview of a comprehensive approach. Retrieved March 7, 2005, from http://www.edc.org/hec/pubs/violence.html.

Lashley, F.R., & deMeneses, M. (2001). Student civility in nursing programs: A national survey. *Journal of Professional Nursing, 17*(2), 81-86.

Mezeske, B.A. (2003). What to do when students weep. *The Teaching Professor, 17*(10), 7.

Pardue, K.T., & Haas, B. (2003). Curriculum considerations for enhancing baccalaureate learning for international students. *Journal of Continuing Education in Nursing, 34*(2), 72-79.

Richardson, V. (2005). The diverse learning needs of students. In D.M. Billings & J.A. Halstead (Eds.), *Teaching in nursing: A guide for faculty* (pp. 21-39). Philadelphia: Saunders.

Selekman, J. (2002). Nursing students with learning disabilities. *Journal of Nursing Education, 41*(8), 334-339.

Sowers, J., & Smith, M.R. (2002). Disability as difference. *Journal of Nursing Education, 41*(8), 331-332.

Sowers, J., & Smith, M.R. (2004). Nursing faculty members' perceptions, knowledge, and concerns about students with disabilities. *Journal of Nursing Education, 43*(5), 213-218.

Thomas, S.P. (2003). Handling anger in the teacher-student relationship. *Nursing Education Perspectives, 24*(1), 17-24.

U.S. Equal Employment Opportunity Commission. (1997). Facts about the Americans with disabilities act. Retrieved January 4, 2005, from http://www.eeoc.gov/facts/fs-ada.html.

Hot Topics in Clinical Nursing Education

To prepare the nurses of tomorrow, today's clinical nursing faculty are expanding the boundaries of practice settings while designing learning experiences that incorporate old and new knowledge and skills sets. Forces within the health care system and the global society have made their mark on nursing education. "Transformations taking place in nursing and nursing education have been driven by major socioeconomic factors, as well as by developments in health care delivery and professional issues unique to nursing" (Heller, Oros, & Durney-Crowley, 2004b). Students must develop enhanced leadership and management skills to respond to the managed care environment, practice skills that reflect and respect the diversity of values and beliefs associated with an increasingly multicultural society, and citizenship skills of civic and social responsibility to meet the needs of population aggregates (Heller et al., 2004b). In response to these needs, faculty are reevaluating pedagogies and clinical environments. Some topics such as ethics and end-of-life care continue to be important to clinical nursing education even as societal norms and health care technology propel them into new contexts. Other issues, such as bioterrorism, are just beginning to be addressed in nursing academic communities. This chapter explores a selection of cutting-edge issues in clinical nursing education.

▓ SKILLS FOR THE MANAGED CARE ENVIRONMENT: LEADERSHIP AND MANAGEMENT

One of the top 10 issues impacting nursing education, according to a recent National League for Nursing (NLN) publication (Heller et al., 2004b), is the high cost of health care generating the challenges of the managed care model. And this issue was seen as the direct stimulus for another: the shift from episodic/acute care to the population-based outcomes of managed care. The results of a cross-sectional survey of more than 350 nurse administrators in the southeastern United States indicate a strong belief that caseload management and supervision competencies are required of baccalaureate graduates in hospital, nursing home, and home health care settings (Utley-Smith, 2004). The results of such research and position papers have lead some authors to take the position that novice nurses from all educational levels should be prepared to work in managed care settings, including being prepared to assume the role of case manager (Barnum, 1999; Dickerson, Sackett, Jones, & Brewer, 2001; Heller et al., 2004b; Utley-Smith, 2004).

It is incumbent upon nursing education to provide theory and practice in the leadership, management, and managed care skills needed by the novice nurse. To accomplish this, nurse educators must examine their curricula, refurbishing them as needed to incorporate both the pertinent new and expanded theory in the classroom and relevant practice in the most applicable clinical settings (Utley-Smith, 2004). In some cases, treasured assumptions about nursing education will have to be reexamined (Barnum, 1999). The clash between an educational preparation for an idealized approach to patient care and the practice realities of the managed care environment echoes the historical disconnection of ivory-towered academia from service settings. "A student who expects the world to correspond with the ideal will inevitably be disappointed. If students are able to work only under ideal circumstances, they have been sadly unprepared for reality" (Barnum, 1999, p. 60).

Theoretical Grasp of Managed Care

In order to work in a health care environment under the managed care model, nursing students must have an understanding of its historical and theoretical bases. Most Americans have some awareness of the staggering fiscal implications of a health care system out of control. It was this concern for cost that served as the primary stimulus for the evolution of managed care. Certainly this model has not resolved all of the financial apprehension associated with health care, but it has slowed the cost escalation. Even so, nearly 15% of the American gross national product is allocated to health care, and more than 40 million people have no health insurance coverage (Heller et al., 2004b). The vision of the managed care environment is one in which there is taut regulation of health care providers, a conceptualization of patients as aggregate groups, and an emphasis on cost containment and increased productivity while endeavoring to preserve quality (Barnum, 1999). The organization of work to be accomplished, the design and implementation of clinical pathways, and how patients perceive and participate in their health care are all aspects of nursing practice impacted by concerns about costs (Heller et al., 2004b).

Characteristics of the managed care model mirror some of the current attitudes and values of academia (Barnum, 1999). In both settings, there is a focus on the consumer; a value system in which quality and quantity are prized; a system of decision making where group norms serve as the foundation; the multidisciplinary and collaborative aspects of a team are fostered; the orientation is on outcomes; and strategic management has replaced management by objectives (Barnum, 1999). Managed care and postsecondary education are both increasingly resource-driven as opposed to goal-driven systems, and the effective use of resources lies at the heart of the strategic plans of both institutions. In today's health care system, work is carried out over time, resources are limited, and creativity and efficiency may extend the available resources (Barnum, 1999); the same could be said of today's academic environment.

The classroom portion of students' nursing education must include the concepts of managed care (Barnum, 1999; Dickerson et al., 2001). Students need to anticipate that the patients they will care for in inpatient settings are more acutely ill than in the past, and with the extension of the life span and the aging of a large portion of the population, care is increasingly complicated by concomitant chronic diseases. Prevention and the management of chronic disease are primarily addressed in outpatient, community-based settings (Heller et al., 2004b). Students must learn managed care terminology and concepts such as "reimbursement mechanisms," "regulation" and "oversight," and "aggregates." Learning how to provide health care to these aggregates will call for students to learn about specific populations in relation to epidemiology, as well as applicable knowledge from biostatistics and the behavioral sciences (Heller et al., 2004b). Classroom active learning activities such as that described by Dickerson et al. (2001) help students move the concepts and terminology to the application level. In this approach, students were provided with a set of guidelines that were followed for the evaluation of existing clinical pathways and then used for the construction of one for a common health problem. Such activities solidify the theoretical aspects of managed care while facilitating the development of critical thinking skills. To reflect the teamwork that is required in the contemporary multidisciplinary, collaborative approach to health care, increased shared educational experiences in the classroom and in the clinical settings will be beneficial to today's nursing students (Barnum, 1999).

Practical Practice Skills for Managed Care

The impact of the need to provide this practice environment on clinical nursing education is profound. Box 17-1 offers some clinical educational approaches for the implementing managed care and supervisory theories and skills. From the onset of their education, nursing students must come to understand that the system they will practice in will place more pressure and stress on their time and attention than they will be capable of addressing unless they have the knowledge and skills that will allow them to attend to the quantity as well as the quality of their care (Barnum, 1999). To meet patient needs within the parameters of today's health care system, students must learn practice methods conducive to improved quality while at the same time being responsive to the complexity of patient care (Heller et al., 2004b). Competencies in supervision and caseload management are as essential for new graduates as are those of interpersonal communication, direct care, computer technology, and health

---

BOX 17-1
Clinical Experiences for Developing the Skills of Managed Care

- Management experiences that include planning, organizing, directing, and controlling; and resources and time management
    - At multiple levels (organizational and direct care)
    - In varied settings (hospitals, nursing homes, and home care settings)
- Opportunities to supervise, delegate, and evaluate others (peers; ancillary personnel)
- Progress from total care of one or two patients to more in number/complexity
- Opportunities to practice the managed care process (environmental resource assessment; prioritizing outcomes)
- Use, critique, and design clinical pathways
- Interdisciplinary practice experiences
- Quality improvement experiences
- Reflective journaling for the purpose of exploring theory and practice experiences
- Management and managed care issues incorporated into clinical conferences

---

promotion (Utley-Smith, 2004). Although there will be variance in the breadth and depth of the knowledge and skills encompassing these competencies, graduates of all levels of educational preparation ought to be ready to put them into practice. One single learning environment cannot encompass all of the knowledge and skills opportunities, but the clinical education experiences of the curriculum taken as a whole should. Nurses are expected to carry out their management skills at the levels of both the health care organization and direct care (Heller et al., 2004b) in hospitals, nursing homes, and home health care settings (Utley-Smith, 2004), so practice experiences should be provided in diverse settings as well.

Supervisory competency for the new nurse entails the capacity to manage the implementation of a plan of care by others, including non-nurse personnel (Utley-Smith, 2004). Previously, the clinical courses within academic nursing curricula have provided students with very few occasions on which they could take on responsibility for ancillary nursing personnel, that is, responsibility for delegating work or supervising its accomplishment (Utley-Smith, 2004). The attainment of beginning competency in supervision requires that students practice all of the skills it encompasses. Students must learn to supervise, delegate, and evaluate, which are all aspects of the management functions: planning, organizing, directing, and controlling (Barnum, 1999; Sullivan & Decker, 2001). Overall, the competency of supervision was most highly prized by the nursing home administrators, compared to those from hospitals or home health care settings, in Utley-Smith's study (2004). Considering the relative numbers of personnel who are subordinate to the supervision of a registered nurse in these settings, this is understandable.

The total care of one or two patients will continue to be a useful learning assignment for nursing students as they gain knowledge of direct care, interpersonal communication, and the application of health promotion principles to individuals and families. However, that purpose needs to be clearly communicated to nursing students. They need to be told that the total, ideal care of one or two patients is an artificial, fabricated practice experience that allows them to attain specific knowledge and skills (Barnum, 1999) and that there is much more to learn. To better learn the expectations that will be placed on them in relation to acuity and complexity, students must be assigned to more than one or two patients at a time, or they must care for patients with more time-consuming needs (Barnum, 1999). The hospital administrators in the Utley-Smith study (2004) indicated an expectation that nurses care for a larger number of patients in a defined period of time; this expectation was shared by administrators of nursing and home health organizations, but not to the same degree.

Competency in caseload management is seen in the ability of the nurse to coordinate care for a specific number of patients; it extends to all of these settings, incorporating time and resource management over a specific period in addition to direct patient care (Utley-Smith, 2004). The managed care process begins with an environmental resource assessment, including staff/personnel and time (Barnum, 1999). Next, the desired outcomes are identified based on the results of the assessment. The final step, which involves prioritizing the chosen outcomes, is of critical import and requires making more choices; what is *essential* must be winnowed from what would be *nice* (Barnum, 1999). The process is carried out at the direct patient care level in order to determine the desired care outcomes for small groups of patients or at the organizational level for the care outcomes of aggregates.

The case management tool, clinical pathways, places the emphasis on the norm for the aggregate (Barnum, 1999). They "provide a student with the equivalent of a ready-made nursing care plan, with the advantage of spelling out what other professionals will do as well" (Barnum, 1999, p. 35). Using clinical pathways during their clinical courses will prepare new graduates for working in managed care environments, where these tools are employed to direct and then evaluate standardized, interdisciplinary interventions across the entire care continuum while improving overall care quality by efficiently using resources (Dickerson et al., 2001). The standardized care outcomes are drawn from applicable practice guidelines and published external benchmarks such as those used in organizational accreditations (Barnum, 1999; Dickerson et al., 2001). Having been introduced to clinical pathways as clinical decision-making tools in the classroom, along with the terminology of managed care, students in clinical courses can progress to their actual use and evaluation.

Beginning with their first clinical course, nursing students can start to apply the knowledge and skills they will need in the managed care environment. Having students assume supervisory positions over their peers is one common approach (Isaacson & Stacy, 2004; O'Neal, 2004). This can be done in the first foundational clinical course, where students might take turns serving as a "resource leader" for the other students, helping with prioritization of care, assisting with care, directing other students to colleagues needing a hand, and answering basic questions (O'Neal, 2004). More advanced students nearing graduation could take on more of the supervisory functions, serving in modified charge nurse positions that incorporate planning, organizing, staffing, directing, and controlling (Isaacson & Stacy, 2004). Students can attend interdisciplinary care meetings; spend a few hours with members of other health care disciplines; participate in quality improvement activities; prepare and present in-service programs; develop and critique time management plans; make personnel assignments; and even participate in the evaluation of others. Clinical reflective journals can focus on integration of theory in which the clinical practice students observe and participate. Clinical conferences can incorporate discussion and critique of time and resource management, concepts of cost/benefit ratios, and issues of cost effectiveness (Barnum, 1999). Practice, conferences, and journals all can be used to explore "organizational, regulatory, political, and interpersonal factors that affect nursing practice and the administration of health care services" (Heller, Drenkard, Esposito-Herr, Romano, Tom, & Valentine, 2004a).

■ CULTURAL COMPETENCY DEVELOPMENT

Population shifts, changes in demographics, and marked increases in societal diversity are all exerting a significant influence on nursing practice, education, and research (Heller et al., 2004b). These alterations "affect the nature and the prevalence of illness and disease, requiring changes in practice that reflect and respect diverse values and beliefs" (Heller et al., 2004b, Changing demographics, 2). The provision of culturally competent care by health care providers is not optional; institutional policies and regulatory agencies mandate it (Dreher & MacNaughton, 2002). In addition to becoming "the mantra of contemporary nursing practice" (Dreher & MacNaughton, 2002, p. 181), cultural competency has become an expected programmatic outcome in nursing education. Faced with inadequate data reflecting outcome attainment and insufficient numbers of faculty with adequate academic or other theoretical preparation to teach culturally competent care (Grant & Letzring, 2003), nursing faculty struggle to determine what and how to teach their students to prepare them for a society that is multiethnic and culturally diverse.

Diversity itself is a construct that evades any consistent definition and is approached in various ways in nursing practice, education, and research (Terhune, 2004). Most often, people are described and classified according to the demographic characteristics of race, ethnicity, gender, and sexual orientation (Machado, 2001). But in reality, cultural groupings evolve from communities and generations of families sharing a wide continuum of conformity to the learned behavioral patterns and beliefs of the groups' traditional cultural norms (Dreher & MacNaughton, 2002). Most people spend their entire lives as members of their referent culture, while holding close to some of its norms, denying others, and adhering to still other cultural values on a situational basis. As we anecdotally well know, the individuals within a cultural group possess a remarkable range of opinions regarding many issues; diversity exists within any group. Dreher and MacNaughton (2002) call the tendency to extrapolate from data drawn from groups of people in order to make broad generalizations about individual members of a culture an "ecologic fallacy." What then occurs "… is that the lived experiences or existential quality of personal experiences are sacrificed for the cultural, social, or global focus" (Kleiman, Frederickson, & Lundy, 2004, p. 251). Far too much is lost in translation. Generalized beliefs applied to individuals are quite accurately defined as stereotypes (Machado, 2001). The next step, when stereotypes are transposed into attitudes, is prejudice. As valuable as constructs such as race and ethnicity may be in the organization of data, the fact is that they can result in the generation of stereotypes (Machado, 2001; Dreher & MacNaughton, 2002). When stereotypes are carried into nursing practice, the resulting care is at minimum inadequate and may even be negligent (Dreher & MacNaughton, 2002).

In their literature review, Grant and Letzring (2003) found the number of publications addressing the incorporation of content related to culture, pedagogical approaches, and evaluation of their effectiveness have increased significantly since the American Nurses Association published a guide for the integration of cultural diversity content into nursing curricula in 1986. Although some programs offered elective international experiences that typically included both theoretical and practice components, most of the educational approaches reported have been classroom-based, with teaching methods involving lectures, videos, panel discussions, case studies, and reflection (Grant & Letzring, 2003). Experiential learning in clinical settings is essential; it is there that the prospect of cultural competency is the most arduous (Dreher & MacNaughton, 2002).

Faculty teaching clinical nursing courses are in a position to guide their students in the clarification and development of attitudes and beliefs about people. Didactic presentation of theory only partially contributes to the skills and knowledge that nursing students acquire during their education; clinical practicum experiences exert a tremendous influence on the eventual practice of novice nurses. For many nursing students, cultural diversity attitudes are learned in exchanges with their faculty, patients, and others in the clinical setting (Paterson, Osborne, & Gregory, 2004). How then can faculty who teach clinical courses best bring about this learning in their students? How can students avoid the pitfall of stereotyping while providing patient care? Box 17-2 summarizes the suggestions presented in the subsequent discussion.

Cultural knowledge is beneficial to students in courses designed for the practice of nursing at the population level—community-based, population-focused interventions, such as preventive care and health promotion projects, or public education programs—but at the individual or family level it only prevents the interpretation of behavior as nonpathologic and does not permit inferences about the behaviors observed (Dreher & MacNaughton, 2002). To assume a

---

BOX 17-2

Suggestions for Enhancing Cultural Sensitivity in Clinical Nursing Courses

- Facilitate students' awareness of their own perspectives, attitudes, and values about people who differ from themselves (e.g., reflective journaling, group discussions).
- Provide an opportunity for male students and those of other cultures to help their peers understand their individual and cultural views (e.g., discussions, group learning experiences).
- Create an environment conducive to dialogue and openness about cultural commonalities and differences.
- Encourage students to attend to the individual patient/family, avoiding generalizing cultural norms (non–community-focused courses).
- Provide opportunities for processing multicultural clinical experiences (verbal or written; individual and group)
- Provide practice experiences:
  - With culturally diverse staff
  - In culturally diverse settings (local, regional, international)
  - With culturally diverse patients/families
  - In community-based, population-focused activities
- Use group learning experiences for enhancing cultural knowledge (e.g., posters, discussion, panel presentations)
- Use written assignments to further cultural sensitivity (e.g., reflective journaling, application of relevant research).
- Design reflective journaling questions to guide application of theory to practice, and exploration of attitudes and beliefs.
- Integrate relevant habits of the mind and skills of critical thinking into learning activities.

---

patient is uncomfortable maintaining eye contact because he is Asian is a disservice to the patient. "Membership in a class is not sufficient as a defining criterion" (Machado, 2001, p. 15). Since individuals within a culture may think and behave differently from one another and from the dictates of their dominant culture, it is clear that in interactions with individuals cultural competency takes the form of sensitivity to potential differences and awareness of one's own cultural perspective. What is termed *cultural competence* "... is really nursing competence ... the capacity to be equally therapeutic with patients from any social or cultural background. The real issue is individualized patient care—the signature of contemporary nursing" (Dreher & MacNaughton, 2002, p. 185).

Cultural sensitivity does not develop overnight; a single course or clinical experience is insufficient. Students must have multiple opportunities to develop an understanding of and respect for diverse cultures, beginning with the exploration of their own values (Sommer, 2001). What nursing students need early in their education is assistance in exploring and understanding their own perspectives, their attitudes and values about ethnicity, race, gender, sexual orientation, and social and economic "otherness." This knowledge serves as their own cultural context, the lens through which they observe those from whom they differ and the vantage point of their interactions with patients as they provide care. "Any attempt to describe a group other than our own is seriously handicapped by our inability to move beyond our own perceptual world; … we may only obtain a glimpse of what that other cultures may truly be like" (Machado, 2001, p. 14). Students will benefit from discussions that occur within the clinical group, but the needed level of self-assessment and evaluation is probably best done initially at the individual level. Reflective journaling is an excellent mechanism for this. Using some well constructed questions to guide their thinking process, students can use the privacy of their written dialogue with faculty to critically analyze how they feel about others who differ from them and even examine the validity of their own beliefs. With this self-awareness, a willingness to be open to others, and a desire to provide quality care, students are poised to explore other health beliefs, especially information that could create barriers to health care. This cultural sensitivity allows nurses to diminish cultural dissonance, enhance the quality of communication, and ultimately generate superior clinical outcomes (Dreher & MacNaughton, 2002).

If both clinical teachers and nursing students were taught to view cultural diversity as relative and occurring in context rather than as a fixed state or identity, it would serve to address the ways in which history, power, and context have influenced how we understand what is right and ideal in nursing and in nursing education (Paterson et al., 2004, Summary).

Beginning with the clinical group itself, faculty can encourage students to see the differences among individual group members and examine some of the minority subcultures that are part of the nursing community. Equality should not be construed to mean "sameness" such that cultural differences evaporate; the challenge of attempting to appreciate these cultural differences while encouraging societal inclusivity has not been resolved. If the clinical group includes male students or students from minority sexual orientation or ethnic groups, they might be invited to share their experiences as students and their perceptions of possible obstacles and facilitators that could effect success in nursing. Afterward, conduct a discussion about noted commonalities and differences.

Following the discussion, students could subsequently be asked to do reflective journaling and perhaps conduct an interview of a nurse who is a member of one of the identified subcultures. Interviews of nurses from subcultures were part of a teaching plan designed by Robinson (2000) for increasing students' cultural sensitivity. Paterson et al. (2004) found that in the context of clinical nursing education, there are " … unwritten and largely invisible expectations of homogeneity in the context of a predominant discourse of equality and cultural sensitivity" (Abstract). The ethnocentrism of educators and practicing nurses is visible in their unwavering belief that their methods are "right" and their utter amazement that others might view things differently (Paterson et al., 2004). Efforts to attract and retain male and ethnic minority students into nursing are a significant component of academic diversity planning (Anthony, 2004; Evans, 2004; O'Lynn, 2004). Having a diverse student body provides a ready arena for enhancing the cultural sensitivity of nursing students. Providing group learning experiences in which small heterogeneous groups of students work collaboratively on projects "…enables students to live out principles of democracy, social equity, and justice" while they learn from one another (Sommer, 2001, p. 278). The creation of an atmosphere in which openness and conversation are encouraged allows faculty and students to discuss their cultural commonalities and differences (Sommer, 2001).

Developing self-awareness and participating in discussions regarding diverse cultures serve as a starting point for the development of cultural sensitivity, but clinical experiences are still essential (Sommer, 2001). Clinical experiences in which one of the goals is the continued development of cultural sensitivity include those in which students are partnered with culturally diverse staff, immersed into culturally diverse clinical settings, provide direct care for individual patients/families from cultures different from their own, and get involved in community-based population-focused activities. Working with nurses from other cultural groups can be beneficial to all students' learning. Also, being partnered with a nurse from the same culture as their own can provide especially valuable role modeling for students of a nondominant culture (e.g., male and international students).

Clinical opportunities are available through some nursing programs for students' experiential learning in other countries (Mill, Yonge, & Cameron, 2005), but most programs with multicultural experiences take advantage of alternative settings within the local region (Grant & Letzring, 2003). For example, Bindler, Allen, and Paul (2004) describe a course for nursing students that included clinical experiences on regional Native American reservation facilities. Many programs place students in clinical settings in which they are exposed to different subcultures as relates to socioeconomic factors, such as free clinics, homeless shelters, and centers for abused women.

In all of these settings, most nursing students have experiences with people different from themselves. Students begin to appreciate that knowing a patient belongs to a certain cultural group can offer hints that may be beneficial to understanding that person, but having this knowledge does not automatically allow the forecast of reactions to the situational contexts or individual patient needs (Kleiman et al., 2004). When they are involved in direct patient care, students need to learn that knowing some of the attitudes and beliefs of patients' cultures does not spontaneously generate a favorable reception by patients or families (Kleiman et al., 2004). The nurse who has only a little knowledge about another culture may draw the patient's ire by making presumptions based on culture. The trust that evolves in the nurse-patient relationship grows out of the caring that is communicated in the nurse's sincere desire and effort to understand the uniquely individual patient.

In community-based courses, populations are the customary unit of intervention and culture is a central concept (Dreher & MacNaughton, 2002). It is in these population-focused courses where students participate in activities related to groups, that cultural knowledge of attitudes, health beliefs and behaviors, taboos, and communication styles associated with the given population are important to planning. "Cultural knowledge provides guidance for social marketing and public education program content, for community-based prevention and health promotion initiatives, and for organizing therapeutic and related services" (Dreher & MacNaughton, 2002, p. 183). In order for activities targeted to specific groups to be successful, students learn that they must use culturally appropriate lines of communication and rely on local expertise. As they learn these lessons, students also must learn the differences in the use of cultural knowledge as it applies to populations and individuals.

In all clinical courses, the seminars/clinical conferences and written assignments can be used to assist in processing culturally diverse experiences and maximizing the learning that occurs. The habits of the mind and critical thinking skills (Scheffer & Rubenfeld, 2000) need to be fostered as part of the teaching strategies of multicultural education (Sommer, 2001) (see Chapter 11). Some of these habits and skills seem designed almost for multicultural education: contextual perspective, inquisitiveness, open-mindedness, and discriminating thought. Incorporating the habits of the mind and skills of critical thinking into group learning experiences and written work provides continuity between students' multicultural learning experiences and their overall clinical experiences. Discussing their clinical experiences in a group of students can generate an amplification of learning. When individual students share an observation or particular experience, their peers are able to build on it, gaining insights and challenging assumptions.

A wide variety of group learning experiences can focus on or incorporate multicultural issues. Students can design informative posters related to various cultural aspects such as spiritualism and diet and their effects on health care delivery. Members of other cultural groups can be invited for panel presentations followed by discussion. Conference time can be used to explore any number of topics, with careful delineation of focus: population or individual. Many of the same topics can be incorporated into written assignments, done individually or by small groups of two or three students. But, unless sharing of the work is included in the teaching plan, the other members of the clinical group are unable to benefit. Regardless of the circumstances, if reflective journaling is part of the course it can be used to help individual students process their clinical experiences, clarify thinking, identify and critique preconceptions, and deepen understanding.

▓ SERVICE-LEARNING EXPERIENCE

Service-learning experiences are being incorporated increasingly into elementary and secondary education, and also into many disciplines in postsecondary education (Cohen & Milone-Nuzzo, 2001; Bailey, Carpenter, & Harrington, 2002;

Miller & Swanson, 2002). These experiences, which bring community service and classroom education together, harken back to the late 18th- and early 19th-century English settlement houses. At that time, university students from Oxford and Cambridge lived among the poor in settlement houses in the expectation they could improve the general learning and civic responsibility of the impoverished. Evolving from this English model, caregivers stationed in Lillian Wald's Henry Street Settlement, established in 1893 in New York City, made home visits to the ill and provided programs for health promotion and disease prevention (Miller & Swanson, 2002). John Dewey, an influential educator of the 20th century, defined the principles of service learning by emphasizing teaching that was democratic, participative, and interactive (Cohen & Milone-Nuzzo, 2001; Bailey et al., 2002). Dewey's educational philosophy included the belief that education must engage with and enlarge experience, be supportive of democracy and the community, and incorporate reflection and the exploration of thinking (John Dewey Society). The connection between education and community service as a pedagogical approach initially waxed and waned in popularity during the latter half of the 20th century, then rebounded in the 1980s and continued to gain momentum into the present (Bailey et al., 2002). Over the years, service-learning opportunities have been developed and supported by various government agencies and educational and community organizations. These structured learning experiences involving both academic programs and community agencies have garnered significant benefits for both organizations. From the standpoint of nursing education, service learning offers connections "... between teaching, research, community service, practice, and the external environment" essential for the preparation of the nurses of tomorrow (Seifer & Vaughn, 2002).

Service-learning applied to nursing is a pedagogical approach that differs in several key ways from clinical experiential learning approaches (Bailey et al., 2002; Seifer, 2002) (Box 17-3). Service-learning is designed to facilitate student engagement with diverse communities (Nokes, Nickitas, Keida, & Neville, 2005). Student learning, the transformation of theory into practice, is the principal focus of traditional clinical practica; in-service learning, student learning and service to the community, are melded (Peterson & Schaffer, 2001;

BOX 17-3

Characteristics of Service-Learning Experiences

- Carried out within the framework of community partnerships
- Goals are collaboratively established, implemented, and evaluated within the partnership
- Reflection is an essential component
- Members of the community partnership have active teaching roles
- Students, faculty, and community agencies mutually benefit

Seifer, 2002). As a pedagogy in which students develop their capabilities as both nurses and citizens, service learning requires academic institutions form distinctive partnerships with community agencies. Within the framework of this partnership, goals are collaboratively established, plans are created, carried out, then evaluated and commemorated by the students and the community partners together (Seifer, 2002). As opposed to traditional clinical education in which faculty design the curricular outcomes and the approaches to their attainment and evaluation, in service learning the students, faculty, and community partners collaborate in determining the service to be provided. This reciprocal relationship is a key defining characteristic of service learning (Bailey et al., 2002; Seifer, 2002). Students "…provide direct community service, learn about the context in which the services are provided, and understand the relationship between the service and their academic course work" (Cohen & Milone-Nuzzo, 2001, p. 31). The student's role differs from that of a volunteer by virtue of the connection to academic expectations and theoretical classroom content (Cohen & Milone-Nuzzo, 2001).

Within the expanded outlook of the community context, students delve into the impact of social, cultural, economic, and political concerns on health, deriving a richer appreciation of the community's strengths and limitations (Nokes et al., 2005). This is accomplished in part through reflection activities. Reflection is an essential aspect of service learning (Cohen & Milone-Nuzzo, 2001; Eyler, 2002; Seifer, 2002; Nokes et al., 2005). "Reflection is the hyphen that links service to learning; … [it] is what transforms service and learning into service-learning" (Eyler, 2002, pp. 453 and 456). The efficacy of reflection as an essential part of service-learning depends on the students' ability in "…creating/clarifying meaning of the experience, thinking, critically analyzing, and connecting community with learning" (Bailey et al., 2002, p. 435). Well crafted reflection activities such as journaling, role playing, group discussions and presentations and written assignments on an ongoing basis throughout the course help students become more astute, examine assumptions more thoroughly, and develop in-depth thinking that goes beyond their initial impressions (Cohen & Milone-Nuzzo, 2001; Bailey et al., 2002; Eyler, 2002).

Another difference between service learning and traditional experiential activities is the roles assumed by faculty and community members. In service learning, individuals within the community partnership take on teaching responsibilities, often in the classroom as well as in the practicum (Cohen & Milone-Nuzzo, 2001; Seifer, 2002). The high degree of involvement of community agency members emphasizes the collaborative nature of service learning. Throughout the experience, students must evaluate not only their own personal growth but also the influence of their labors on the community (Miller & Swanson, 2002). The mutuality of benefits for all stakeholders in the partnership is a major feature of service learning (Cohen & Milone-Nuzzo, 2001).

Policies at both the community agencies and academic institutions may be revised as practices are challenged; relationships between faculty and community representatives are enriched; quality and quantity of community services are increased; and research ventures are stimulated (Peterson & Schaffer, 2001; Cohen & Milone-Nuzzo, 2001; Miller & Swanson, 2002). Faculty may choose agencies they are already involved with as sites for student service learning; this may increase their interest and engagement in service learning (Bailey et al., 2002). It is possible for faculty to integrate all aspects of their academic role (teaching, service, scholarship) into service-learning experiences (Peterson & Schaffer, 2001; Miller & Swanson, 2002).

Student benefits derived from service-learning experiences are most often anecdotally reported, and evidence-based evaluations are limited. A partial list of the advantages of service learning for students described in the literature includes refined communication and interpersonal skills; increased critical thinking skills; improved technical understanding; experience with community building; improved academic performance; clarification of values; enhanced leadership skills; revised understanding and appreciation of career options; commitment to life-long service involvement; increased cultural competency and civic engagement; stimulation of creativity; a heightened sense of caring; expanded understanding of social policy and social justice (Cohen & Milone-Nuzzo, 2001; Peterson & Schaffer, 2001; Carter & Dunn, 2002; Herman & Sassatelli, 2002; Holloway, 2002; Miller & Swanson, 2002; Redman & Clark, 2002; Nokes et al., 2005).

Service learning, by definition, occurs within a community context. Most often applied in nursing in community-based/population-focused clinical courses (Miller & Swanson, 2002; Erickson, 2004; Schoener & Hopkins, 2004; Nokes et al., 2005), it has been incorporated into nursing curricula in a variety of fashions. Service learning has been used as the means to facilitate the integration of principles of social justice (Herman & Sassatelli, 2002; Redman & Clark, 2002). Graduate, baccalaureate, and associate degree nursing programs have incorporated service-learning opportunities into their curricula (Holloway, 2002; Seifer & Vaughn, 2002; Erickson, 2004; Falk-Rafael, Ward-Griffin, Laforet-Fliesser, & Beynon, 2004). It has been applied to faith-based collaboration between religious academic and community institutions (Herman & Sassatelli, 2002). Service-learning has been the organizing feature of a psychiatric nursing course (Warren, Donaldson, & Whaley, 2005) and a collaborative course with the discipline of health education (Mayne & Glascoff, 2002) and has been used as the vehicle for health disparity research in an undergraduate social science class (Hanks, 2003).

Two texts are especially valuable in providing guidance both at the broad curricular level and in the application of service-learning within nursing courses:

Norbeck, J., Connolly, C., & Koerner, J. (Eds.). (1998). *Caring and community: Concepts and models for service-learning in nursing*. Washington, DC: American Association for Higher Education.

Poirrier, G. (2001). *Service-learning: Curricular applications in nursing*. Sudbury, MA and New York: Jones and Bartlett and National League for Nursing.

In addition to a wide selection of journal publications regarding service-learning theory and applications, the literature also provides a listing of relevant

---

BOX 17-4
Websites Relevant to Service Learning and Higher Education

▓ The Center for the Health Professions, University of California, San Francisco: http://futurehealth.ucsf.edu/
▓ National Service-Learning Cooperative Clearinghouse: http://www.servicelearning.org/
▓ Corporation for National and Community Service: http://www.cns.gov/
▓ Campus Compact: http://www.compact.org/
▓ NetAid: http://www.netaid.org/
▓ RAND report on combining service and learning in higher education: http://www.rand.org/publications/MR/MR998/
▓ National Service-Learning Clearinghouse http://www.servicelearning.org/lib_svcs/bibs/he_bibs/syllabi/index.php

---

websites (Cohen & Milone-Nuzzo, 2001) that can be verified and supplemented by searching the web (Box 17-4). Eyler (2002) shares suggestions for the incorporation of reflection activities, including an organizational tool and a "reflection map" for faculty use in course planning. Bailey et al. (2002) offers more ideas about the inclusion of reflection activities and emphasizes the importance of preparing structure for journaling and questions to guide group reflection discussion.

SUMMARY

The future of nursing practice is inextricably tied to changes in the global society as well as to those within the health care system. Based on identified trends, nurses will have to enter the practice arena with enhanced management and leadership skills, an awareness of and appreciation for the diversity of humankind, and a civic-mindedness encompassing their local, national, and worldwide communities. All of these can and should be addressed within clinical practica as a part of their nursing education.

REFLECTION EXERCISE 17

Reflecting on the Role of Cultural Values and Attitudes Upon Teaching

How does your own cultural perspective affect how you interact (or will interact) with students whose perspectives are different?

The first step in addressing cultural sensitivity with nursing students is facilitating their awareness of their own cultural beliefs and how these beliefs impact their interactions with others who bring their own values and attitudes to the interaction. As the teacher, it is important to model this cultural awareness.

Imagine you are about to enter a room with a group of 10 students for your first meeting with them. As you walk into the room, you scan the group.

Jot down your immediate reactions (thoughts and feelings) to each of the students described below:

Female, white, appears in her late 50's

Two males: one white, mid-20's, tall, muscular build, ponytail, sandals, Hawaiian shirt; one Asian, fine boned, sitting off to the side of the rest of the group

Two black females: one early 40's, short and significantly overweight; the other early 20's, tall, hair in cornrows with beads

Two young white females, appearing to be right out of high school, slim and stylishly dressed, talking animatedly with one another

White female, early 30's, clothing appears clean but shabby, face appears careworn and haggard, hands noticeably tremulous

Two white females, both in their late 20's, dressed in clearly out of date clothing, speaking to one another in a language other than English

Now, go back over what you have written. Look at your initial reactions to these students.

◆ Did you draw conclusions about them based on what you "saw"?

◆ How do you think your own cultural perspective affected your responses and conclusions?

◆ Are there assumptions about gender, race/ethnicity, and social/economic class embedded in your responses and conclusions?

◆ How might you use what you have learned about your own perspectives to develop the students' cultural sensitivity in this first meeting?

References

Anthony, A.S. (2004). Gender bias and discrimination in nursing education: Can we change it? *Nurse Educator, 29*(3), 121-125.

Bailey, P.A., Carpenter, D.R., & Harrington, P. (2002). Theoretical foundations of service-learning in nursing education. *Journal of Nursing Education, 41*(10), 433-436.

Barnum, B.S. (1999). *Teaching nursing in the era of managed care.* New York: Springer.

Bindler, R., Allen, C., & Paul, R. (2004). Native American learning: An integrative model. *Journal of Nursing Education, 43*(5), 237-240.

Carter, J., & Dunn, B. (2002). A service-learning partnership for enhanced diabetes management. *Journal of Nursing Education, 41*(10), 450-452.

Cohen, S.S., & Milone-Nuzzo, P. (2001). Advancing health policy in nursing education through service learning. *Advances in Nursing Science, 23*(3), 28-40.

Dickerson, S.S., Sackett, K., Jones, J.M., & Brewer, C. (2001). Guidelines for evaluating tools for clinical decision making. *Nurse Educator, 26*(5), 215-220.

Dreher, M., & MacNaughton, N. (2002). Cultural competence in nursing: Foundation or fallacy? *Nursing Outlook, 50*(5), 181-186.

Erickson, G.P. (2004). Community health nursing in a nonclinical setting: Service-learning outcomes of undergraduate students and clients. *Nurse Educator, 29*(2), 54-57.

Evans, B.C. (2004). Application of the caring curriculum to education of Hispanic/Latino and American Indian nursing students. *Journal of Nursing Education, 43*(5), 219-228.

Eyler, J. (2002). Reflecting on service: Helping nursing students get the most from service-learning. *Journal of Nursing Education, 41*(10), 453-456.

Falk-Rafael, A.R., Ward-Griffin, C., Laforet-Fliesser, Y., & Beynon, C. (2004). Teaching nursing students to promote the health of communities. *Nurse Educator, 29*(2), 63-67.

Grant, L.F., & Letzring, T.D. (2003). Status of cultural competence in nursing education: A literature review. *Journal of Multicultural Nursing and Health, 9*(2), 6-13.

Hanks, C. (2003). Health disparities research and service learning. *Journal of Multicultural Nursing and Health, 9*(3), 18-23.

Heller, B.R., Drenkard, K., Esposito-Herr, M.B., Romano, C., Tom, S., & Valentine, N. (2004a). Educating nurses for leadership roles. *Journal of Continuing Education in Nursing, 35*(5), 203-210.

Heller, B.R., Oros, M.T., & Durney-Crowley, J. (2004b). The future of nursing education: Ten trends to watch. National League for Nursing—Nursing Education Perspectives. Retrieved October 27, 2004, from http://www.nln.org/nlnjournal/infotrends.htm.

Herman, C., & Sassatelli, J. (2002). DARING to Reach the Heartland: A collaborative faith-based partnership in nursing education. *Journal of Nursing Education, 41*(10), 443-445.

Holloway, A.S. (2002). Service-learning in community college nursing education. *Journal of Nursing Education, 41*(10), 440-442.

Isaacson, J.J., & Stacy, A.S. (2004). Nursing students in an expanded charge nurse role: A real clinical management experience. *Nursing Education Perspectives, 25*(6), 292-296.

John Dewey Society for the Study of Education and Culture. Retrieved April 7, 2005, from http://www.johndeweysociety.org/

Kleiman, S., Fredrickson, K., & Lundy, T. (2004). Using an eclectic model to education students about cultural influences on the nurse-patient relationship. *Nursing Education Perspectives, 25*(5), 249-253.

Machado, G.A. (2001). Cultural sensitivity and stereotypes. *Journal of Multicultural Nursing and Health, 7*(2), 13-15.

Mayne, L., & Glascoff, M. (2002). Service learning: Preparing a healthcare workforce for the next century. *Nurse Educator, 27*(4), 191-195.

Mill, J.E., Yonge, O.J., & Cameron, B.L. (2005). Challenges and opportunities of international clinical practica. *International Journal of Nursing Education Scholarship, 2*(1), Article 18. Retrieved November 27, 2005, from http://www.bepress.com/ijnes/vol2/iss1/art18.

Miller, M.P., & Swanson, E. (2002). Service learning and community health nursing: A natural fit. *Nursing Education Perspectives, 23*(1), 30-33.

Nokes, K.M., Nickitas, D.M., Keida, R., & Neville, S. (2005). Does service-learning increase cultural competency, critical thinking, and civic engagement? *Journal of Nursing Education, 44*(2), 65-70.

Norbeck, J., Connolly, C., & Koerner, J. (Eds.). (1998). *Caring and community: Concepts and models for service-learning in nursing.* Washington, DC: American Association for Higher Education.

O'Lynn, C.D. (2004). Gender-based barriers for male students in nursing education programs: Prevalence and perceived importance. *Journal of Nursing Education, 43*(5), 229-236.

O'Neal, C. (2004). Creating leadership skills in fundamental courses. *Journal of Nursing Education, 43*(11), 524.

Paterson, B.L., Osborne, M., & Gregory, D. (2004). How different can you be and still survive? Homogeneity and difference in clinical nursing education. *International Journal of Nursing Education Scholarship, 1*(1), Article 2. Retrieved December 3, 2004, from http://www.bepress.com/ijnes/vol1/iss1/art2.

Peterson, S.J., & Schaffer, M.A. (2001). Service-learning: Isn't that what nursing education has always been? *Journal of Nursing Education, 40*(2), 51-52.

Poirrier, G. (2001). *Service-learning: Curricular applications in nursing.* Sudbury, MA and New York: Jones and Bartlett and National League for Nursing.

Redman, R.W., & Clark, L. (2002). Service-learning as a model for integrating social justice in the nursing curriculum. *Journal of Nursing Education, 41*(10), 446-449.

Robinson, J.H. (2000). Increasing students' cultural sensitivity: A step toward greater diversity in nursing. *Nurse Educator, 25*(3), 131-135.

Scheffer, B.K., & Rubenfeld, M.F. (2000). A consensus statement on critical thinking in nursing. *Journal of Nursing Education, 39*(8), 352-359.

Schoener, L., & Hopkins, M.L. (2004). Service learning: A tuberculosis screening clinic in an adult residential care facility. *Nurse Educator, 29*(6), 242-245.

Seifer, S.D. (2002). From placement site to partnership: The promise of service-learning. *Journal of Nursing Education, 41*(10), 431-432.

Seifer, S.D., & Vaughn, R.L. (2002). Partners in Caring and Community: Service-learning in nursing education. *Journal of Nursing Education, 41*(10), 437-439.

Sommer, S. (2001). Multicultural nursing education. *Journal of Nursing Education, 40*(6), 276-278.

Sullivan, E.J., & Decker, P.J. (2001). *Effective leadership and management in nursing* (5th ed.). Upper Saddle River, NJ: Prentice-Hall.

Terhune, C. (2004). From desegregation to diversity: How far have we really come? *Journal of Nursing Education, 43*(5), 195-196.

Utley-Smith, Q. (2004). 5 competencies needed by new baccalaureate graduates. *Nursing Education Perspectives, 25*(4), 166-170.

Warren, B.J., Donaldson, R., & Whaley, M. (2005). Service learning: An adjunct to therapeutic communication and critical thinking skills for baccalaureate nursing students. *Journal of Nursing Education, 44*(3), 147.

UNIT V

Endings and Beginnings

CHAPTER 18

Assessing Student Learning Outcomes: Evaluation and Grading

Assessing the attainment of the educational outcomes for a clinical practicum is considerably more challenging than making similar determinations for a classroom theory course where evaluation of cognitive knowledge is the focus (Walsh & Seldomridge, 2005). In the clinical setting, students are expected to reach a specified level of competency in all the domains of knowledge: cognitive, psychomotor, and affective. Issues of safety, judgment, and adaptability also must be considered, because they are so important in preparing students to enter a practice discipline (Walsh & Seldomridge, 2005). Measurement of clinical performance and the determination of clinical course grades have generated

---

BOX 18-1
Educational Evaluation and Grading

Evaluation

Purpose: Feedback to the student regarding goal attainment.

Informal evaluation: Routine feedback provided during and immediately following student learning experiences.

Formal evaluation: More structured synopsis of performance, according to course objectives, provided at the following times:

- Midpoint of the term, along with suggestions for attaining growth within the course (formative)
- Conclusion of the course, including a summarization of attainment of course objectives and recommendations for future growth

Grading

Purpose: Conversion of evaluative content into a stylized format for standardized communication within academia.

---

tremendous concern and debate among nursing faculty for decades (Tanner, 2004). In reviewing the recent nursing literature regarding clinical evaluation issues, unfairness and subjectivity of faculty and instruments, inconsistencies in the resulting allocation of grades, student preoccupation with grades, grade inflation, and the potential deleterious effects of evaluation on the faculty-student relationship are reiterated time and again (Wiles & Bishop, 2001; Wishnia, Yancy, Silva, & Kern-Manwaring, 2002; Reising & Devich, 2004; Scanlon & Care, 2004; Tanner, 2004; Walsh & Seldomridge, 2005). Assumptions regarding evaluation and grading must be questioned and new avenues explored, but the work of evaluating today's students must proceed simultaneously. A basic understanding of clinical evaluation and grading is essential for the novice faculty (Box 18-1).

■ CLOSING THE CLINICAL TEACHING-LEARNING LOOP

In the classic model of the teaching-learning process, the four steps of assessment, planning, implementation, and evaluation progress sequentially and circularly, each step informing the next, with the results of evaluation providing new assessment data. When conceptualized in this stylized fashion, the emphasis in each step has traditionally been on the role of a powerful and controlling teacher and the learner has been cast in a passive role. In reality, the teaching-learning process is dynamic and fluid; its components coexist and interact freely with one another. The classic perspective is also incongruent with today's learning paradigm; a dynamic model is based on a more egalitarian and interdependent relationship between student and teacher as senior learner. Together, the clinical coach and student determine the short-term learning goals that will propel the student toward the long-term educational outcomes of the course. Learning experiences are selected, students evaluate their learning, and faculty provide evaluative feedback along the way. Throughout the course, despite the most sincere efforts by both parties, an undercurrent of imbalance in the teacher-student relationship is inevitable because of an innate power disparity: teachers routinely make the final determination regarding grades. Ultimately, the end-point of the course is reached, and although students should contribute to these final evaluations as well, the legal and ethical responsibility of ascertaining the degree to which students have met the educational goals of the course rests with the clinical faculty member.

▓ WHERE DOES LEARNING END AND EVALUATION BEGIN?

Although it is often suggested that at the beginning of a clinical course, evaluation is "set… aside in preference for teaching" (Walsh & Seldomridge, 2005, p. 167), the reality is that evaluation of learning is ongoing from the initiation of the course (Jeffries & Norton, 2005). There is no discrete end of learning and beginning of evaluation. Conceptualizing the evaluative aspects as a part of a dynamic and intertwined teaching-learning process implies that there are different types of evaluation. Informal evaluation is made available through the feedback faculty provide to students moment-to-moment and day-to-day regarding performance in the clinical setting, in group learning experiences, and in written assignments. Formal course evaluations reflect the extent to which students have met the objectives of the course and are provided at least twice during the term, as a midpoint progress report to guide learning for the remainder of the term and a final evaluation at the conclusion of the course.

How then are students to learn, to make errors and approximations, when they are continuously being evaluated? This is a question often posed by students, and sometimes even by faculty. Embedded in the question is a philosophic posture regarding the evaluation of clinical practicum: is the student's final clinical evaluation a reflection solely of performance at the end of the term, or is it a compilation of data collected throughout the term illustrating a pattern of improvement, growth, and ultimate attainment of course objectives? It is essential that faculty teaching clinical courses understand the position of the nursing program regarding evaluation and that they communicate that stance clearly to their students. The position taken may vary between the clinical courses within a curriculum, although there should be a rationale for this approach, and it must be communicated to the students. But consistency within a course is essential. Faculty teaching different sections of the same clinical course must approach evaluation in the same way; otherwise, grounds for accusations of inequity would be valid. When teaching a course such as Advanced Cardiac Life Support, in which there is a final practical and written examination, final student evaluations are based on the results of these examinations. All of the students' prior efforts during the course are purely for learning purposes, with informal feedback being provided. Unsatisfactory performance cannot be determined until the end of the course. However, in most clinical courses, a single inclusive final practical examination is not possible. Faculty simply are not physically able to have every student in a clinical group demonstrate the attainment of all of the course objectives at the same time at the conclusion of the course. More commonly, clinical courses incorporate established "minifinal" evaluations related to aspects of the course objectives intermittently throughout the course. For instance, an accurate and thorough newborn assessment may be a required component of a maternity nursing clinical course. As students rotate through the newborn nursery, they are expected to meet this requirement. If a student fails to satisfactorily meet this expectation initially, faculty typically permit the student to have another opportunity in the clinical setting or perhaps through a simulation in the learning resource center (LRC). For other aspects of course objectives, data are most commonly accrued, patterns and progression demonstrated. Whatever the circumstances, faculty must be clear about how and when evaluation is to occur, and they must communicate that to their students.

SUBJECTIVITY IN EVALUATION

In teaching, all evaluation is grounded in the professional judgment of the teacher, and no mortal judgment is truly objective. Using the objectives of the course, knowledge of the content area, and their own beliefs and values, faculty collect and judge samples of student performance. In a didactic course, given all of the possible questions that might be asked on an examination, faculty use their judgment to determine what is key content and which questions best address that content. Although commonly referred to as "objective" tests, subjectivity imbues these written examinations. In the clinical setting, all the knowledge, experiences, and values of each faculty member impact what data are collected and especially how those data are interpreted. What students really mean when they complain that faculty are not objective in evaluating them is that they have a sense of unfairness. Whereas objectivity in evaluation cannot be provided, fairness in didactic and clinical courses certainly can. In order to assure fairness in clinical evaluation, faculty can take a number of actions. Students too have contributions to make. All activities discussed in this chapter that foster fairness in clinical evaluation are summarized at its conclusion in Box 18-3 on p. 289.

PROLOGUE TO EVALUATION

Fairness is engendered within open and trusting relationships between faculty and students. Every action faculty take in establishing and nurturing relationships with students will facilitate fairness in evaluation. Faculty must take the time to examine the course objectives and ascertain the specific behaviors they describe (Zuzelo, 2000). Before the students can understand the course objectives, they must be understood and clearly articulated to them by their faculty. Sharing with the students course objectives that are clearly written, and telling them how, when, and where they will be evaluated, is also integral to providing fair evaluations (Zuzelo, 2000; Jeffries & Norton, 2005). For instance, if data will be collected from agency staff and/or clientele, students should be informed of this.

Fairness in evaluation is demonstrated by establishing performance standards that have been developed from the course objectives, communicating them clearly from the beginning of the course, and then applying them equally and consistently to all students in the clinical group. The course evaluation tool must be shared with the students, and they should be given the opportunity to discuss it and ask questions. Providing students with the evaluation tool gives them a "road map" to success in the course. Help students understand that evaluation is naturally subjective, and describe how fairness will be protected. Students need to know that they will be evaluated in terms of their attainment of the course objectives and not in relation to the abilities of the other students in the group (Zuzelo, 2000).

The method by which the evaluation will be transformed into a grade for the course should be clear to faculty and students alike. From the beginning of the course, students should know the criteria on which their grade is to be based (Tanner, 2004). Formal evaluations at the conclusion of the course should contain no surprises; everything addressed should have already been brought to the student's attention through informal feedback methods and opportunities to address weaknesses should have been provided. Lastly, faculty should review the rules and regulations of the nursing program related to the evaluation and grading processes and the mechanisms for assuring students' due process rights (Zuzelo, 2000).

■ EVALUATION VERSUS GRADING

Evaluation and grading are different but related concepts. Unfortunately, both faculty and students routinely view them synonymously (Tanner, 2004; Bourke & Ihrke, 2005). Informal evaluation (feedback) and formal evaluative progress reports guide and motivate learning. The evaluative process "...is a means of appraising data...rendering judgment by pointing out strengths and weaknesses" and examining the data through a comparison to performance standards (Bourke & Ihrke, 2005, p. 443). In a clinical course, the grade symbol allocated at the time of the final course evaluation reflects an effort to convert this otherwise highly qualitative data into a quantitative format that can be more easily communicated and used within academia (Scanlan & Care, 2004).

Evaluation and grading are fraught with difficulties, and the limitations associated with evaluation are compounded when they are carried over into the allocation of grades. The lack of clearly delineated standards of performance for nursing students and other validity and reliability concerns regarding the instruments used for evaluation brings into question the data on which grades are based (Walsh & Seldomridge, 2005). There has been an assumption that the motivational impact of evaluation is transposed into the grades students earn, that students will work harder in order to obtain higher grades, but this assumption is increasingly being challenged (Scanlan & Care, 2004). At a societal level, grade inflation distorts the validity of the grade by inaccurately communicating the degree of mastery of the course content, yet the pressures placed upon faculty to bestow high grades has never been greater (Scanlan & Care, 2004; Walsh & Seldomridge, 2005).

Nursing programs use one of two general approaches to assigning clinical course grades: a scale of letters or numbers (e.g., A, B, C, or 1, 2, 3), often with gradations to provide greater discrimination, or a dichotomous system of Pass/Fail or Satisfactory/Unsatisfactory. Even when the former system is used, little discrimination in clinical grading may occur if, as one study reports, the vast majority of students are given grades of B+ or above (Scanlan & Care, 2004). In an effort to provide recognition for exceptional accomplishment within a pass/fail grading system, some faculty have chosen to insert a level above pass/ satisfactory into their instruments. Faculty and students may fail to recognize "Pass" as a grade, because it is not included in the calculation of grade point and cannot be accurately converted into an alphanumeric system. It has been reported that the decision to make clinical course grades pass/fail is grounded in the belief that subjectivity, unfairness, and stress for both faculty and students are reduced with this approach (Wiles & Bishop, 2001). However, others take the position that pass/fail grading is subjective in nature (Wishnia et al., 2002). These stances are both reflections of a lack of theoretical understanding of grading and the innate subjectivity in evaluation. The system may certainly be arbitrary or poorly delineated, but subjectivity is not a property of a grading system.

The application of a pass/fail grading system also raises the serious concern that students may see these clinical courses as ultimately less valuable, therefore less important to prepare for or energetically participate in. Such a concern evolves from the assumption that grades, as opposed to interest in the course content, are the primary motivator for learning. In some programs, courses are combined and students receive a single grade ostensibly reflecting performance in both the theory and clinical components. Other programs incorporate contracting between faculty and student into the clinical grade determination (Wiles & Bishop, 2001).

A thorough exploration of the methods of grade calculation, and the theoretical, individual, and organizational problems associated with grading, is beyond the scope of this text. These matters should be a part of faculty discussions and curricular development within nursing programs. Consistency within a nursing program in the approach to grading is desirable; consistency among faculty within each clinical course is essential.

■ TYPES OF FORMAL STUDENT EVALUATION

There are two types of formal evaluation of student performance in the clinical setting: formative and summative. Each type of formal evaluation serves a specific purpose and occurs at a designated point during the course (Bourke & Ihrke, 2005; Jeffries & Norton, 2005).

Formal Formative Evaluation

Formal formative evaluation is a summation of all of the informal evaluative feedback that has been provided up to a given point during the learning process. It would be accurate to say that what has been differentiated in this text as "feedback" could be labeled formative evaluation, because it is provided to students during the course as the student is learning. But in practice, formative evaluation is a more global appraisal of the student's progress toward meeting the objectives of the course that is provided at the midpoint in the course. The evaluative instrument that will be employed at the end of the course is used to present the data. Noting this differentiation is beneficial to faculty and students alike; it provides a demarcation between evaluation during learning (feedback) and evaluation as a progress report (formative). This is a time for the faculty member and student to meet and discuss the student's progress in the course, identify strengths and limitations, distinguish deficiencies, and explore the learning experiences needed during the remainder of the course in order to attain the course outcomes.

Another important purpose of formative evaluation is to give students the opportunity to experience the application of the evaluative tool used in the course. Student performance up to this point is synthesized and formatted to conform to the course evaluation tool. Specific illustrative examples of the student's work should be incorporated to enhance the student's understanding of the data and the conclusions drawn from them. When current data are used for formative evaluation, the distortion of data that can occur over time is avoided (Bourke & Ihrke, 2005).

Faculty and student need to find a quiet time and place to review the formative evaluation and make learning plans for the rest of the term. Suggestions in Chapter 13 for how to phrase feedback to students can be applied to evaluation as well. Formative evaluation should not be seen as being an accurate prediction of the student's ultimate outcome in the course (Bourke & Ihrke, 2005). A student may be making unsatisfactory progress and ultimately succeed in meeting the course objectives, or vice versa. Students need to know this too, lest they become overly discouraged or complacent. The temptation to rush through the formative evaluation experience, given the demands on both faculty and student, should be resisted; in the teaching-learning process, formative evaluation is ultimately far more important than the final course evaluation! Plan sufficient time to fulfill this role well; half an hour is a good general time frame.

Summative Evaluation

Summative evaluation is the student's final clinical evaluation, carried out at the conclusion of the teaching-learning process of the course. All student work should be completed, reviewed by faculty, and incorporated in the summative evaluation. To be meaningful and effective, as with formative evaluation, enough time must be allocated for the summative evaluation. The student's performance is measured against the standards generated from the course objectives as delineated on the evaluation tool. The summative evaluation is also used to determine the student's grade in the course. Strengths and limitations are typically identified in a summative evaluation, but for an entirely different purpose. They are used by students in the teaching-learning processes of subsequent clinical courses or as graduates preparing to enter clinical practice. Students may be encouraged to consider their future academic or career goals based on this evaluation. If a student fails to achieve course objectives at the minimal level required to pass, deficiencies must be clearly delineated. As with formative evaluation, privacy should be assured and adequate time for discussion provided.

▓ FRAMEWORKS FOR EVALUATIVE MEASUREMENT

The frameworks for measurement in educational evaluation are the same ones used in the conduct of referencing measurement in research: norm-referenced and criterion-referenced (Burns & Grove, 2005). These frameworks differ in terms of the referent to which the student's performance is compared. There are also different concerns regarding validity and reliability of instruments derived from each measurement framework. Many of the methods of recording student performance during the clinical experience that are discussed in a subsequent section are incorporated into the actual design format of these instruments. An in-depth discussion of measurement is best provided in a research or instrumentation text; the presentation in this text is intended only as an overview.

Norm-Referenced Measurement

The referent in norm-referenced measurement is a norm group (Burns & Grove, 2005). Applied to clinical evaluation, each student's performance is measured against that of the other students in the clinical group, or the norm for all students in the clinical course, or some standardized norm measure. If evaluation in a clinical group is performed by ranking the students in terms of their relative performance, norm-referenced measurement has been used. The National League for Nursing Achievement Test is one example of a norm-referenced measure (Waltz, Strickland, & Lenz, 1984). The individual student's score derives its meaning when compared to the scores of all of the nursing students who took the test at the time. Other tests, such as the Minnesota Multiphasic Personality Inventory (MMPI) are standardized norm-referenced measures (Burns & Grove, 2005). Standardization is achieved by using data drawn from many thousands of individuals to generate indices such as mean score and standard deviation that are reflective of the population measured. Norm-referenced measurement provides the maximal discrimination between students, so it possesses a high degree of variance and generates a classic bell-shaped curve (Waltz et al., 1984). Because the distribution of scores is symmetrical, the number of students with high scores equals the number of those with low scores, and the potential for course failure is very real. The performance goals in clinical nursing education are drawn from real-world practice expectations rather than the performance of student peer groups. Because of this, norm-referenced measurement is far more useful in research than in clinical education.

Criterion-Referenced Measurement

In criterion-referenced measurement, the referent is the predetermined criterion or performance standard that has been delineated in terms of goal behaviors (Burns & Grove, 2005). This form of measurement is far more suited to clinical nursing education because of the specific cognitive, psychomotor, and affective abilities that are required for nursing practice. "Instruction and evaluation of nursing students in the clinical setting is highly amenable to the use of criterion-referenced measures because of the emphasis placed on the application of knowledge and skills,…what a person is able to do rather than on how the person compares with others" (Waltz et al., 1984, p. 162). These are the reasons for the movement from norm- to criterion-referenced measurement in clinical evaluation, not the oft-presented assumption that this approach reduces subjectivity in evaluation. Subjectivity is not a property of any well-constructed tool; it is intrinsic in the judgments of the user. Those who embrace this assumption (Reising & Devich, 2004) and those who are unable to see the skewed distribution of clinical alphanumeric grades as a function of criterion-referenced measurement (Scanlon & Care, 2004) contribute to the general lack of understanding of the subject of evaluation. Rather than determining that the student's performance is "average" as a norm-referenced measure does, a criterion-referenced tool allows the evaluator to judge clinical performance in relation to standards derived from the course objectives. Used in a wide variety of evaluative research activities, criterion-referenced measures for clinical nursing education have gained credibility over the past four decades and are now the customary approach. For a criterion-referenced tool, the establishment of performance standards is most imperative and necessitates the determination of critical behaviors for each course objective (Waltz et al., 1984). The instrument can be designed from a mastery perspective in which the student either succeeds or fails to demonstrate the specified behaviors. Mastery learning has its place and is commonly used in clinical practice for agency orientation programs or skills review testing. A clinical course in which evaluation results in a pass/fail grade could justifiably use a mastery-based criterion-referenced tool. But such an approach fails to provide the student with guidance or motivation for learning. To accomplish the determination of the degree to which a student's performance approximates the performance standard, the components of the evaluation tool must be especially sensitive and discriminating (Waltz et al., 1984). In order to provide the student with guidance and motivation for learning, and to attain accuracy in awarding alphanumeric grades, the criteria/standards and degrees of attainment must be clearly articulated for both students and faculty. Unfortunately, this is rarely the case (Walsh & Seldomridge, 2005).

Faculty have endeavored to design criterion-referenced tools for the clinical courses they teach, or they have elected to use ready-made instruments with documented validity and reliability indicators. If the latter approach is used, caution must be exercised to assure that the standards used are congruent with the objectives of the course. If faculty develop their own instruments, guidelines for instrument development should be followed, and validity and reliability should always be determined. And, if they chose to use tools developed elsewhere, permission must be obtained, and validity and reliability must be reassessed regardless of whether modifications to the tool are made because of changes in setting and sample (Waltz et al., 1984).

Tools assume a variety of formats and incorporate an array of data sources (see discussion below) depending on the course objectives, the standards that have been established, and the grading system to which the results must be applied. The trend in clinical practice for documentation by exception has been applied to student evaluation in clinical courses in one nursing program, resulting in increased satisfaction in the evaluation process among both students and faculty (Wishnia et al., 2002). Some nursing programs have incorporated a single instrument to be used in clinical courses across the entire curriculum (Reising & Devich, 2004). While this may not be feasible or appropriate for every nursing program, there is value in the use of the same or similar format for all clinical courses within a program; the increased familiarity this approach could produce among the nursing students would likely facilitate both the evaluation process and the student-faculty relationship. Included in the Clinical Toolbox (Chapter 20, pp. 369-370) are examples of standards established for use in a pass/fail and a graded clinical course.

▓ EVALUATIVE DATA SOURCES

Faculty may obtain data from many different sources for use in their formal evaluations. As in nursing research, the process of data triangulation, obtaining data from multiple sources, increases the accuracy of the conclusions drawn (Burns & Grove, 2005). Meaningful input from as many different sources as possible not only enhances the validity of the evaluation, it provides richness and detail to the student's entire learning experience. If a nontraditional model of clinical instruction is being used, all the parties involved in teaching have some role in contributing data for evaluation even if they do not meet with the student and deliver the formal evaluation (see Chapter 3).

Faculty Observations

Although they contribute by far the greatest amount of data to student evaluations in most clinical courses, faculty observations often are not given sufficient

---

BOX 18-2
Evaluative Data Sources

- Faculty observations
- Written assignments
- Student entries in clinical records
- Oral communication
  - With peers
  - With patients
  - With agency personnel
  - With faculty
- Self-evaluations
- Agency personnel

consideration or credibility. Faculty collect observational data on student performance in the clinical setting, from real-time simulations, and from videotaped performances in the LRC. At times, faculty observe completely as nonparticipants; the students' are not even aware they are present. Other times, faculty observe students as active participants in the learning experience, perhaps as they assist in the performance of a skill. Most of the time faculty participate as passive observers, in that students know their faculty are present and watching. In both of these situations, the faculty member's personality and the quality of the relationship with the given student will inevitability affect how the student performs.

As in the conduct of qualitative research, the relationship between observer (faculty) and those observed (students) influences those being observed to some degree (Burns & Grove, 2005). The influence that student awareness of faculty presence has on performance can be significant. Simply by being present, faculty can change student behavior; in qualitative research, this is considered a source of bias (Burns & Grove, 2005). Students also have "bad days" when their performance is impacted by factors beyond their control, rendering their performance "atypical." The accuracy of faculty judgments about student performance under both of these circumstances is considered suspect; this supports the concern of faculty and students about the fairness of evaluation. Faculty can address this concern in two fashions: (1) faculty observations are distilled into patterns of performance and (2) faculty ultimately make their judgments from data collected from multiple sources. When a student is calculating the dosage of a drug as faculty directly observe, feedback is provided. If the student repeatedly makes the same type of error, or consistently makes errors of many types, faculty can justifiably conclude the student's math calculation skills are inadequate and problematic. If the student also demonstrates difficulties in medication calculation on written tests, as well as when observed by staff, the conclusion of student ineptitude is further validated. Establishing patterns of student behavior and using multiple data sources provide further support for fairness in evaluation.

For the most part, faculty observations tend to be of an unstructured nature. Unstructured observations are most amenable to situations when faculty assume some participant role (Waltz et al., 1984). In unstructured observation, there is no prior planning, and observations are made spontaneously without consideration of what will be the specific focus (Burns & Grove, 2005). The flexibility and spontaneity of unstructured observations must be balanced with the potential randomness of the data obtained. Unable to attend to everything going on at the time, novice faculty especially may be left with no real usable data. Establishing at least a minimal amount of structure in advance will ultimately result in more valuable data from observations (Burns & Grove, 2005). When the focus is shared in advance with the student, this approach also can do a great deal to assuage performance anxiety (Bourke & Ihrke, 2005). Observations of videotapes or skill performance in the LRC tend to have the most structure. But even in busy clinical settings, determining that the focus of the observation is to be the student's cardiovascular assessment or the determination of a patient's risk for falling allows a more targeted appraisal and results in better data collection. Serendipitous data can be tremendously helpful, but without an original focus, it simply does not exist!

Written Assignments and Student Documentation in Clinical Records

Students' written work provides a significant amount of data that can be used for formal evaluations. The written feedback provided on assignments should be summarized, its relationship to course objectives and specific behavioral standards noted, and then recorded for later inclusion in formal evaluations, specifically formative ones. Data from students' reflective journals should not be used because the purpose of this assignment is to enhance students' self-awareness; but it could be included in a general fashion by way of discussing the students' critical thinking skills and insight if this has been made clear to students in advance (see discussion regarding evaluation of reflective journaling in Chapter 15).

In many clinical courses, students document their assessments, care, and evaluations of that care in patient records. Routine feedback is provided to assist the students' learning and guide the development of documentation skills. When formal evaluations are provided, the students' progress (formative) and achievement of (summative) performance standards related to documentation should be included. Again, faculty must maintain records of the routine feedback provided with applicable examples.

Oral Communication

Students' oral communication skills are routinely addressed in clinical course objectives. Feedback should be appropriately provided as part of learning experiences, and then summarized for formal evaluations. Progress toward the established behavior standards for oral communication should be included in formative evaluations, and their achievement should be included in the summative ones.

Data related to student communication abilities with peers, patients, agency personnel, and faculty are all important elements that should be included in formal evaluations. The student's oral communication with peers can be noted during group learning experiences (clinical conferences) and in the clinical setting. Communication with patients is integral to successful clinical practice and justifiably receives the most attention in student evaluations. As with observations, these data are often inaccurate reflections of the students' actual abilities if obtained when faculty are present during the exchanges. If it is at all possible to listen in on some student-patient discussions, including instances of patient teaching, this information can be used to correct or validate other data collected when faculty are present. It is essential faculty tell students and agency personnel in advance if this technique is to be used. Students' oral communication with agency personnel is an important contribution to their developing relationships with each other and a harbinger of how they will function with colleagues in their eventual practice. And finally, the students' communication with faculty provide evaluative data that are important. Usually verbal exchanges with faculty are examined in relation to their content (e.g., the students' critical thinking skills, safety assessments, and understanding and application of theory) and applied to the appropriate standards. For objectives related specifically to communication skills, oral communication with faculty can be evaluated according to standards of clarity, accuracy, and timeliness.

Student Self-Evaluations

In accordance with adult learning theories, cognitive learning theories, humanism (caring), and postmodern schools of educational thought, students should have the opportunity to take an active role in their entire learning process, including the evaluation of their performance. Self-evaluation is an important skill for practicing nurses, and students can learn and refine their skills through clinical practice courses. Students' self-evaluations can become increasingly insightful and accurate over the course of the nursing program when they have been provided beforehand with some structure to guide the process and feedback from faculty to assist them in learning.

Ideally, students should evaluate their performance as it relates to the course objectives and the established standards on a weekly basis and use the results, combined with faculty feedback, to guide their future learning experiences in the course. Having been introduced to the formal evaluative instrument at the onset of the course, and practiced weekly self-evaluation, students are well prepared to contribute to both formative and summative evaluations. If these are submitted to the faculty in advance, the student's input can be incorporated into the faculty-prepared evaluation or appended to it. Advanced knowledge of the student's perspective also can serve to alert faculty of potential areas of discordance prior to meeting with the student. Following the formal formative and summative evaluation meetings, students should be provided with a copy of the completed tool either as a matter of policy or upon request. Legally, a student's signature on the evaluation tool conveys only that it has been read; agreement or disagreement is not acknowledged.

Often evaluative tools are designed to include a section set aside for student response to the faculty evaluation. The purpose of this is very different than the student's self-evaluation. It provides an outlet for the student's rebuttal or concurrence with what has been written by the faculty. However, students are not significantly contributing to their evaluation if this is the only opportunity they have to comment on the evaluation. At the moment, in the glow of a positive evaluation or the angst of one that is perceived as less so, what the student writes has little meaning or value and reflects little concerted thought. If a student is distressed by the evaluation and/or the accompanying grade, the student should be directed to the grievance procedure outlined in the student handbook (see Chapter 8).

In the search for additional mechanisms by which students can contribute to formal evaluations, creative approaches are being explored in the literature.

For instance, Clark, Owen, and Tholcken (2004) designed, tested, and published a scale for measuring student perceptions of their clinical competence. Using Bandura's self-efficacy theory related to efficacy expectations as the theoretical framework, these faculty designed a scale for student self-report of their level of confidence with and interpretation of the importance of specific items drawn from the course objectives. The data obtained for individual students were used in formative evaluations, and aggregate data results supplemented evaluation of the course by faculty.

Agency Personnel

General information regarding the preparation of agency personnel for students' arrival is presented in Chapter 9. The staff in the clinical agency spend a considerable amount of time working closely with students, often more so than faculty. Their contribution to student evaluations can be tremendously valuable. However, in order for the data to be meaningful, faculty must supply them with direction regarding the course expectations, what data to collect, and how to document student performance.

Staff need to know what the expectations are for the level of student in the course. Expectations of students in their first clinical course are understandably quite different that those of students nearing completion of a program of study. Delineation of clear expectations is especially important if students from more than one program or at differing levels of a program in the agency are being evaluated at the same time. Agency staff also can find the beginning of a term to be quite challenging in terms of student evaluation because the performance stage of the students who have just completed the course will be upper most in their minds. This could set the stage for an unfair comparison of the beginning students.

Usefulness of the evaluative data provided by various agency personnel is increased when a single approach to documentation is followed. Content will differ with the course and whether the personnel are registered nurses or other staff (e.g., social workers, dietitians, volunteers, day care workers). The approach should allow for rapid recording; checklists or scales are best, with an area on the form for the inclusion of optional narrative data. Although critical incident recordings can result in excellent data, the process is too time consuming for routine use. Personnel should sign the form so that follow-up or clarification can be obtained. Faculty will have to determine whether orientation to the form is necessary or whether the directions for its use are sufficiently clear to assure quality data.

As useful as their input is, agency staff will likely tire of providing feedback if it is requested too frequently or if one person must give information regarding several students at a time. The quality of the data often will be affected adversely in such circumstances. One approach to this conundrum is sampling—occasionally choosing a day when agency input is obtained for all students. Whoever is working most closely with a student should be asked to provide the data; this will increase the accuracy of the information obtained.

If students choose who to ask for an evaluation, they will naturally ask the person they believe will give the most positive information; this will skew the data and make it less representative of the students' performances.

RECORDING DATA

To be most meaningful, data should be recorded systematically, at the time it is collected (during clinical time) or as soon afterward as possible (Burns & Grove, 2005). This can be a very time-consuming process; however, there are some approaches that are more time-efficient but still help maintain the accuracy of the data. These formats are most commonly paper and pencil recording methods, but technologic advances also have impacted faculty record-keeping. Handheld computers are being used to increase the accuracy of clinical documentation (Lehman, 2003). The basic software provided by the manufacturer allows writing and editing entries much like the larger notebook, laptop, and desktop computers. Additional facilitative software programs are available online, often free of charge (www.PalmGear.com and www.handmark.com). Lehman (2003) emphasizes other beneficial features of handheld computers including sizable memory (roughly 8 megabytes); the ability to back up and preserve data on larger home computer systems; availability of reference software such as drug manuals (www.ePocrates.com); currency, legibility, and consistency of documentation; and portability (weight about 6 ounces and pocket-size).

Anecdotal Notes

The quickly jotted notations of clinical observations must later be "fleshed out" as anecdotal notes to add detail and specificity to the data. This step is essential to the validity of observational data. The detail provided by quality anecdotal notes can be used to provide instructive examples for students in their formal evaluations. To facilitate data organization in the clinical setting, faculty may consider preparing a weekly template for each student listing the course objectives and providing space below each one for notations. This can help to jog the memory when notes are later transcribed. Such a template also increases validity by providing consistent documentation among students. Anecdotal notes should always be used, but other recording devices also can be used (Tomey, 2000). Chapter 8 provides a more detailed discussion of anecdotal note-taking.

Checklists

Checklists document that a skill was performed, an objective met, or a behavior observed (Tomey, 2000; Bourke & Ihrke, 2005; Burns & Grove, 2005). They can be designed to record the frequency of a specified observation or when the requisite steps in the performance of a skill have been acceptably carried out. For a norm-referenced evaluation instrument and/or a course culminating in a pass/fail grade, a checklist approach for documentation is sufficient because the level of performance beyond satisfactory is immaterial. However, during formative evaluation, a student would be told only what has and has not been accomplished; how close the student may be to achieving the standards would

Date: _____		
Student: _____		
Course objective: Promotes patient safety		
Sample Standards	**Observed**	**Comments**
Administers medications according to the Five Rights		
Performs a safety assessment		
Notifies staff/faculty of changes in patient status that may impact safety		

FIGURE 18-1 ▪ Example of a documentation checklist.

not be determined by using a checklist only. A comment column can be added for quick notations that can be converted later into anecdotal notes. A scale also can be incorporated in order to quantify the quality of the performance.

Scales

Scales offer more sensitive data than the usual dichotomous data provided by a checklist (Burns & Grove, 2005). Both checklists and rating scales can be used to judge experiential outcomes (Waltz et al., 1984). They can also both be employed by an external evaluator (i.e., faculty or staff) or for student self-evaluation. Scales can be created for most cognitive, psychomotor, and affective skills as long as the requisite standards can be clearly described. There are several types of scales, but they are all composed of clinical standards paired with some form of graduated measurement scale. The degree to which the student's performance approximates each standard is determined and marked on the scale. When this approach is used to design a criterion-referenced clinical course evaluation instrument, the resulting discrimination can provide the basis for an alphanumeric course grade.

Likert scales are the most commonly used scaling technique (Burns & Grove, 2005) and are highly amenable to recording data for use in clinical evaluation. Scales are usually composed of four to six levels of quality. The quality descriptors used must be clear to the evaluator and often are defined on the form. As in the documentation of patient care, terms such as "good" and "well" are insufficiently accurate descriptors without definitions as to the intended interpretation. The extreme anchor points on the scale are typically some derivative of unsatisfactory and exceptional, with the labels of points between them connoting degrees of accomplishment. In this case, midpoint on the scale would denote satisfactory (passing) attainment of the standard. Columns are often added to track behaviors not observed, times when insufficient data are available to make a qualitative judgment or specific aspects are deemed as inadequate or stellar. When recording is done for the purpose of providing weekly feedback and compiling information for formative evaluations, scale results can provide valuable guidance for student learning. Progression and patterns of performance can be identified; consideration can be given to the following aspects of learning:

- Approximation to the standard
- Quality of performance
- Assistance required

The other common approaches to scaling are semantic differentials and visual analogue scales. They also can be theoretically adapted for use in recording data for clinical evaluation, but they are self-report tools so could be used only by students in self-evaluation. Semantic differentials, originally developed for the measurement of attitudes and beliefs, are now often used in research for the measurement of various interpretations of concepts (Waltz et al., 1984; Burns & Grove, 2005). Using bipolar adjectives as anchors for a continuum (e.g., good/bad, positive/negative, active/passive), the respondent selects a position

Competency delineations used in evaluation:

- Independent (I)
- Requires supervision (S)
- Requires assistance (A)
- Marginal (M)
- Dependent (D) No/insufficient data (ND)

Course objective: Critically analyzes and applies relevant research, theories, and concepts from the professional literature in the practice of leadership and management in nursing.

Sample Standard	I	S	A	M	D	ND
Applies relevant findings in the conduct of supervisory role in the given clinical setting. Comments:						

FIGURE 18-2 ■ Example of documentation with a Likert scale. (Adapted from Bondy, K.N. [1983]. Criterion-referenced definitions for rating scales in clinical evaluation. *Journal of Nursing Education, 22*, 376-382.)

from 5 to 7 scaled steps between the extremes. Visual analogue (magnitude) scales use a design format similar to that of semantic differentials. The maximal and minimal levels or degrees of the concept form the anchors (e.g., no shortness of breath/greatest possible shortness of breath) and the respondent marks a point along a 100-mm continuum line. The resulting measurement of the distance from the left anchor to the marked response provides data that are more finely discriminated than can be obtained with semantic differentials (Burns & Grove, 2005).

▨ DEALING WITH HUMAN RANDOM AND SYSTEMATIC ERROR

The accuracy (validity) and consistency (reliability) of evaluation are affected by the potential for error. Attempts are made to control these errors during the design of the evaluation tools, but error also can occur due to factors external to the instruments themselves. These types of errors serve as grounds for student complaints of unfairness in evaluation. There are actions faculty can take to reduce these errors and their impact on the quality of student clinical evaluations.

Random errors in evaluation occur inconsistently and unpredictably and can impact reliability by tainting the observations at the time (Waltz et al., 1984). For example, if a clinical faculty member has a headache or a cold or is taking antihistamines for allergies, random error can occur. Or a student's performance today may be different than it was yesterday or will be tomorrow due to anxiety, illness, or even ambient temperature and time of day! The existence of possible random error supports the sampling approach to data collection, the examination of the data for patterns of performance, and the use of multiple data sources.

Systematic error primarily affects validity and is the degree to which the evaluative tool measures standards or objectives other than those for which it was intended (Burns & Grove, 2005). Systematic error in the use of a tool occurs when data collection is biased in a way that does not change during repeated observations and data recordings. There are two sources of human systematic error in clinical evaluation. This type of error may be a reflection of the underlying attitudes, beliefs, and values of an individual evaluator. Beliefs related to gender, age, ethnicity, or physical or mental health might even subtly affect how student performance is viewed. If a clinical faculty believes men simply do not make good nurses, the validity of the data recorded about their performance is suspect because of systematic error. This form of systematic error can result in bestowing "halos or horns" on students when they do not actually exist (Tomey, 2000). Consciously bringing potential sources of bias to the foreground will allow faculty to make concerted efforts to address and control them. The other source of systematic error occurs when there are inconsistencies between the clinical faculty in a single course in terms of how the objectives or standards are interpreted. This is an especially important issue when student clinical evaluation requires discrimination in terms of levels of performance. There are also methods to reduce this source of human systematic error. All faculty involved in a clinical course can benefit from group norming activities. Using the evaluation tool and examples of data collected using the recording tools employed by faculty in the course, each course objective and accompanying standards can be discussed. Does the standard requiring conforming to the five rights in the administration of medications include proper documentation? If not, where is this aspect of the safety objective addressed? For forms of clinical performance documentation and evaluation tools that discriminate between levels of performance, what does each level look like? Is it possible to create a grading rubric that would be beneficial to both faculty and students? Both of these approaches can reduce systematic error and help to make student clinical evaluations more fair.

▓ LEGAL AND ETHICAL ISSUES OF CLINICAL EVALUATION AND GRADING

Ethically as well as legally, faculty teaching clinical courses are obligated to endeavor to be fair and just in evaluating their students' performance (Scanlan, Care, & Gessler, 2001). Issues related to due process, unsafe clinical performance, and failing students have been addressed elsewhere in this text (Chapter 8). As with other aspects related to teaching and learning, the quality of the relationship between teacher and student is integral to effective evaluation. Both students and faculty must be clear about when formal evaluations are to occur, what data sources are to be used, and how data will be collected and recorded. Concerted faculty efforts to identify and control bias and other sources of error likewise support fairness and justice in clinical evaluations. Facilitating active student involvement in the process, obtaining data from multiple sources, and using methods to record data that retain accuracy also contribute to the provision of evaluations that are fair, equitable, and meaningful.

BOX 18-3

Activities to Enhance Fairness in Evaluation

- Establish and maintain open, trusting student-faculty relationships
- Understand the course objectives and standards
- Fully inform the students on the following aspects of evaluation:
  - Explain the subjectivity of evaluation
  - Describe how fairness will be attained
  - Explain the meaning of course objectives and standards
  - Review the course evaluation tool (allow discussion and questions)
  - Inform as to when, where, and how evaluative data will be collected
  - Explain the basis of grading
- Provide quality feedback
- Encourage student participation in evaluation
- Apply course standards equally and consistently
- Avoid comparing one student's performance to others
- Use multiple sources for evaluative data
- Sample data and analyze for performance patterns
- Perform a self-assessment for sources of bias
- Participate in faculty group activities to facilitate interfaculty consistency in evaluation

SUMMARY

Formal evaluation in clinical courses is derived from students' patterns of performance as they progress toward and attain the course objectives. Everything faculty know about themselves, their students, teaching and learning, their nursing programs' curriculum, and the clinical course they are teaching culminate in this final aspect of the teaching-learning process. Formal summative evaluation of student attainment of learning outcomes meets curricular and accreditation requirements and guides the grading required by society and academic institutions. But these are all of secondary importance; formal clinical evaluations contribute to the preparation of tomorrow's nurses. Practicing nurses establish goals for their professional growth and determine benchmarks for measuring their progress. As they participate in their clinical evaluations in the academic setting, students are learning the content and process of evaluation that they will continue to apply in practice. Even as we evaluate, we teach!

REFLECTION EXERCISE 18

Reflecting on Evaluation

Think back to your experiences with formal evaluation during your initial nursing education. Most likely specifics have faded, but the emotions linger. Reflect on those feelings.

◆ What were they generally?

◆ Can you recall differences in how you felt in different clinical courses? What evoked these differing responses? Was it related to the approach of the faculty? Your feelings about the course? Your feelings about being evaluated? Something else?

◆ What actions on the part of the faculty would have made evaluation a more positive experience? Consider how you might use this knowledge as you assume a clinical faculty role.

A source of systematic error in evaluation is the attitudes, beliefs, and values of the faculty member. Spend some time and effort critically examining yours about people in general and nurses specifically in relation to age, gender, ethnicity (especially the case of English being a second language), size (height and weight, especially overweight/obesity), mental and physical disability or illness (depression, bipolar, OCD, attention deficient disorders, eating disorders, diabetes, epilepsy, asthma, and histories of alcohol or drug abuse are most common).

◆ What expectations would you have about these people's performance? How might that impact how you evaluate them? What can you do differently during evaluation in light of your clarification experience?

References

Bourke, M.P., & Ihrke, B.A. (2005). The evaluation process: An overview. In D.M. Billings & J.A. Halstead (Eds.), *Teaching in nursing: A guide for faculty* (2nd ed.). (pp. 443-464). Philadelphia: Saunders.

Burns, N., & Grove, S.K. (2005). *The practice of nursing research: Conduct, critique, and utilization* (5th ed.). Philadelphia: Saunders.

Clark, M.C., Owen, S.V., & Tholcken, M.A. (2004). Measuring student perceptions of clinical competence. *Journal of Nursing Education, 43*(12), 548-554.

Jeffries, P.R., & Norton, B. (2005). Selecting learning experiences to achieve curriculum outcomes. In D.M. Billings & J.A. Halstead (Eds.), *Teaching in nursing: A guide for faculty* (2nd ed.). (pp. 187-212). Philadelphia: Saunders.

Lehman, K. (2003). Clinical nursing instructors' use of handheld computers for student recordkeeping and evaluation. *Journal of Nursing Education, 42*(1), 41-42.

Reising, D.L., & Devich, L.E. (2004). Comprehensive practicum evaluation across a nursing program. *Nursing Education Perspectives, 25*(3), 114-116.

Scanlan, J.M., & Care, W.D. (2004). Grade inflation: Should be we concerned? *Journal of Nursing Education, 43*(10), 475-478.

Scanlan, J.M., Care, W.D., & Gessler, S. (2001). Dealing with the unsafe student in clinical practice. *Nurse Educator, 26*(1), 23-27.

Tanner, C.A. (2004). Practical issues in measurement and evaluation. *Journal of Nursing Education, 43*(10), 435.

Tomey, A.M. (2000). Testing techniques: Performance assessment. *Nurse Educator, 25*(2), 59-60, 98.

Walsh, C.M., & Seldomridge, L.A. (2005). Clinical grades: Upward bound. *Journal of Nursing Education, 44*(4), 162-168.

Waltz, C.F., Strickland, O., & Lenz, E.R. (1984). *Measurement in nursing research*. Philadelphia: F.A. Davis.

Wiles, L.L., & Bishop, J.F. (2001). Clinical performance appraisal: Renewing graded clinical experiences. *Journal of Nursing Education, 40*(1), 37-39.

Wishnia, G.S., Yancy, P., Silva, J., & Kern-Manwaring, N. (2002). Evaluation by exception for nursing students. *Journal of Nursing Education, 41*(11), 495-497.

Zuzelo, P.R. (2000). Clinical probation: Supporting the at-risk student. *Nurse Educator, 25*(5), 216-218.

CHAPTER 19

The Teacher as Student: Evaluation and Career Development

The academic term grows to a close. Final evaluative student conferences are completed; institutional grades have been submitted; notes of appreciation have been sent to the clinical agencies. As the students progress to their next clinical course or graduate and enter nursing practice, the time has arrived for teachers-as-students to evaluate their own performance as clinical faculty and consider future opportunities for growth. This chapter explores these topics; reflection exercises are imbedded within the text to assist in their unique application for each individual faculty member.

The development of teachers is a recursive pursuit (McKeachie, 2002). Even the most experienced teacher needs to continue to learn. In nursing education, "signal change is all around us, defining not only what we teach, but also how we teach our students" (Heller, Oros, & Durney-Crowley, 2004). "Teachability" should be innate in teachers. Teachability, says John C. Maxwell (1999), is a striving to grow, learn, and perfect one's craft, regardless of vocation. As a trait of clinical faculty, teachability drives development as a teacher and fuels a continual enthusiasm for the profession. For teachers, there is no true terminal goal, no real summative evaluation. Evaluating teaching is inseparable from learning how to improve teaching, and there are many sources of input to tap and resources to explore. But to begin with, novice clinical faculty must determine the goals to which they aspire.

ACADEMIC CAREER DEVELOPMENT

Once the decision is made to remain in academia, each nursing faculty member must consider the trajectory that academic career will take. Several options are available, but they are not all available at every academic institution. The personal fit of every potential avenue should be considered, because each route will differ in terms of requirements and opportunities. These will then govern decisions regarding professional practice development, academic and continuing education, and development as a clinical educator. The requisite for doctoral education for some of these options is a key factor to be considered.

As presented in Chapter 1, depending on the degrees offered and the mission of the institution, several choices for a career in academia are available. Instructors who want to work in academia only part-time while remaining in clinical practice may have no options other than term or yearly appointments that offer no opportunity for further academic career advancement. As full-time instructors, faculty may be offered longer renewable, temporary appointments that last several years and include the possibility of advancing in rank, such as to the level of Senior Instructor.

Many nursing programs now offer *clinical-track* appointments with accompanying ranks and requirements (Assistant, Associate, and Full Professor). These positions may allow the selection of a less than full-time appointment. In addition to teaching obligations, usually in clinical courses, clinical-track appointments also involve scholarship productivity expectations and service responsibilities to the academic institution and the larger practice communities at regional, state, and/or national levels. The amount of time allocated for clinical practice and the term of appointment vary. Associate and/or Full Professor ranks may require doctoral education, and expectations for scholarly productivity typically increase as well. Master's education has been described as a personal and professional evolution through the enhancement of values and attitudes initially attained at the baccalaureate educational level (Cragg & Andrusyszyn, 2005). Doctoral education leads not only to even more career options but also to changes of a truly radical nature in one's view of the world–in general and in nursing. Routinely, the other avenue for an academic career is a *tenure-track* position. Again, requirements for appointment vary, especially in terms of academic degrees. Expectations for teaching, service, and scholarship can differ markedly, based on the institution's mission. Many tenure-track appointments provide little if any release time for clinical practice, so if faculty desire to continue to practice, it must be done during weekends or academic breaks. The American Association of University Professors (AAUP) addressed the major aspects of tenure in their 1940 document "Statement of Principles on Academic Freedom and Tenure," which is reproduced in the "Clinical Toolbox" (see Chapter 20, p. 317).

Appointments in which research is the primary role expectation (research scientist) are available at a few institutions, usually those designated as Carnegie Research–extensive. These positions are offered to academics with well developed and funded programs of research.

To help clarify what direction to take an academic career, consider what primary emphasis in addition to teaching is most desirable to personally, —that of scholar, that of practitioner, or some combination of teacher-scholar-practitioner. Making this decision will facilitate the selection of the type of academic institution to aspire to and will identify what additional education or other preparation will be required. Talk to colleagues about their decisions, and listen to their stories. Consider what brings joy and challenge professionally and how the other aspects of your personal life will fit best into the big picture of a career in academia.

REFLECTION EXERCISE 19

Academic Career Development

Take the time to seriously consider where you want your professional and personal lives to be in 10 years. Once these goals are clearer, work backwards to create a timeline that can serve as a career development roadmap. Nothing is set in stone; reexamine your goals, timeline, and progress annually. Use the following questions to help guide your thinking:

- Do you want to remain, at least part-time, in academia?
- What role, in addition to teacher, is most attractive to you: practitioner, scholar, or practitioner-scholar?
- What are your goals for your personal life outside of your career?
- Are there others whose life plans also need to be considered (e.g., spouse, significant other, children, parents)?
- How do you feel about pursuing doctoral education?
- Are you open to moving to another location to pursue your career and/or education?
- Has talking with colleagues in academia shed new light on your options? If so, how?

PROFESSIONAL PRACTICE DEVELOPMENT

Regardless of what decision is made about academic career development, as long as teaching clinical courses is a part of their role, faculty must consider how to maintain currency and relevance in professional practice. Clinical faculty are on the cutting edge of practice, in touch with the technology, changing roles and expectations in nursing, and health care trends. It is not possible to maintain this connection only by teaching clinical courses. How clinical competency and currency are to be maintained is often hotly debated among faculty, with strong personal biases and assumptions forming the foundations of such arguments. Academic institutions also may have specifically delineated expectations of faculty in this area.

Some faculty sustain and enhance their clinical knowledge and skills while supplementing their academic salaries by practicing nursing part-time during the academic term (e.g., weekends and breaks), or for longer blocks of time between terms. Certainly with the evolution of nursing practice, graduate nurses will need new knowledge and skills, but the elements of assessment, communication, time management, and clinical judgment are in no danger of becoming obsolete. Clinical practice has the added advantage of helping faculty stay in touch with how it feels to be a staff nurse (Didham, 2003), which is beneficial to continued teambuilding efforts in clinical agencies. Maintaining clinical practice in some form may be required for faculty by the academic program.

At the very least, faculty should be routinely reading relevant nursing practice journals and attending clinically based continuing education programs whenever possible. Release time and funding are significant barriers for faculty wishing to attend continuing education programs and conferences. These issues are the source of a great deal of frustration for nursing faculty who both want and need to learn. Some nursing programs offer reduced enrollment costs or educational funds to assist with the expenses incurred when attending continuing education programs or conferences, especially if these are required for maintaining certifications. Faculty can access a wide range of journals through the library at the academic institution or the clinical agencies. Many publications are available in print and also online, and others are only accessible electronically. Online nursing discussion groups can be a stimulating and thought-provoking approach to include in the clinical faculty's armamentarium of professional practice development choices.

Ultimately, the impetus for "…personal growth and development come(s) from within. Personal professional growth is not defined, imposed, demanded, or actualized through external authority" (Dyer & Fontaine, 1995, p. 28). Maxwell's (1999) teachability maxim is integral to professional practice development. Clearly, if faculty truly want to excel in teaching clinical courses tomorrow, they must be teachable today.

REFLECTION EXERCISE 20

Professional Practice Development

Didham (2003) addresses the need for nurse educators to reflect on nursing and their own nursing practice to provide guidance for their teaching. She suggests the answers to the following questions be considered to begin this process:

◆ "What do I value about being a nurse?

◆ How would I define my own nursing practice?

◆ What messages do I transmit to my students, knowingly and unknowingly, about the practice of nursing?" (p. 485).

To provide focus on professional practice development, reflect on these questions:

◆ What aspects of professional practice peak your interest?

◆ Is maintaining expertise in the clinical setting while working in academia an attractive choice? If so, where and how might you accomplish this?

◆ What nursing practice publications are most applicable to your clinical teaching focus? Where can you access them? Create a plan for reading that would facilitate currency in your knowledge base (e.g., go to the school's library one evening a month to read the latest issues).

◆ What options for practice-focused continuing education/conferences are available to you (e.g., subject matter, location, cost)? What resources are available to make these possible (i.e., funding, travel assistance)?

▨ CLINICAL EDUCATOR DEVELOPMENT

All too often even those faculty who have taught clinical courses for many years believe that maintaining their clinical practice knowledge and skills are sufficient to being good clinical nursing teachers. They focus on reading a few practice-related journals and attending the occasional practice-related continuing education program, while totally ignoring the need to develop as a teacher. This is an even more pressing concern given the number of faculty teaching clinical courses who have had no formal preparation in education to begin with. Most nursing faculty are less prepared in the theoretical bases of education than kindergarten teachers! This blind spot in faculty development cannot continue to be perpetuated if the scholarship of nursing education is to become visible and curricular innovation is to continue. The ever-shortening half-life of knowledge and the changing health care system dictate nurse educators' continued learning in order to revolutionize clinical education (Yoder-Wise, 2000; Tanner, 2002). Not only must faculty be open to the new developments within the nursing discipline, they must also be attuned to the emerging knowledge regarding teaching and learning (McKeachie, 2002). Maintaining (or developing) currency in the practice of teaching, refining techniques, and expanding theoretical knowledge in both nursing education and higher education are essential (Neese, 2003).

The development of scholarly teaching begins when nursing faculty examine their teaching effectiveness, move to expand their teaching knowledge base, and progress toward contributing to the curriculum; these actions culminate ultimately in faculty making valuable contributions to the educational knowledge base that is drawn from this process (Allen & Field, 2005). An aspiration to be a scholarly teacher should be a part of the novice clinical faculty member's overall career plan.

In a position statement issued in 2001, the National League for Nursing addressed the complexity and multiple facets of lifelong learning for nursing faculty. Responding to the limited numbers of faculty with knowledge of teaching and learning principles, recommendations were provided for both faculty and institutional administrators. One of the topic areas specifically identified was clinical teaching and evaluation. The resources available to assist faculty in the development of the education aspect of their clinical nursing educator role are significant. Beginning with an individual self-assessment, the trek includes collecting input from students and colleagues, reading educational literature from other relevant disciplines as well as nursing, and attending conferences devoted to educational development.

▓ REFLECTING ON TEACHING

Honest self-appraisal is the starting point for the process of cultivating the skills of clinical teaching (Lichtman et al., 2003). Using this skill, faculty begin to learn how to teach by learning from their own teaching (Neese, 2003). In the "About This Book" section of this text, the reader is encouraged to begin the journaling process, incorporating personal reflection and thoughts about the exercises provided and recording clinical teaching stories. The intent of this journaling experience is to encourage systematic and critical reflection on assumptions, thoughts, and experiences to assist in learning from the teaching experience. The dilemmas, disappointments, and victories that arise in teaching provide occasions for reflection and professional growth (Shellenbarger, Palmer, Labant, & Kuzneski, 2005). The accuracy and consistency of self-assessment improves with practice (like any skill!). The reflective process can help to identify learning needs (Westberg & Jason, 2001). Making oneself open to self-assessment is a basic requirement to learning about teaching (Neese, 2003). Solitary reflection allows faculty to scrutinize their teaching and query themselves, during and following their teaching experiences. Used for formative reflection, questions such as "what happened?" "so what?" and "now what?" guide the clinical faculty, whereas summative reflection focuses more on what can be improved or done differently (Shellenbarger et al., 2005). If used alone, solitary journaling in regard to teaching and reflection are inadequate because they expose only one facet of teaching; at the same time, journal reflections can expose elements not accessible by any other means.

REFLECTION EXERCISE 21

Reflecting on Teaching—Self-Assessment

Read through the notations made in your teaching journal, or think back over the past term. With the following questions as a guide, certain experiences will be especially meaningful in contributing to and directing growth as a teacher. * *Record responses in order to clarify them and have them available for future reference.*

◆ What teaching experiences resulted in moments of pure joy in teaching, times of engagement with students and affirmation as a teacher? Were there commonalities that characterized them?

◆ What teaching experiences made you feel inadequately prepared or anxious? Reflect on these, and see whether you can extract areas requiring further growth from them.

◆ With the benefit of your learning to this point, what things would you do differently as a clinical teacher?

As honestly as possible, complete the following statements*:

◆ The most important thing I've learned about nursing students is...

◆ The most important thing I've learned about teaching is...

◆ The most important thing I've learned about myself is...

◆ The assumptions I had regarding teaching and learning that have been confirmed are...

◆ The assumptions I had regarding teaching and learning that have been challenged are...

◆ Now, I wonder about...

◆ And, now I want to know (more) about...

Think analytically about these questions, again recording your responses†

◆ "Do I want to be a teacher?"

◆ How can I become a better teacher?

◆ What kind of teacher do I need to become?" (p. 486).

*Adapted from Brookfield, S.D. (1995). *Becoming a critically reflective teacher.* San Francisco: Jossey-Bass.
†From Didham, P. (2003). From the tower into the trenches: A nurse educator's reflections on the knowledge of experience. *Journal of Nursing Education, 42*(11), 485-487. Reprinted with permission from SLACK Incorporated.

▓ SEEING TEACHING THROUGH STUDENTS' EYES

"Students can be valuable learning resources if educators are willing to listen" (Neese, 2003, p. 261). Examining teaching through the lens of students' perspectives allows faculty to tap into how students experience the teaching-learning process (Brookfield, 1995). If we truly want to grow as teachers and make nursing education responsive to the changes ahead, it will take more than a refocus on nursing education research; it is essential that we listen to our students' stories about their educational experiences (Fitzpatrick, 2005). Typically, the only expression of the students' perspectives made available to faculty are the results of evaluations mandated by the academic institution. These are insufficient in providing information about the effects of teaching and areas needing growth, and the information they provide may in fact be an inaccurate reflection of the clinical learning experience. Collected at the conclusion of a course and therefore only summative in nature, these evaluations are often nothing more than indexes of student satisfaction (Brookfield, 1995). Educational research has substantiated that students can indeed determine whether they are learning; therefore, if tools are well designed, student ratings are valid (McKeachie, 2002). Interestingly, it also has been determined that, unless the course is simply too difficult for the students, challenging courses tend to receive higher ratings (McKeachie, 2002). But even as summative evaluations, the data generated by these tools are inadequate in their representation of teaching effectiveness. "Teaching is an art. Consequently, it should be judged as other art forms— for the passion and beauty of the performance and the meaningfulness of the message conveyed" (Fitzpatrick, 2004, p. 109). Measures of student satisfaction, how much they liked faculty, "leave us in the dark regarding the dynamics and rhythms of their learning" (Brookfield, 1995, p. 93).

In order to obtain input from students about teaching, faculty must build on the value of feedback and evaluation in learning that they have instilled. Clinical faculty provide students with informal and formal evaluation as they learn to be nurses; students should be encouraged to provide faculty with informal and formal evaluation as they learn to be more effective teachers. Within the student-faculty relationship, and the ideal of a caring environment in nursing education, mutual growth and development is valued. Students should know that their faculty want to grow, as do they, and that meaningful evaluation facilitates that process. This is a reflection of authenticity in the relationship. The same suggestions for providing feedback to students (Chapter 13) should be given to students as an aid in evaluating their faculty: timeliness, specificity, and balance. Excellence in nursing education is found in faculty and students working and learning together, listening to one another (Ironside, 2005). Learning to provide quality evaluation is a part of developing the professional nursing role.

Institutional evaluations may address the course and its content, the presentation and teaching of the faculty, or both. Course evaluations are useful for curricular assessment; teacher evaluations are routinely used for administrative decisions related to salary, retention, and tenure. Valid and reliable instruments are hard to find. Because of the way the tools are designed, students are often unclear as to what they are evaluating—the course or the teacher. Some academic institutions even use a single format for evaluation throughout all disciplines, believing that the results will permit comparisons of teaching effectiveness in a chemistry class to that in an English class. The deficiencies in this assumption are clear: although there are commonalities, there are stark differences best addressed in evaluations with at least some discipline-specific items. Even if an evaluation tool is developed for use within a given nursing program, it often is not amenable for use in clinical courses. What faculty teaching clinical nursing courses need are evaluation tools that permit student evaluation regarding their teaching within the clinical context. And feedback provided during the course as well as evaluation at its conclusion is most valuable for ongoing faculty growth.

Feedback from students can be obtained in a variety of ways. If students are writing reflective journals, they can be asked to periodically address one or two key questions within this medium, or their responses can be submitted to faculty separately. Faculty can pose questions such as the following:

What did I do this (day, week) that was most beneficial to your learning?
Is there something specific I could do that would help you learn better?
What suggestion(s) do you have that could help me grow in my teaching as
    a clinical faculty member?

One suggested approach is then to examine the feedback for themes; summarize them, and present the results to the group of students for discussion (McKeachie, 2002). This can be an opportunity to share changes that will be made and differences in opinion and what they communicate about student differences in learning styles and personal needs. It seems there is always one student who wants more guided assistance and another who requests faculty back off!

Requesting formative evaluation of teaching at the time of midterm evaluations can allow the collection of a broader range of data. Clinical faculty may use a qualitative or quantitative approach, or a combination of both, and the input from students may be anonymous or signed. Open-ended items may be just as useful as or even more so than closed ones (McKeachie, 2002). If the tool used for summative teaching evaluation provides faculty with useful information, perhaps it could be used for formative purposes as well. The "Clinical Toolbox" (see Chapter 20, p. 371) provides some examples of formative teaching evaluations.

When the course is completed, summative evaluative data are collected from students according to institutional policies and procedures. Because the primary purpose of these evaluations is often for use in administrative personnel decisions, their value for furthering faculty development can be limited (McKeachie, 2002). The academic program may use some standard teaching evaluation or one that has been designed specifically for use in clinical courses (see "Clinical Toolbox," p. 373). If the format of the tool does not lend itself to the clinical teaching context, much of what was previously requested for formative teaching evaluations can be modified and used to supplement summative evaluations. Faculty should not hesitate to deviate from a standard tool by adding items that are more appropriate to their use (McKeachie, 2002). Two other creative suggestions offered by Brookfield (1995) could be used to supplement institutional summative teaching evaluations. Students can be asked to jot down suggestions for what they would like to see added or deleted from the course. In a clinical course, this could include written assignments, group learning activities, or specific clinical learning experiences. Another approach is to ask students in the group to write a letter of advice to the faculty member's next group of students that includes suggestions for how to survive and thrive in the course. These "letters to successors" can provide valuable information to faculty and can be incorporated into the course orientation for subsequent students.

Student evaluations of teaching do not always yield affirmation and well-worded constructive criticism. There are times when some students use this opportunity to dump gunnysacks of vitriolic commentaries they have been previously unable or unwilling to share with their faculty. This can occur even when structured tools are used for formative and summative evaluation. In a group of ten students, such a response from even one student can be upsetting, and faculty are often saddened to learn that any student harbored this degree of antipathy. At times like this, turning to other colleagues for support is helpful.

It is wise to try to use this as a learning experience as well, examining the criticism for any possible valid critique that could be used for faculty development.

Faculty should know that their students are observing them closely (Brookfield, 1995). "(W)hat we do as teachers has enormous significance in the eyes of our students" (p. 112). Students in the clinical setting see their faculty as role models of the profession. It is primarily from their clinical faculty that neophyte nurses learn the attitudes, values, and norms of the profession.

How you model in your own life a continuous engagement in learning determines very significantly the extent to which students take learning seriously. And the only way you'll know how well you're modeling these values and processes is by seeing your actions through students' eyes (p. 113). Evaluation of the teaching of clinical faculty and the identification of avenues for further development would be sorely incomplete without input from the students.

REFLECTION EXERCISE 22

Seeing Teaching Through Students' Eyes

◆ What are your beliefs about student feedback/evaluations of teachers? On what assumptions are these beliefs built?

◆ What has been your experience in giving feedback to teachers and evaluating them? How might this affect you now, being in the role of teacher?

◆ Considering the clinical course you teach, or will be teaching (i.e., content, site, level of student), what feedback questions might you pose to students about your teaching? For formal formative evaluation? For formal summative evaluation?

COLLEAGUES' PERCEPTIONS OF TEACHING

Given the multiple demands on nursing faculty time, obtaining peer evaluations and assistance in the development of clinical teaching can be a challenging project. The value of peer visitations partially depends on their purpose (McKeachie, 2002). Unfortunately, when peer clinical visitations do occur, they are often for the purpose of securing information for administrative use rather than for faculty development. Recommendations for growth are provided with hesitation if they must be incorporated into administrative personnel evaluations for use in salary, retention, promotion, or tenure considerations. This information may be offered in discussions with colleagues following the visitation. McKeachie (2002) reports a colleague from Berkeley has found retired faculty to be a useful resource for classroom visitations because they are not involved in administrative personnel decisions and possess expertise in teaching within the discipline. Nursing programs could look to their emeritus faculty to provide feedback for the development of clinical faculty as well.

Valuable insights are often gleaned from discourse with other clinical faculty within the academic program. Both neophytes and experts can affirm the commonalities of experience, contribute to critical discourse, and participate in reflection. Reflection carried out individually may be superficial; reflection conducted in concert with colleagues can provoke deeper understanding and insight (Shellenbarger et al., 2005). These conversations necessitate "a moral and political culture characterized by an openness to diverse perspectives and ideologies, and a respectful acknowledgement of the importance of each person's contribution, irrespective of seniority or status" (Brookfield, 1995, p. 140). This process is called by many different names in the literature: "cognitive coaching" (Dyer & Fontaine, 1995), "critical conversations about teaching" (Brookfield, 1995), "participative inquiry" (Mahara & Jones, 2005) and "teaching circles" (Shellenbarger et al., 2005) to name a few. By any name or design, these discussions allow faculty to examine their practices in terms of the thinking and assumptions behind them, explore new approaches to teaching and evaluation, and find novel methods to analyze and address the challenges of instruction.

"Teacher talk is often obsessed with the failings of administrators, the obstructive nature of colleagues…, or the annoying loutishness and intellectual limitations of students" (Brookfield, 1995, p. 142). This is not the type of discourse that will help advance nurse educators' lifelong learning! Establishing some ground rules as to content, process, and confidentiality will help those involved remain on task. Mutual trust and respect are essential for success. If beliefs and practices are to be explored in a meaningful fashion, all those involved must try to avoid being judgmental or defensive (Dyer & Fontaine, 1995).

Brookfield (1995) suggests several basic activities to initiate discussion: reflective inventory (Box 19-1) and personal assumptions inventory (Box 19-2). To provide ongoing grist for discussion, Brookfield suggests participants be encouraged to bring critical incidents describing teaching peaks and valleys from which general common themes can be extracted (e.g., resistance to learning, dealing with student errors, approaches to providing feedback, responding to teaching-learning moments). Shellenbarger et al. (2005) suggest the creation of reflection

---

BOX 19-1
Guidelines for Reflective Inventory

Participants take turns introducing themselves by offering their responses to the following questions:
- What am I proudest of in my work as a teacher?
- What would I like my students to say about me when I'm out of the room?
- What do I most need to learn about in my teaching?
- What do I worry most about in my work as a teacher?
- When do I know I've done good work?
- What's the mistake I've made that I've learned the most from?

From Brookfield, S.D. (1995). *Becoming a critically reflective teacher*. San Francisco: Jossey-Bass.

BOX 19-2
Guidelines for Personal Assumptions Inventory

Participants complete the following sentences and initiate the conversation by reading some of them aloud:

- I know I've done good work when…
- I know I've done bad work when…
- I feel best about my work when…
- I feel worst about my work when…
- The last time I saw really good teaching was when…
- The best learning experience I've ever seen students involved in was when…

From Brookfield, S.D. (1995). *Becoming a critically reflective teacher*. San Francisco: Jossey-Bass.

---

maps to provide structure for individual and group reflection before, during, and after a course is taught. These informal, semistructured collegial conversations can be scheduled as brown bag lunches or any other venue that will permit as many clinical faculty to attend as possible. Nursing programs often have routine journal clubs or research meetings; surely conversations to support and stimulate growth in teaching are of equal import. These meetings also can help faculty identify topics for faculty development workshops.

Collegial evaluations and suggestions for further development of clinical teaching knowledge and skills can be obtained not only from other faculty but also from the personnel in the clinical agencies. Input may be obtained throughout the term, at its conclusion, or both. Clinical staff may be approached to provide verbal feedback or given opportunities to respond in writing with a more structured form. The academic program may have a form for colleague evaluation that can be used. These personnel can proffer information about how they were prepared for the students' arrival, lines of communication with faculty, and their observations of student-faculty interactions. Faculty who have requested feedback from personnel in clinical settings indicated in one study that the information they received both confirmed their beliefs regarding teaching and exposed things about their teaching they had not previously thought about (Scanlan, 2001).

Guidance in faculty development that comes from colleagues has an even wider scope than within each nursing program. Colleges and Universities commonly have internal programs to aid in improving teaching. As a common goal across disciplines, the development of teaching skills is often the focus of campus-wide workshops. Attending these conferences is valuable to the learning of new and seasoned faculty alike (Lichtman et al., 2003; Mann, 2004). By meeting with colleagues from other diverse disciplines to learn how to enhance their teaching, nursing faculty are likely to discover problems common to all courses as well as new skills.

Moving beyond the boundaries of the academic institution, accessing experts in teaching and nursing education at regional, national, and even international levels is becoming increasingly possible. Online courses allow faculty to study and learn at their leisure. The opportunity to network with nurse educators and those in other disciplines is made possible by physically attending conferences or attending teleconferences and via the Internet through listservs, chat rooms, and educator databases. The ease with which educators on every continent can learn from one another will only continue to escalate!

REFLECTION EXERCISE 23
Colleagues' Perceptions of Teaching

◆ If you wanted to obtain the most useful feedback on your clinical teaching from the personnel at the clinical site, how might you do that (e.g., who would you ask, when and how would you request input, what specific information would you ask for)?

◆ If a colleague were to come to observe your clinical teaching, on what would you ask that the focus be (e.g., skills instruction, feedback to students, clinical queries)? What questions about your teaching would you pose?

◆ Imagine you are going to participate in a teacher talk conversation with some clinical faculty colleagues. Prepare for the experience by returning to Boxes 19-1 and 19-2 and writing your responses to the activities.

▓ EXPLORING THE EDUCATIONAL LITERATURE

In addition to reading about issues and advances in nursing practice, faculty teaching clinical courses (and didactic ones!) should endeavor to learn about teaching through reading educational literature. Brookfield (1995) calls educational literature the "lens of theory" and tells us that it "can help us investigate the hunches, instincts, and tacit knowledge that shape our practice,...suggest different possibilities,...understand better what we already do and think,...(and) suggest new and provocative ways of seeing ourselves and our practice" (p. 185).

Every academic discipline has journals and books that deal with teaching and learning, and nursing is no exception. Nursing education literature provides a forum for the dissemination of knowledge regarding creative and novel approaches to clinical teaching and learning, student evaluation, issues and trends, and evidence-based education. Scan the index of the library of the nursing program or request the assistance of the library personnel to locate books with information on clinical nursing education. Two of the most recent publications to look for are as follows:

Diekelmann, N.L. (Ed.). (2003). *Teaching the practitioners of care: New pedagogies for the health professions.* Madison, WI: University of Wisconsin Press.
Lowenstein, A.J., & Bradshaw, M.J. (Eds.). (2001). *Fuzzard's innovative teaching strategies in nursing.* Gaithersburg, MD: Aspen.

Be on the lookout for information related to education issues within research and practice-focused journals as well. As with practice-focused journals, many nursing education journals are available online. Nursing education literature spans the world; some of the most widely available include the following:

International Journal of Nursing Education Scholarship
Journal of Nursing Education
Journal of Continuing Education in Nursing
Nurse Education Today
Nurse Educator
Nursing Education Perspectives
Annual Review of Nursing Education

If they explore the literature regarding teaching, faculty tend to focus on teaching within their own discipline, rarely venturing into other landscapes (Weimer, 2000). This is truly unfortunate, because journals and books from the educational literature of other disciplines can provide information of immeasurable value to faculty teaching clinical nursing courses. These materials reflect educational philosophy, psychology, and research from around the world. Nurse educators make far too little use of these magnificent resources that can be a source of knowledge both innovative and inspirational. Again, no effort is made to be all-inclusive; the following suggestions are intended to be representative only:

Journals

Adult Education Quarterly
British Journal of Educational Psychology
Educational Psychologist
Innovative Higher Education
Journal of Educational Psychology
Journal of Educational Research
Journal of Higher Education
National Teaching and Learning Forum
New Directions for Higher Education
The Teaching Professor

Books

Brookfield, S.D. (1995). *Becoming a critically reflective teacher*. San Francisco: Jossey-Bass.

Livsey, R.C., & Palmer, P.J. (1999). *The courage to teach: A guide for reflection and renewal*. San Francisco: Jossey-Bass.

McKeachie, W.J. (2002). *McKeachies's teaching tips: Strategies, research, and theory for college and university teachers* (11th ed.). Boston: Houghton Mifflin.

Palmer, P.J. (1998). *The courage to teach: Exploring the inner landscape of a teacher's life*. San Francisco: Jossey-Bass.

Delving into the educational literature allows clinical faculty to reaffirm their practice, identify educational universals, stimulate collegial dialogue, and emerge from the rut of groupthink. It contributes immeasurably to lifelong learning.

REFLECTION EXERCISE 24

Exploring the Educational Literature

Locate recent issues of any general education and nursing education journals. Read the editors' columns, if the journals have them. Scan the table of contents and select one article from each journal. After you have read them, reflect on their impact on you as a teacher and/or your teaching. You might use the following questions to guide your thinking:

◆ What surprised you? Why?

◆ How did what you read relate to what you have learned and reflected on while reading this book?

◆ What are the clinical teaching practice implications of what you read?

◆ What new questions did your reading engender? Where might you go to look for answers?

■ THE TEACHING PORTFOLIO

Just as portfolios are being increasingly developed by students to document the progression of their learning, so too teaching portfolios are a common approach to recording faculty accomplishments and development. They are dynamic creations, documenting growth over time in the advancement of knowledge and skills in teaching. In master's and doctoral nursing programs with an educational focus, preparation of teaching portfolios is a common student requirement. They may be written on paper stored in a 3-ring notebook or incorporated into the electronic medium of a web page to include graphics, videos, and even multimedia presentations. Some academic institutions require teaching portfolios and use them in combination with student and colleague evaluations as an approach to faculty evaluation and development (Appling, Naumann, & Berk, 2001). The teaching portfolio format may be institutionally dictated, but the general components appear fairly universal: an individual philosophy of teaching and learning; description of teaching responsibilities; discussion of teaching methods; future development goals; participation in activities such as workshops and conferences; current curriculum vitae; scholarly productions including presentations and publications. Box 19-3 lists some references regarding the preparation and use of teaching portfolios. A teaching portfolio begun now can be a viable tool for a future academic career.

■ CERTIFICATION AS AN ACADEMIC NURSE EDUCATOR

Those who choose to teach nursing in academic settings are also advanced practice nurses (National League for Nursing, 2005). Advanced practice nurses possess focused education and practice experience in their area of expertise, and this is most certainly true of nurse educators. Advanced practice in many other nursing specialty areas is formally acknowledged through a certification process, and this option is also available for academic nurse educators.

BOX 19-3
Selected References Regarding the Preparation of a Teaching Portfolio

Center for Instructional Development and Research. University of Washington, Seattle, WA. *Developing a teaching portfolio*. Retrieved July 1, 2005, from http://depts.washington.edu/cidrweb/PortfolioTools.htm

Center for Teaching Effectiveness, University of Texas at Austin. *Preparing a teaching portfolio: A guidebook*. Retrieved July 1, 2005, from http://www.utexas.edu/academic/cte/teachfolio.html

Griffith Institute for Higher Education. Griffith University, Australia. *Teaching portfolios: Compiling your teaching portfolio*. Retrieved July 1, 2005, from http://www.griffith.edu.au/text/centre/gihe/teachinglearning/portfolios/portfolio_guidelines3.htm

Herteis, E.M. *Teaching portfolios at the University of Saskatchewan, Canada*. Retrieved July 1, 2005, from http://www.usask.ca/tlc/teaching_portfolios/index.html

Oermann, M.H. (1999). Developing a teaching portfolio. *Journal of Professional Nursing, 14*(4), 224-228.

Reece, S.M., Pearce, S.W., Melillo, K.D., & Deaudry, M. (2001). The faculty portfolio: Documenting the scholarship of teaching. *Journal of Professional Nursing, 17*(4), 180-186.

The opportunity to sit for the certification examination requires application through the National League for Nursing (http://www.nln.org/). Simply preparing for the examination will expand the faculty member's knowledge base because a valuable list of resources is provided. A satisfactory result on the examination culminates in the designation of Certified Nurse Educator (CNE). Depending on the applicant's educational preparation, which does not have to include graduate level education course work, between 2 to 4 years of full-time academic teaching experience is required to qualify for the examination. This certification step should be part of every nurse educator's career plan, regardless of clinical practice focus.

■ CONTRIBUTING TO THE SCHOLARSHIP OF CLINICAL NURSING EDUCATION

Nursing education is a nascent field of study. Since the call for curricular revolution in the late 1980s (Bevis, 1988; Bevis & Watson, 1989), innovation endeavors in nursing education have primarily focused on global curricular changes, new approaches to classroom education, and efforts toward establishing evidence-based educational practices. Even so, significant change has been slow in coming. The ongoing transformations in society at-large and the health care system specifically, escalate the need for alterations in how nursing students learn to practice in clinical settings as well (see "Ten Trends to Watch," Box 19-4; Heller et al., 2004). As a part of developing an academic career, each clinical nursing faculty has an obligation to contribute in some way to the scholarship

> **BOX 19-4**
> **The Future of Nursing Education: Ten Trends to Watch**
>
> - Changing demographics and increasing diversity
> - The technological explosion
> - Globalization of the world's economy and society
> - The era of the educated consumer, alternative therapies and genomics, and palliative care.
> - Shift to population-based care and the increasing complexity of patient care
> - The cost of health care and the challenge of managed care
> - Impact of health policy and regulation
> - The growing need for interdisciplinary education for collaborative practice
> - The current nursing shortage/opportunities for lifelong learning and workforce development
> - Significant advances in nursing science and research
>
> Adapted from The future of nursing education: ten trends to watch. *Nursing and Health Care Perspectives*, Vol. 21, Number 1, 2000. National League for Nursing *(Nursing Education Perspectives)*.

of clinical nursing education. Participating in this process does not have to be arduous; indeed it can be spirited and fun! What is required above all is curiosity and enthusiasm for learning. Clinical faculty must talk and listen, critically read, and share their experiences and insights in writing.

It is essential that faculty "rethink clinical education in order to design new methods that meet students' needs to learn practice and that prepare graduates to thrive in today's healthcare environments" (National League for Nursing, 2003). To accomplish this, clinical faculty must examine the assumptions behind how they currently teach (Diekelmann, 2005), and they must talk with and listen to one another—faculty, clinicians, preceptors, researchers, and students (Diekelmann, Ironside, & Gunn, 2005; Ironside, 2005). In order to design the research that will contribute to the educational knowledge base, all nursing faculty must question their educational practices and scrutinize the assumptions they are built on (Ferguson & Day, 2005). Our faculty colleagues, clinical colleagues, and our students have much to teach us and we have much to learn. Narrative pedagogy, nursing research's unique contribution to nursing education, arose from the study of all of the participants in its educational processes (see Chapter 2). Now, like an anfractuous pendulum, narrative pedagogy informs and reforms the educational experience of all those involved. Learning to share perspectives in order to gain insights and alternative viewpoints, clinical nurse educators must continue to dialogue with all those involved to create a new vision of the future.

Faculty teaching nursing in clinical settings are the pathfinders of reform in nursing education (Diekelmann et al., 2005). Bringing their students to the front lines of practice, clinical faculty can see for themselves the changes occurring in health care, in the environments themselves, in those who are served, and those who provide services. They can identify the unique contexts of the community served by the nursing program, bringing that knowledge back to curriculum committees and faculty discussion groups for use in guiding programmatic evolution (Ferguson & Day, 2005). "A scholarship of teaching embraces the concept of always holding open and problematic the identification of essential content as an ever-present, contextual, political conversation" (Diekelmann, 2002, p. 382). Most commonly, the exhortation for openness to change in nursing education is applied broadly to curricula—the content presented and methods employed in nursing classrooms. But it is most certainly applicable to the clinical classroom as well. Clinical faculty must also respond to the call for reformation by providing practice opportunities for students' to integrate their new knowledge in such areas as technology, health economics, and disaster management, as well as maintaining an emphasis on evidence-based nursing practice (National League for Nursing, 2005).

As clinical faculty make an effort to help students apply evidence-based practices, so too must they attempt to support and contribute to evidence-based education. "The term *evidence-based nursing education* involves the use of best evidence to justify particular teaching or curricular interventions, considering the needs of individual learners, the professional judgment of nurse educators, and the resource costs of the interventions" (Ferguson & Day, 2005, p. 110). If evidence-based teaching is to occur, research to identify the knowledge to be used to guide nursing education is essential. There is no doubt that nurse educators are positioned to be leaders in this research (Yonge et al., 2005). Clinical faculty can participate in the fostering of evidence-based nursing education by suggesting and evaluating alternative approaches to clinical instruction (Diekelmann, 2005), identifying areas for innovation (Murray, 2004) and topics for research (Ferguson & Day, 2005), supporting one another in novel teaching approaches, and experimenting with innovative activities themselves (Diekelmann et al., 2005). Even innovations in the methods by which faculty can share their experiential wealth will contribute to the scholarship of teaching. The simple suggestion that the first 15 minutes of faculty meetings be devoted to a faculty member sharing a pragmatic teaching approach can be stimulating and intellectually refreshing (Diekelmann et al., 2005). There is much to learn from the efforts behind the creation and support of evidence-based practice, not only in nursing but also in other health care disciplines such as medicine, where the gap between knowledge generation and its incorporation into practice averages 17 years (Ferguson & Day, 2005). It has been nearly two decades since visionaries raised the hue and cry for the reconceptualization of nursing education and yet clinical nursing education has changed very little.

As clinical faculty seek to grow professionally, they must critically review the available research in nursing education (Diekelmann, 2005), and look to the implications for clinical nursing education of research in other disciplines (Ferguson & Day, 2005). But much of the pedagogical scholarship can be overlooked as such because it addresses teachers' "ideas" and "tips" extracted from the experience of teaching and couched in an anecdotal format. Given the esteem academia in general places on inquiry, the deficiency of scholarship related to teaching is especially unfortunate (Weimer, 2000). Presented in the guise of simplicity, and therefore notably undervalued as scholarship, articles of this sort must be elevated, ratcheted up so as to provide meaningful contributions to the knowledge base of nursing education. The wisdom found in the practice of teachers is unique and valuable, but readers must examine the theoretical or empirical principles underlying this practice, critically evaluating what can be viewed as experiential scholarship (Weimer, 2000). Efforts to accomplish this are underway. In the fall of 2004, the *Journal of Nursing Education* initiated a new feature—"Syllabus selections: Innovative learning activities" (Tanner, 2004). This venue is a place to share specific novel approaches to teaching grounded in the existent pedagogies of theory and practice. It is hoped that this will build on the scholarship of teaching. The resulting publications can stimulate faculty discussion within and between nursing programs. So, share the wealth and contribute to the scholarship of clinical nursing education!

REFLECTION EXERCISE 25

Reflection on the Scholarship of Clinical Nursing Education

Consider your experiences in teaching in the clinical nursing setting.

◆ What have you seen or experienced in your clinical context that could be fodder for faculty discussions in the nursing program? What would others benefit from knowing about practice, practitioners, students, or the recipients of care?

◆ If you were asked to share some innovative approach to clinical instruction with your colleagues, what might it be? Is there something you've tried that worked well, or that lead you to consider other approaches?

◆ Critically examine an anecdotal "teaching tip" from the literature. Now, read a selection from the *Journal of Nursing Education's* "Syllabus Selections." How could the anecdotal material be elevated to a more scholarly level? What questions do you have about clinical teaching that you haven't seen addressed in the literature? What might you do with these questions next?

SUMMARY

The teachability of faculty teaching clinical nursing courses is the critical ingredient to their long-term success. Determining the road to follow to advance their academic careers will provide direction for that teachability to be actualized. Developing professional practice expertise is certainly one aspect of lifelong learning, but so too is building on knowledge and skills as an educator; there are abundant resources available for both. Fulfilling the role of clinical educator includes exploring avenues by which each faculty can make contributions to the scholarship of nursing education. Ultimately, there is no end to the role of teacher-as-student.

References

Allen, M.N., & Field, P.A. (2005). Scholarly teaching and scholarship of teaching: Noting the difference. *International Journal of Nursing Education Scholarship, 2*(1), Article 12. Retrieved September 12, 2005, from http://www.bepress.com/ijnes/vol2/iss1/art12.

Appling, S.E., Naumann, P.L., & Berk, R.A. (2001). Using a faculty evaluation triad to achieve evidence-based teaching. *Nursing and Health Care Perspectives, 22*(5), 247-251.

Bevis, E.O. (1988). New directions for a new age. In *Curriculum Revolution: Mandate for change.* (pp. 27-52). New York: National League for Nursing.

Bevis, E.O., & Watson, J. (1989). *Toward a caring curriculum: A new pedagogy for nursing.* New York: National League for Nursing.

Brookfield, S.D. (1995). *Becoming a critically reflective teacher.* San Francisco: Jossey-Bass.

Cragg, C.E., & Andrusyszyn, M. (2005). The process of Master's education in nursing: Evolution or revolution? *International Journal of Nursing Scholarship, 2*(1), Article 21. Retrieved September 12, 2005, from http://www.bepress.com/ijnes/vol2/iss1/art21.

Didham, P. (2003). From the tower into the trenches: A nurse educator's reflections on the knowledge of experience. *Journal of Nursing Education, 42*(11), 485-487.

Diekelmann, N. (2002). "She asked this simple question": Reflecting and the scholarship of teaching. *Journal of Nursing Education, 41*(9), 381-382.

Diekelmann, N. (2005). Creating an inclusive science for nursing education. *Nursing Education Perspectives, 26*(2), 64-65.

Diekelmann, N.L., Ironside, P.M., & Gunn, J. (2005). Recalling the curriculum revolution: Innovation with research. *Nursing Education Perspectives, 26*(2), 70-77.

Dyer, J., & Fontaine, O. (1995). Can a zebra change its spots? Some reflections on cognitive coaching; [1]. *Education Canada, 35*(1), 28-32.

Ferguson, L., & Day, R.A. (2005). Evidence-based nursing education: Myth or reality? *Journal of Nursing Education, 44*(3), 107-115.

Fitzpatrick, J.J. (2004). Evaluating teaching effectiveness. *Nursing Education Perspectives, 25*(3), 109.

Fitzpatrick, J.J. (2005). Can we "escape fire" in nursing education? *Nursing Education Perspectives, 26*(4), 205.

Heller, B.R., Oros, M.T., & Durney-Crowley, J. (2004). The future of nursing education: Ten trends to watch. National League for Nursing—*Nursing Education Perspectives.* Retrieved October 27, 2004, from http://www.nln.org/nlnjournal/infotrends.htm.

Ironside, P.M. (2005). The experiences of nursing teachers, students, and clinicians. *Nursing Education Perspectives, 26*(2), 78-85.

Lichtman, R., Burst, H.V., Campau, N., Carrington, B., Diegmann, E.K., Hsia, L., et al. (2003). Pearls of wisdom for clinical teaching: Expert educators reflect. *Journal of Midwifery and Women's Health, 48*(6), 455-463.

Mahara, M.S., & Jones, J.A. (2005). Participatory inquiry with a colleague: An innovative faculty development process. *Journal of Nursing Education, 44*(3), 124-130.

Mann, A.S. (2004). Eleven tips for the new college teacher. *Journal of Nursing Education, 43*(9), 389-390.

Maxwell, J.C. (1999). *The 21 indispensable qualities of a leader: Becoming the person others will want to follow.* Nashville, TN: Thomas Nelson.

McKeachie, W.J. (2002). *McKeachie's teaching tips: Strategies, research, and theory for college and university teachers* (11th ed.). Boston: Houghton Mifflin.

Murray, J.P. (2004). *Innovation in nursing education.* Nursing Education Perspectives, 25(1), 2.

National League for Nursing. (2001). Position statement: *Lifelong learning for nursing faculty*. Retrieved June 28, 2005, from http://www.nln.org/aboutnln/PositionStatements/lifelonglearning01.htm.

National League for Nursing. (2003). Position statement: *Innovation in nursing education: A call to reform*. Retrieved June 28, 2005, from http://www.nln.org/aboutnln/PostionStatements/innovation.htm.

National League for Nursing. (2005). Position statement: *Transforming nursing education*. Retrieved June 28, 2005, from http://www.nln.org/aboutnln/positionstatements/transforming052005.pdf.

Neese, R. (2003). A transformational journey from clinician to educator. *Journal of Continuing Education, 34*(6), 258-262.

Scanlan, J.M. (2001). Learning clinical teaching: Is it magic? *Nursing and Health Care Perspectives, 22*(5), 240-246.

Shellenbarger, T., Palmer, E.A., Labant, A.L., & Kuzneski, J.L. (2005). Use of faculty reflection to improve teaching. *Annual Review of Nursing Education, 3*, 343-357.

Tanner, C.A. (2002). Clinical education, circa 2010. *Journal of Nursing Education, 41*(2), 51-52.

Tanner, C.A. (2004). Help is on the way: JNE's new feature, syllabus selections. *Journal of Nursing Education, 43*(9), 383-384.

Weimer, M. (2000). Better scholarship "on" teaching. *Journal of Nursing Education, 39*(5), 195-196.

Westberg, J., & Jason, H. (2001). *Fostering reflection and providing feedback: Helping others learn from experience*. New York: Springer.

Yoder-Wise, P.S. (2000). Continuing to gain knowledge. *Journal of Continuing Education in Nursing, 31*(3), 100.

Yonge, O.J., Anderson, M., Profetto-McGrath, J., Olson, J.K., Sillen, D.L., Boman, J., et al. (2005). An inventory of nursing education research. *International Journal of Nursing Education Scholarship, 2*(1), Article 11. Retrieved September 12, 2005, from http://www.bepress.com/ijnes/vol2/iss1/art11.

Clinical Educator Resources

CHAPTER 20

Clinical Toolbox

American Association of University Professors 1940 Statement of Principles on Academic Freedom and Tenure With 1970 Interpretive Comments

(Discussed in Chapter 7)
In 1940, following a series of joint conferences begun in 1934, representatives of the American Association of University Professors and of the Association of American Colleges (now the Association of American Colleges and Universities) agreed upon a restatement of principles set forth in the 1925 Conference Statement on Academic Freedom and Tenure. *This restatement is known to the profession as the 1940* Statement of Principles on Academic Freedom and Tenure.

The 1940 Statement is printed below, followed by Interpretive Comments as developed by representatives of the American Association of University Professors and the Association of American Colleges in 1969. The governing bodies of the two associations, meeting respectively in November 1989 and January 1990, adopted several changes in language in order to remove gender-specific references from the original text.

The purpose of this statement is to promote public understanding and support of academic freedom and tenure and agreement upon procedures to ensure them in colleges and universities. Institutions of higher education are conducted for the common good and not to further the interest of either the individual teacher[1] or the institution as a whole. The common good depends upon the free search for truth and its free exposition.

Academic freedom is essential to these purposes and applies to both teaching and research. Freedom in research is fundamental to the advancement of truth. Academic freedom in its teaching aspect is fundamental for the protection of the rights of the teacher in teaching and of the student to freedom in learning. It carries with it duties correlative with rights.[1][2]

Tenure is a means to certain ends; specifically: (1) freedom of teaching and research and of extramural activities, and (2) a sufficient degree of economic security to make the profession attractive to men and women of ability. Freedom and economic security, hence, tenure, are indispensable to the success of an institution in fulfilling its obligations to its students and to society.

Academic freedom

Teachers are entitled to full freedom in research and in the publication of the results, subject to the adequate performance of their other academic duties; but research for pecuniary return should be based upon an understanding with the authorities of the institution.

Teachers are entitled to freedom in the classroom in discussing their subject, but they should be careful not to introduce into their teaching controversial matter which has no relation to their subject.[2] Limitations of academic freedom because of religious or other aims of the institution should be clearly stated in writing at the time of the appointment.[3]

From American Association of University Professors, *Policy Documents and Reports*, 9th ed. (Washington, D.C.), 2001, 3-7.
1. The word "teacher" as used in this document is understood to include the investigator who is attached to an academic institution without teaching duties.
2. Boldface numbers in brackets refer to Interpretive Comments which follow.

Continued

American Association of University Professors 1940 Statement of Principles on Academic Freedom and Tenure With 1970 Interpretive Comments—cont'd

College and university teachers are citizens, members of a learned profession, and officers of an educational institution. When they speak or write as citizens, they should be free from institutional censorship or discipline, but their special position in the community imposes special obligations. As scholars and educational officers, they should remember that the public may judge their profession and their institution by their utterances. Hence they should at all times be accurate, should exercise appropriate restraint, should show respect for the opinions of others, and should make every effort to indicate that they are not speaking for the institution.[4]

Academic tenure

After the expiration of a probationary period, teachers or investigators should have permanent or continuous tenure, and their service should be terminated only for adequate cause, except in the case of retirement for age, or under extraordinary circumstances because of financial exigencies.

In the interpretation of this principle it is understood that the following represents acceptable academic practice:

The precise terms and conditions of every appointment should be stated in writing and be in the possession of both institution and teacher before the appointment is consummated.

Beginning with appointment to the rank of full-time instructor or a higher rank,[5] the probationary period should not exceed seven years, including within this period full-time service in all institutions of higher education; but subject to the proviso that when, after a term of probationary service of more than three years in one or more institutions, a teacher is called to another institution, it may be agreed in writing that the new appointment is for a probationary period of not more than four years, even though thereby the person's total probationary period in the academic profession is extended beyond the normal maximum of seven years.[6] Notice should be given at least one year prior to the expiration of the probationary period if the teacher is not to be continued in service after the expiration of that period.[7]

During the probationary period a teacher should have the academic freedom that all other members of the faculty have.[8]

Termination for cause of a continuous appointment, or the dismissal for cause of a teacher previous to the expiration of a term appointment, should, if possible, be considered by both a faculty committee and the governing board of the institution. In all cases where the facts are in dispute, the accused teacher should be informed before the hearing in writing of the charges and should have the opportunity to be heard in his or her own defense by all bodies that pass judgment upon the case. The teacher should be permitted to be accompanied by an advisor of his or her own choosing who may act as counsel. There should be a full stenographic record of the hearing available to the parties concerned. In the hearing of charges of incompetence the testimony should include that of teachers and other scholars, either from the teacher's own or from other institutions.

American Association of University Professors 1940 Statement of Principles on Academic Freedom and Tenure With 1970 Interpretive Comments—cont'd

Teachers on continuous appointment who are dismissed for reasons not involving moral turpitude should receive their salaries for at least a year from the date of notification of dismissal whether or not they are continued in their duties at the institution.[9]

Termination of a continuous appointment because of financial exigency should be demonstrably bona fide.

1940 Interpretations

At the conference of representatives of the American Association of University Professors and of the Association of American Colleges on November 7–8, 1940, the following interpretations of the 1940 *Statement of Principles on Academic Freedom and Tenure* were agreed upon:

That its operation should not be retroactive.

That all tenure claims of teachers appointed prior to the endorsement should be determined in accordance with the principles set forth in the 1925 *Conference Statement on Academic Freedom and Tenure*.

If the administration of a college or university feels that a teacher has not observed the admonitions of paragraph (c) of the section on Academic Freedom and believes that the extramural utterances of the teacher have been such as to raise grave doubts concerning the teacher's fitness for his or her position, it may proceed to file charges under paragraph 4 of the section on Academic Tenure. In pressing such charges, the administration should remember that teachers are citizens and should be accorded the freedom of citizens. In such cases the administration must assume full responsibility, and the American Association of University Professors and the Association of American Colleges are free to make an investigation.

1970 Interpretive comments

Following extensive discussions on the 1940 Statement of Principles on Academic Freedom and Tenure with leading educational associations and with individual faculty members and administrators, a joint committee of the AAUP and the Association of American Colleges met during 1969 to reevaluate this key policy statement. On the basis of the comments received, and the discussions that ensued, the joint committee felt the preferable approach was to formulate interpretations of the Statement in terms of the experience gained in implementing and applying the Statement for over thirty years and of adapting it to current needs.

The committee submitted to the two associations for their consideration the following "Interpretive Comments." These interpretations were adopted by the Council of the American Association of University Professors in April 1970 and endorsed by the Fifty-sixth Annual Meeting as Association policy.

Continued

American Association of University Professors 1940 Statement of Principles on Academic Freedom and Tenure With 1970 Interpretive Comments—cont'd

1970 Interpretive comments—cont'd

In the thirty years since their promulgation, the principles of the 1940 *Statement of Principles on Academic Freedom and Tenure* have undergone a substantial amount of refinement. This has evolved through a variety of processes, including customary acceptance, understandings mutually arrived at between institutions and professors or their representatives, investigations and reports by the American Association of University Professors, and formulations of statements by that association either alone or in conjunction with the Association of American Colleges. These comments represent the attempt of the two associations, as the original sponsors of the 1940 *Statement*, to formulate the most important of these refinements. Their incorporation here as Interpretive Comments is based upon the premise that the 1940 *Statement* is not a static code but a fundamental document designed to set a framework of norms to guide adaptations to changing times and circumstances.

Also, there have been relevant developments in the law itself reflecting a growing insistence by the courts on due process within the academic community which parallels the essential concepts of the 1940 *Statement*; particularly relevant is the identification by the Supreme Court of academic freedom as a right protected by the First Amendment. As the Supreme Court said in *Keyishian v. Board of Regents*, 385 U.S. 589 (1967), "Our Nation is deeply committed to safeguarding academic freedom, which is of transcendent value to all of us and not merely to the teachers concerned. That freedom is therefore a special concern of the First Amendment, which does not tolerate laws that cast a pall of orthodoxy over the classroom."

The numbers refer to the designated portion of the 1940 *Statement* on which interpretive comment is made.

The Association of American Colleges and the American Association of University Professors have long recognized that membership in the academic profession carries with it special responsibilities. Both associations either separately or jointly have consistently affirmed these responsibilities in major policy statements, providing guidance to professors in their utterances as citizens, in the exercise of their responsibilities to the institution and to students, and in their conduct when resigning from their institution or when undertaking government-sponsored research. Of particular relevance is the *Statement on Professional Ethics*, adopted in 1966 as Association policy. (A revision, adopted in 1987, may be found in AAUP, *Policy Documents and Reports*, 9th ed. [Washington, DC, 2001], 133–134.)

The intent of this statement is not to discourage what is "controversial." Controversy is at the heart of the free academic inquiry which the entire statement is designed to foster. The passage serves to underscore the need for teachers to avoid persistently intruding material which has no relation to their subject.

Most church-related institutions no longer need or desire the departure from the principle of academic freedom implied in the 1940 *Statement*, and we do not now endorse such a departure.

American Association of University Professors 1940 Statement of Principles on Academic Freedom and Tenure With 1970 Interpretive Comments—cont'd

1970 Interpretive comments—cont'd

This paragraph is the subject of an interpretation adopted by the sponsors of the 1940 *Statement* immediately following its endorsement which reads as follows:

If the administration of a college or university feels that a teacher has not observed the admonitions of paragraph (c) of the section on Academic Freedom and believes that the extramural utterances of the teacher have been such as to raise grave doubts concerning the teacher's fitness for his or her position, it may proceed to file charges under paragraph 4 of the section on Academic Tenure. In pressing such charges, the administration should remember that teachers are citizens and should be accorded the freedom of citizens. In such cases the administration must assume full responsibility, and the American Association of University Professors and the Association of American Colleges are free to make an investigation.

Paragraph (c) of the section on Academic Freedom in the 1940 *Statement* should also be interpreted in keeping with the 1964 "Committee A Statement on Extramural Utterances" (*Policy Documents and Reports*, 32), which states inter alia: "The controlling principle is that a faculty member's expression of opinion as a citizen cannot constitute grounds for dismissal unless it clearly demonstrates the faculty member's unfitness for his or her position. Extramural utterances rarely bear upon the faculty member's fitness for the position. Moreover, a final decision should take into account the faculty member's entire record as a teacher and scholar."

Paragraph 5 of the *Statement on Professional Ethics* also deals with the nature of the "special obligations" of the teacher. The paragraph reads as follows:

As members of their community, professors have the rights and obligations of other citizens. Professors measure the urgency of other obligations in the light of their responsibilities to their subject, to their students, to their profession, and to their institution. When they speak or act as private persons they avoid creating the impression of speaking or acting for their college or university. As citizens engaged in a profession that depends upon freedom for its health and integrity, professors have a particular obligation to promote conditions of free inquiry and to further public understanding of academic freedom.

Both the protection of academic freedom and the requirements of academic responsibility apply not only to the full-time probationary and the tenured teacher, but also to all others, such as part-time faculty and teaching assistants, who exercise teaching responsibilities.

5. The concept of "rank of full-time instructor or a higher rank" is intended to include any person who teaches a full-time load regardless of the teacher's specific title.*

---

*For a discussion of this question, see the "Report of the Special Committee on Academic Personnel Ineligible for Tenure," *Policy Documents and Reports*, 88–91.

Continued

American Association of University Professors 1940 Statement of Principles on Academic Freedom and Tenure With 1970 Interpretive Comments—cont'd

1970 Interpretive comments—cont'd

6. In calling for an agreement "in writing" on the amount of credit given for a faculty member's prior service at other institutions, the *Statement* furthers the general policy of full understanding by the professor of the terms and conditions of the appointment. It does not necessarily follow that a professor's tenure rights have been violated because of the absence of a written agreement on this matter. Nonetheless, especially because of the variation in permissible institutional practices, a written understanding concerning these matters at the time of appointment is particularly appropriate and advantageous to both the individual and the institution.**

7. The effect of this subparagraph is that a decision on tenure, favorable or unfavorable, must be made at least twelve months prior to the completion of the probationary period. If the decision is negative, the appointment for the following year becomes a terminal one. If the decision is affirmative, the provisions in the 1940 *Statement* with respect to the termination of service of teachers or investigators after the expiration of a probationary period should apply from the date when the favorable decision is made.

The general principle of notice contained in this paragraph is developed with greater specificity in the *Standards for Notice of Nonreappointment*, endorsed by the Fiftieth Annual Meeting of the American Association of University Professors (1964). These standards are:

Notice of nonreappointment, or of intention not to recommend reappointment to the governing board, should be given in writing in accordance with the following standards:

(a) *Not later than March 1 of the first academic year of service*, if the appointment expires at the end of that year; or, if a one-year appointment terminates during an academic year, at least three months in advance of its termination.

(b) *Not later than December 15 of the second academic year of service*, if the appointment expires at the end of that year; or, if an initial two-year appointment terminates during an academic year, at least six months in advance of its termination.

(c) At least twelve months before the expiration of an appointment after two or more years in the institution.

Other obligations, both of institutions and of individuals, are described in the *Statement on Recruitment and Resignation of Faculty Members*, as endorsed by the Association of American Colleges and the American Association of University Professors in 1961.

**For a more detailed statement on this question, see "On Crediting Prior Service Elsewhere as Part of the Probationary Period," *ibid.*, 100–101.

American Association of University Professors 1940 Statement of Principles on Academic Freedom and Tenure With 1970 Interpretive Comments—cont'd

1970 Interpretive comments—cont'd

8. The freedom of probationary teachers is enhanced by the establishment of a regular procedure for the periodic evaluation and assessment of the teacher's academic performance during probationary status. Provision should be made for regularized procedures for the consideration of complaints by probationary teachers that their academic freedom has been violated. One suggested procedure to serve these purposes is contained in the *Recommended Institutional Regulations on Academic Freedom and Tenure*, prepared by the American Association of University Professors.

9. A further specification of the academic due process to which the teacher is entitled under this paragraph is contained in the *Statement on Procedural Standards in Faculty Dismissal Proceedings*, jointly approved by the American Association of University Professors and the Association of American Colleges in 1958. This interpretive document deals with the issue of suspension, about which the 1940 *Statement* is silent.

The 1958 *Statement* provides: "Suspension of the faculty member during the proceedings is justified only if immediate harm to the faculty member or others is threatened by the faculty member's continuance. Unless legal considerations forbid, any such suspension should be with pay." A suspension which is not followed by either reinstatement or the opportunity for a hearing is in effect a summary dismissal in violation of academic due process.

The concept of "moral turpitude" identifies the exceptional case in which the professor may be denied a year's teaching or pay in whole or in part. The statement applies to that kind of behavior which goes beyond simply warranting discharge and is so utterly blameworthy as to make it inappropriate to require the offering of a year's teaching or pay. The standard is not that the moral sensibilities of persons in the particular community have been affronted. The standard is behavior that would evoke condemnation by the academic community generally.

American Association of University Professors Statement on Professional Ethics

(Discussed in Chapter 7)
The statement which follows, a revision of a statement originally adopted in 1966, was approved by the Association's Committee on Professional Ethics, adopted by the Association's Council in June 1987, and endorsed by the Seventy-third Annual Meeting.

Introduction

From its inception, the American Association of University Professors has recognized that membership in the academic profession carries with it special responsibilities. The Association has consistently affirmed these responsibilities in major policy statements, providing guidance to professors in such matters as their utterances as citizens, the exercise of their responsibilities to students and colleagues, and their conduct when resigning from an institution or when undertaking sponsored research. The *Statement on Professional Ethics* that follows sets forth those general standards that serve as a reminder of the variety of responsibilities assumed by all members of the profession.

In the enforcement of ethical standards, the academic profession differs from those of law and medicine, whose associations act to ensure the integrity of members engaged in private practice. In the academic profession the individual institution of higher learning provides this assurance and so should normally handle questions concerning propriety of conduct within its own framework by reference to a faculty group. The Association supports such local action and stands ready, through the general secretary and the Committee on Professional Ethics, to counsel with members of the academic community concerning questions of professional ethics and to inquire into complaints when local consideration is impossible or inappropriate. If the alleged offense is deemed sufficiently serious to raise the possibility of adverse action, the procedures should be in accordance with the 1940 *Statement of Principles on Academic Freedom and Tenure*, the 1958 *Statement on Procedural Standards in Faculty Dismissal Proceedings*, or the applicable provisions of the Association's *Recommended Institutional Regulations on Academic Freedom and Tenure*.

The statement

1. Professors, guided by a deep conviction of the worth and dignity of the advancement of knowledge, recognize the special responsibilities placed upon them. Their primary responsibility to their subject is to seek and to state the truth as they see it. To this end professors devote their energies to developing and improving their scholarly competence. They accept the obligation to exercise critical self-discipline and judgment in using, extending, and transmitting knowledge. They practice intellectual honesty. Although professors may follow subsidiary interests, these interests must never seriously hamper or compromise their freedom of inquiry.

From American Association of University Professors, *Policy Documents and Reports*, 9th ed. (Washington D.C.), 2001, 133-134.

**American Association of University Professors
Statement on Professional Ethics—cont'd**

The statement—cont'd

2. As teachers, professors encourage the free pursuit of learning in their students. They hold before them the best scholarly and ethical standards of their discipline. Professors demonstrate respect for students as individuals and adhere to their proper roles as intellectual guides and counselors. Professors make every reasonable effort to foster honest academic conduct and to ensure that their evaluations of students reflect each student's true merit. They respect the confidential nature of the relationship between professor and student. They avoid any exploitation, harassment, or discriminatory treatment of students. They acknowledge significant academic or scholarly assistance from them. They protect their academic freedom.

3. As colleagues, professors have obligations that derive from common membership in the community of scholars. Professors do not discriminate against or harass colleagues. They respect and defend the free inquiry of associates. In the exchange of criticism and ideas professors show due respect for the opinions of others. Professors acknowledge academic debt and strive to be objective in their professional judgment of colleagues. Professors accept their share of faculty responsibilities for the governance of their institution.

4. As members of an academic institution, professors seek above all to be effective teachers and scholars. Although professors observe the stated regulations of the institution, provided the regulations do not contravene academic freedom, they maintain their right to criticize and seek revision. Professors give due regard to their paramount responsibilities within their institution in determining the amount and character of work done outside it. When considering the interruption or termination of their service, professors recognize the effect of their decision upon the program of the institution and give due notice of their intentions.

5. As members of their community, professors have the rights and obligations of other citizens. Professors measure the urgency of these obligations in the light of their responsibilities to their subject, to their students, to their profession, and to their institution. When they speak or act as private persons, they avoid creating the impression of speaking or acting for their college or university. As citizens engaged in a profession that depends upon freedom for its health and integrity, professors have a particular obligation to promote conditions of free inquiry and to further public understanding of academic freedom.

American Nurses' Association Code of Ethics for Nurses With Interpretive Statements

(Discussed in Chapter 7)

Provision 1: *The nurse, in all professional relationships, practices with compassion and respect for the inherent dignity, worth, and uniqueness of every individual, unrestricted by considerations of social or economic status, personal attributes, or the nature of health problems.*

Respect for human dignity

A fundamental principle that underlies all nursing practice is respect for the inherent worth, dignity, and human rights of every individual. Nurses take into account the needs and values of all persons in all professional relationships.

Relationships to patients

The need for health care is universal, transcending all individual differences. The nurse establishes relationships and delivers nursing services with respect for human needs and values, and without prejudice. An individual's lifestyle, value system, and religious beliefs should be considered in planning health care with and for each patient. Such consideration does not suggest that the nurse necessarily agrees with or condones certain individual choices, but that the nurse respects the patient as a person.

The nature of health problems

The nurse respects the worth, dignity, and rights of all human beings irrespective of the nature of the health problem. The worth of the person is not affected by disease, disability, functional status, or proximity to death. This respect extends to all who require the services of the nurses for the promotion of health, the prevention of illness, the restoration of health, the alleviation of suffering, and the provision of supportive care to those who are dying.

The measures nurses take to care for the patient enable the patient to live with as much physical, emotional, social, and spiritual well-being as possible. Nursing care aims to maximize the values that the patient has treasured in life and extends supportive care to the family and significant others. Nursing care is directed toward meeting the comprehensive needs of patients and their families across the continuum of care. This is particularly vital in the care of patients and their families at the end of life to prevent and relieve the cascade of symptoms and suffering that are commonly associated with dying.

Nurses are leaders and vigilant advocates for the delivery of dignified and humane care. Nurses actively participate in assessing and assuring the responsible and appropriate use of interventions in order to minimize unwarranted or unwanted treatment and patient suffering. The acceptability and importance of carefully considered decisions regarding resuscitation status, withholding and withdrawing life-sustaining therapies, forgoing medically provided nutrition and hydration, aggressive pain and symptom management and advance directives are increasingly evident. The nurse should provide interventions to relieve pain and other symptoms in the dying patient even when those interventions entail risks of hastening death.

American Nurses' Association Code of Ethics for Nurses With Interpretive Statements—cont'd

The nature of health problems—cont'd

However, nurses may not act with the sole intent of ending a patient's life even though such action may be motivated by compassion, respect for patient autonomy, and quality of life considerations. Nurses have invaluable experience, knowledge, and insight into care at the end of life and should be actively involved in related research, education, practice, and policy development.

1.4 The right to self-determination

Respect for human dignity requires the recognition of specific patient rights, particularly, the right of self-determination. Self-determination, also known as autonomy, is the philosophical basis for informed consent in health care. Patients have the moral and legal right to determine what will be done with their own person; to be given accurate, complete, and understandable information in a manner that facilitates an informed judgment; to be assisted with weighing the benefits, burdens, and available options in their treatment, including the choice or no treatment; to accept, refuse, or terminate treatment without deceit, undue influence, duress, coercion, or penalty; and to be given necessary support throughout the decision-making and treatment process. Such support would include the opportunity to make decisions with family and significant others and the provision of advance and support from knowledgeable nurses and other health professionals. Patients should be involved in planning their own health care to the extent they are able and choose to participate.

Each nurse has the obligation to be knowledgeable about the moral and legal rights of all patients to self-determination. The nurse preserves, protects, and supports these interests by assessing the patient's comprehension of both the information presented and the implications of decisions. In situations in which the patient lacks the capacity to make a decision, a designated surrogate decision-maker should be consulted. The role of the surrogate is to make decisions as the patient would, based on the patient's previously expressed wishes and known values. In the absence of a designated surrogate decision-maker, decisions should be made in the best interest of the patient, considering the patient's personal values to the extent that they are known. The nurse supports patient self-determination by participating in discussions with surrogates, providing guidance and referral to other resources as necessary, and identifying and addressing problems in the decision-making process. Support of autonomy in the broadest sense also includes recognition that people of some cultures place less weight on individualism and choose to defer to family or community values in decision-making. Respect not just for the specific decision but also for the patient's method of decision-making is consistent with the principle of autonomy.

Individuals are interdependent members of the community. The nurse recognizes that there are situations in which the right to individual self-determination may be outweighed or limited by the rights, health and welfare of others, particularly in relation to public health considerations.

Continued

American Nurses' Association Code of Ethics for Nurses With Interpretive Statements—cont'd

1.4 The right to self-determination—cont'd
Nonetheless, limitation of individual rights must always be considered a serious deviation from the standard of care, justified only when there are no less restrictive means available to preserve the rights of others and the demands of justice.

1.5 Relationships with colleagues and others
The principle of respect for persons extends to all individuals with whom the nurse interacts. The nurse maintains compassionate and caring relationships with colleagues and others with a commitment to the fair treatment of individuals, to integrity-preserving compromise, and to resolving conflict. Nurses function in many roles, including direct care provider, administrator, educator, researcher, and consultant. In each of these roles, the nurse treats colleagues, employees, assistants, and students with respect and compassion. This standard of conduct precludes any and all prejudicial actions, any form of harassment or threatening behavior, or disregard for the effect of one's actions on others. The nurse values the distinctive contribution of individuals or groups, and collaborates to meet the shared goal of providing quality health services.

Provision 2: *The nurse's primary commitment is to the patient, whether an individual, family, group or community.*
2.1 Primacy of the patient's interests
The nurse's primary commitment is to the recipient of nursing and health care services—the patient—whether the recipient is an individual, a family, a group, or a community. Nursing holds a fundamental commitment to the uniqueness of the individual patient; therefore, any plan of care must reflect that uniqueness. The nurse strives to provide patients with opportunities to participate in planning care, assures that patients find the plans acceptable, and supports the implementation of the plan. Addressing patient interests requires recognition of the patient's place in the family or other networks of relationship. When the patient's wishes are in conflict with others, the nurse seeks to help resolve the conflict. Where conflict persists, the nurse's commitment remains to the identified patient.

2.2 Conflict of interest for nurses
Nurses are frequently put in situations of conflict arising from competing loyalties in the workplace, including situations of conflicting expectations from patients, families, physicians, colleagues, and in many cases, health care organizations and health plans. Nurses must examine the conflicts arising between their own personal and professional values, the values and interests of others who are also responsible for patient care and health care decisions, as well as those of patients. Nurses strive to resolve such conflicts in ways that ensure patient safety, guard the patient's best interests, and preserve the professional integrity of the nurse.

Situations created by changes in health care financing and delivery systems, such as incentive systems to decrease spending, pose new possibilities of conflict between economic self-interest and professional integrity.

American Nurses' Association Code of Ethics for Nurses With Interpretive Statements—cont'd

2.2 Conflict of interest for nurses—cont'd

The use of bonuses, sanctions, and incentives tied to financial targets are examples of features of health care systems that may present such conflict. Conflicts of interest may arise in any domain of nursing activity including clinical practice, administration, education, or research. Advanced practice nurses who bill directly for services and nursing executives with budgetary responsibilities must be especially cognizant of the potential for conflicts of interest. Nurses should disclose to all relevant parties (e.g., patients, employers, colleagues) any perceived or actual conflict of interest and in some situations should withdraw from further participation. Nurses in all roles must seek to ensure that employment arrangements are just and fair and do not create an unreasonable conflict between patient care and direct personal gain.

2.3 Collaboration

Collaboration is not just cooperation, but it is the concerted effort of individuals and groups to attain a shared goal. In health care, that goal is to address the health needs of the patient and the public. The complexity of health care delivery systems requires a multi-disciplinary approach to the delivery of services that has the strong support and active participation of all the health professions. Within this context, nursing's unique contribution, scope of practice, and relationship with other health professionals needs to be clearly articulated, represented, and preserved. By its very nature, collaboration requires mutual trust, recognition, and respect among the health care team, shared decision-making about patient care, and open dialogue among all parties who have an interest in and a concern for health outcomes. Nurses should work to assure that the relevant parties are involved and have a voice in decision-making about patient care issues. Nurses should see that the questions that need to be addressed are asked and that the information needed for informed decision-making is available and provided. Nurses should actively promote the collaborative multi-disciplinary planning required to ensure the availability and accessibility of quality health services to all persons who have needs for health care.

Intraprofessional collaboration within nursing is fundamental to effectively addressing the health needs of patients and the public. Nurses engaged in non-clinical roles, such as administration or research, while not providing direct care, nonetheless are collaborating in the provision of care through their influence and direction of those who do. Effective nursing care is accomplished through the interdependence of nurses in differing roles—those who teach the needed skills, set standards, manage the environment of care, or expand the boundaries of knowledge used by the profession. In this sense, nurses in all roles share a responsibility for the outcomes of nursing care.

Continued

American Nurses' Association Code of Ethics for Nurses With Interpretive Statements—cont'd

2.4 Professional boundaries

When acting within one's role as a professional, the nurse recognizes and maintains boundaries that establish appropriate limits to relationships. While the nature of nursing work has an inherently personal component, nurse-patient relationships and nurse-colleague relationships have, as their foundation, the purpose of preventing illness, alleviating suffering, and protecting, promoting, and restoring the health of patients. In this way, nurse-patient and nurse-colleague relationships differ from those that are purely personal and unstructured, such as friendship. The intimate nature of nursing care, the involvement of nurses in important and sometimes highly stressful life events, and the mutual dependence of colleagues working in close concert all present the potential for blurring of limits to professional relationships. Maintaining the authenticity and expressing oneself as an individual, while remaining within the bounds established by the purpose of the relationship, can be especially difficult in prolonged or long-term relationships. In all encounters, nurses are responsible for retaining their professional boundaries. When those professional boundaries are jeopardized, the nurse should seek assistance from peers or supervisors or take appropriate steps to remove her/himself from the situation.

Provision 3: *The nurse promotes, advocates for, and strives to protect the health, safety and rights of the patient.*

3.1 Privacy

The nurse safeguards the patient's right to privacy. The need for health care does not justify unwanted intrusion into the patient's life. The nurse advocates for an environment that provides for sufficient physical privacy, including auditory privacy for discussions of a personal nature and policies and practices that protect the confidentiality of information.

3.2 Confidentiality

Associated with the right to privacy, the nurse has a duty to maintain confidentiality of all patient information. The patient's well-being could be jeopardized and the fundamental trust between patient and nurse destroyed by unnecessary access to data or by the inappropriate disclosure of identifiable patient information. The rights, well-being, and safety of the individual patient should be the primary factors in arriving at any professional judgment concerning the disposition of confidential information received from or about the patient, whether oral, written, or electronic. The standard of nursing practice and the nurse's responsibility to provide quality care require that relevant data be shared with those members of the health care team who have a need to know. Only information pertinent to a patient's treatment and welfare is disclosed, and only to those directly involved with the patient's care. Duties of confidentiality, however, are not absolute and may need to be modified in order to protect the patient, other innocent parties, and in circumstances of mandatory disclosure for public health reasons.

Information used for purposes of peer review, third-party payments, and other quality improvement or risk management mechanisms may be disclosed only under defined policies, mandates, or protocols.

American Nurses' Association Code of Ethics for Nurses With Interpretive Statements—cont'd

3.2 Confidentiality—cont'd

These written guidelines must assure that the rights, well-being, and safety of the patient are protected. In general, only that information directly relevant to a task or specific responsibility should be disclosed. When using electronic communications, special effort should be made to maintain data security.

3.3 Protection of participants in research

Stemming from the right of self-determination, each individual has the right to choose whether or not to participate in research. It is imperative that the patient or legally authorized surrogate receive sufficient information that is material to an informed decision, to comprehend that information, and to know how to discontinue participation in research without penalty. Necessary information to achieve an adequately informed consent includes the nature of participation, potential harms and benefits, and available alternatives to taking part in the research. Additionally, the patient should be informed of how the data will be protected. The patient has the right to refuse to participate in research or to withdraw at any time without fear of adverse consequences or reprisal.

Research should be conducted and directed only by qualified persons. Prior to implementation, all research should be approved by a qualified review board to ensure patient protection and the ethical integrity of the research. Nurses should be cognizant of the special concerns raised by research involving vulnerable groups, including children, prisoners, students, the elderly, and the poor. The nurse who participates in research in any capacity should be fully informed about both the subject's and the nurse's rights and obligations in the particular research study and in research in general. Nurses have the duty to question and, if necessary, to report and to refuse to participate in research they deem morally objectionable.

3.4 Standards and review mechanisms

Nursing is responsible and accountable for assuring that only those individuals who have demonstrated the knowledge, skill, practice experiences, commitment, and integrity essential to professional practice are allowed to enter into and continue to practice within the profession. Nurse educators have a responsibility to ensure that basic competencies are achieved and to promote a commitment to professional practice prior to entry of an individual into practice. Nurse administrators are responsible for assuring that the knowledge and skill of each nurse in the workplace are assessed prior to the assignment of responsibilities requiring preparation beyond basic academic programs.

The nurse has a responsibility to implement and maintain standards of professional nursing practice. The nurse should participate in planning, establishing, implementing, and evaluating review mechanisms designed to safeguard patients and nurses, such as peer review processes or committees, credentialing processes, quality improvement initiatives, and ethics committees. Nurse administrators must ensure that nurses have access to and inclusion on institutional ethics committees.

Continued

American Nurses' Association Code of Ethics for Nurses With Interpretive Statements—cont'd

3.4 Standards and review mechanisms—cont'd

Nurses must bring forward difficult issues related to patient care and/or institutional constraints upon ethical practice for discussion and review. The nurse acts to promote inclusion of appropriate others in all deliberations related to patient care.

Nurses should also be active participants in the development of policies and review mechanisms designed to promote patient safety, reduce the likelihood of errors, and address both environmental systems factors and human factors that present increased risk to patients. In addition, when errors to occur, nurses are expected to follow institutional guidelines in reporting errors committed or observed to the appropriate supervisory personnel and for assuring responsible disclosure of errors to patients. Under no circumstances should the nurse participate in, or condone through silence, either an attempt to hide an error or a punitive response that serves only to fix blame rather than correct the conditions that led to the error.

3.5 Acting on questionable practice

The nurse's primary commitment is to the health, well-being, and safety of the patient across the life span and in all settings in which health care needs are addressed. As an advocate for the patient, the nurse must be alert to and take appropriate action regarding any instances of incompetent, unethical, illegal, or impaired practice by any member of the health care team or the health care system or any action on the part of others that places the rights or best interests of the patient in jeopardy. To function effectively in this role, nurses must be knowledgeable about the Code of Ethics, standards of practice of the profession, relevant federal, state, and local laws and regulations, and the employing organization's policies and procedures.

When the nurse is aware of inappropriate or questionable practice in the provision or denial of health care, concern should be expressed to the person carrying out the questionable practice. Attention should be called to the possible detrimental affect upon the patient's well-being or best interests as well as the integrity of nursing practice. When factors in the health care delivery system or health care organization threaten the welfare of the patient, similar action should be directed to the responsible administrator. If indicated, the problems should be reported to an appropriate higher authority within the institution or agency, or to an appropriate external authority.

There should be established processes for reporting and handling incompetent, unethical, illegal, or impaired practice within the employment setting so that such reporting can go through official channels, thereby reducing the risk of reprisal against the reporting nurse. All nurses have a responsibility to assist those who identify potentially questionable practice. State nurses associations should be prepared to provide assistance and support in the development and evaluation of such processes and reporting procedures. When incompetent, unethical, illegal, or impaired practice is not corrected within the employment setting and continues to jeopardize patient well-being and safety, the problem

American Nurses' Association Code of Ethics for Nurses With Interpretive Statements—cont'd

3.5 Acting on questionable practice—cont'd

should be reported to other appropriate authorities such as practice committees of the pertinent professional organizations, the legally constituted bodies concerned with licensing of specific categories of health workers and professional practitioners, or the regulatory agencies concerned with evaluating standards or practice. Some situations may warrant the concern and involvement of all such groups. Accurate reporting and factual documentation, and not merely opinion, undergird all such responsible actions. When a nurse chooses to engage in the act of responsible reporting about situations that are perceived as unethical, incompetent, illegal, or impaired, the professional organization has a responsibility to provide the nurse with support and assistance and to protect the practice of those nurses who choose to voice their concerns. Reporting unethical, illegal, incompetent, or impaired practices, even when done appropriately, may present substantial risks to the nurse; nevertheless, such risks do not eliminate the obligation to address serious threats to patient safety.

3.6 Addressing impaired practice

Nurses must be vigilant to protect the patient, the public, and the profession from potential harm when a colleague's practice, in any setting, appears to be impaired. The nurse extends compassion and caring to colleagues who are in recovery from illness or when illness interferes with job performance. In a situation where a nurse suspects another's practice may be impaired, the nurse's duty is to take action designed both to protect patients and to assure that the impaired individual receives assistance in regaining optimal function. Such action should usually begin with consulting supervisory personnel and may also include confronting the individual in a supportive manner and with the assistance of others or helping the individual to access appropriate resources. Nurses are encouraged to follow guidelines outlined by the profession and policies of the employing organization to assist colleagues whose job performance may be adversely affected by mental or physical illness or by personal circumstances. Nurses in all roles should advocate for colleagues whose job performance may be impaired to ensure that they receive appropriate assistance, treatment, and access to fair institutional and legal processes. This includes supporting the return to practice of the individual who has sought assistance and is ready to resume professional duties.

If impaired practice poses a threat or danger to self or others, regardless of whether the individual has sought help, the nurse must take action to report the individual to persons authorized to address the problem. Nurses who advocate for others whose job performance creates a risk for harm should be protected from negative consequences. Advocacy may be a difficult process and the nurse is advised to follow workplace policies. If workplace policies do not exist or are inappropriate—that is, they deny the nurse in question access to due legal process or demand resignation—the reporting nurse may obtain guidance from the professional association, state peer assistance programs, employee assistance program, or a similar resource.

Continued

American Nurses' Association Code of Ethics for Nurses With Interpretive Statements—cont'd

Provision 4: *The nurse is responsible and accountable for individual nursing practice and determines the appropriate delegation of tasks consistent with the nurse's obligation to provide optimum patient care.*

4.1 Acceptance of accountability and responsibility

Individual registered nurses bear primary responsibility for the nursing care that their patients receive and are individually accountable for their own practice. Nursing practice includes direct care activities, acts of delegation, and other responsibilities such as teaching, research, and administration. In each instance, the nurse retains accountability and responsibility for the quality of practice and for conformity with standards of care.

Nurses are faced with decisions in the context of the increased complexity and changing patterns in the delivery of health care. As the scope of nursing practice changes, the nurse must exercise judgment in accepting responsibilities, seeking consultation, and assigning activities to others who carry out nursing care. For example, some advanced practice nurses have the authority to issue prescription and treatment orders to be carried out by other nurses. These acts are not acts of delegation. Both the advanced practice nurse issuing the order and the nurse accepting the order are responsible for the judgments made and accountable for the actions taken.

4.2 Accountability for nursing judgment and action

Accountability means to be answerable to oneself and others for one's own actions. In order to be accountable, nurses act under a code of ethical conduct that is grounded in the moral principles of fidelity and respect for the dignity, worth, and self-determination of patients. Nurses are accountable for judgments made and actions taken in the course of nursing practice, irrespective of health care organizations' policies or providers' directives.

4.3 Responsibility for nursing judgment and action

Responsibility refers to the specific accountability or liability associated with the performance of duties of a particular role. Nurses accept or reject specific role demands based upon their education, knowledge, competence, and extent of experience. Nurses in administration, education, and research also have obligations to the recipients of nursing care. Although nurses in administration, education, and research have relationships with patients that are less direct, in assuming the responsibilities of a particular role, they share responsibility for the care provided by those whom they supervise and instruct. The nurse must not engage in practices prohibited by law or delegate activities to others that are prohibited by the practice acts of other health care providers.

Individual nurses are responsible for assessing their own competence. When the needs of the patient are beyond the qualifications and competencies of the nurse, consultation and collaboration must be sought from qualified nurses, other health professionals, or other appropriate sources. Educational resources should be sought by nurses and provided by institutions to maintain and advance the competence of nurses. Nurse educators act in collaboration with

American Nurses' Association Code of Ethics for Nurses With Interpretive Statements—cont'd

4.3 Responsibility for nursing judgment and action—cont'd
their students to assess the learning needs of the student, the effectiveness of the teaching program, the identification and utilization of appropriate resources, and the support needed for the learning process.

4.4 Delegation of nursing activities
Since the nurse is accountable for the quality of nursing care given to patients, nurses are accountable for the assignment of nursing responsibilities to other nurses and the delegation of nursing care activities to other health care workers. While delegation and assignment are used here in a generic moral sense, it is understood that individual states may have a particular legal definition of these terms.

The nurse must make reasonable efforts to assess individual competence when assigning selected components of nursing care to other heath care workers. This assessment involves evaluating the knowledge, skills, and experience of the individual to whom the care is assigned, the complexity of the assigned tasks, and the health status of the patient. The nurse is also responsible for monitoring the activities of these individuals and evaluating the quality of the care provided. Nurses may not delegate responsibilities such as assessment and evaluation; they may delegate tasks. The nurse must not knowingly assign or delegate to any member of the nursing team a task for which that person is not prepared or qualified. Employer policies or directives do not relieve the nurse of responsibility for making judgments about the delegation and assignment of nursing care tasks.

Nurses functioning in management or administrative roles have a particular responsibility to provide an environment that supports and facilitates appropriate assignment and delegation. This includes providing appropriate orientation to staff, assisting less experienced nurses in developing necessary skills and competencies, and establishing policies and procedures that protect both the patient and nurse from the inappropriate assignment or delegation of nursing responsibilities, activities, or tasks.

Nurses functioning in educator or preceptor roles may have less direct relationships with patients. However, through assignment of nursing care activities to learners they share responsibility and accountability for the care provided. It is imperative that the knowledge and skills of the learner be sufficient to provide the assigned nursing care and that appropriate supervision be provided to protect both the patient and the learner.

Provision 5: *The nurse owes the same duties to self as to others, including the responsibility to preserve integrity and safety, to maintain competence, and to continue personal and professional growth.*
5.1 Moral self-respect
Moral respect accords moral worth and dignity to all human beings irrespective of their personal attributes or life station. Such respect extends to oneself as well; the same duties that we owe to others we owe to ourselves. Self-regarding duties refer to a realm of duties that primarily concern oneself and include professional growth and maintenance of competence, preservation of wholeness of character, and personal integrity.

Continued

American Nurses' Association Code of Ethics for Nurses With Interpretive Statements—cont'd

5.2 Professional growth and maintenance of competence

Though it has consequences for others, maintenance of competence and ongoing professional growth involves the control of one's own conduct in a way that is primarily self-regarding. Competence affects one's self-respect, self-esteem, professional status, and the meaningfulness of work. In all nursing roles, evaluation of one's own performance coupled with peer review, is a means by which nursing practice can be held to the highest standards. Each nurse is responsible for participating in the development of criteria for evaluation of practice and for using those criteria in peer and self-assessment.

Continual professional growth, particularly in knowledge and skill, requires a commitment to lifelong learning. Such learning includes, but is not limited to, continuing education, networking with professional colleagues, self-study, professional reading, certification, and seeking advanced degrees. Nurses are required to have knowledge relevant to the current scope and standards of nursing practice, changing issues, concerns, controversies, and ethics. Where the care required is outside of the competencies of the individual nurse, consultation should be sought or the patient should be referred to others for appropriate care.

5.3 Wholeness of character

Nurses have both personal and professional identities that are neither entirely separate, nor entirely merged, but are integrated. In the process of becoming a professional, the nurse embraces the values of the profession, integrating them with personal values. Duties to self involve an authentic expression of one's own moral point-of-view in practice. Sound ethical decision-making requires the respectful and open exchange of views between and among all individuals with relevant interests. In a community of moral discourse, no one person's view should automatically take precedence over that of another. Thus the nurse has a responsibility to express moral perspectives, even when they differ from those of others, and even when they might not prevail.

This wholeness of character encompasses relationships with patients. In situations where the patient requests a personal opinion from the nurse, the nurse is generally free to express an informed personal opinion as long as this preserves the voluntariness of the patient and maintains appropriate professional and moral boundaries. It is essential to be aware of the potential for undue influence attached to the nurse's professional role. Assisting patients to clarify their own values in reaching informed decisions may be helpful in avoiding unintended persuasion. In situations where nurses' responsibilities included care for those whose personal attributes, condition, lifestyle, or situation is stigmatized by the community and are personally unacceptable, the nurse still renders respectful and skilled care.

American Nurses' Association Code of Ethics for Nurses With Interpretive Statements—cont'd

5.4 Preservation of integrity

Integrity is an aspect of wholeness of character and is primarily a self-concern of the individual nurse. An economically constrained health care environment presents the nurse with particularly troubling threats to integrity. Threats to integrity may include a request to deceive a patient, to withhold information, or to falsify records, as well as verbal abuse from patients or coworkers. Threats to integrity also may include an expectation that the nurse will act in a way that is inconsistent with the values or ethics of the profession, or more specifically a request that is in direct violation of the Code of Ethics. Nurses have a duty to remain consistent with both their personal and professional values and to accept compromise only to the degree that it remains an integrity-preserving compromise. An integrity-preserving compromise does not jeopardize the dignity or well-being of the nurse or others. Integrity-preserving compromise can be difficult to achieve, but it is more likely to be accomplished in situations where there is an open forum for moral discourse and an atmosphere of mutual respect and regard.

Where nurses are placed in situations of compromise that exceed acceptable moral limits or involve violations of the moral standards of the profession, whether in direct patient care or any other forms of nursing practice, they may express their conscientious objection to participation. Where a particular treatment, intervention, activity, or practice is morally objectionable to the nurse, whether intrinsically so or because it is inappropriate for the specific patient, or where it may jeopardize both patients and nursing practice, the nurse is justified in refusing to participate on moral grounds. Such grounds exclude personal preference, prejudice, convenience, or arbitrariness. Conscientious objection may not insulate the nurse against formal or informal penalty. The nurse who decides not to take part on the grounds of conscientious objection must communicate this decision in appropriate ways. Whenever possible, such a refusal should be made known in advance and in time for alternate arrangements to be made for patient care. The nurse is obliged to provide for the patient's safety, to avoid patient abandonment, and to withdraw only when assured that alternative sources of nursing care are available to the patient.

Where patterns of institutional behavior or professional practice compromise the integrity of all its nurses, nurses should express their concern or conscientious objection collectively to the appropriate body or committee. In addition, they should express their concern, resist, and seek to bring about a change in those persistent activities or expectations in the practice setting that are morally objectionable to nurses and jeopardize either patient or nurse well-being.

Continued

American Nurses' Association Code of Ethics for Nurses With Interpretive Statements—cont'd

Provision 6: *The nurse participates in establishing, maintaining, and improving health care environments and conditions of employment conducive to the provision of quality health care and consistent with the values of the profession through individual and collective action.*

6.1 Influence of the environment on moral virtues and values

Virtues are habits of character that predispose persons to meet their moral obligations; that is, to do right. Excellences are habits of character that predispose a person to do a particular job or task well. Virtues such as wisdom, honesty, and courage are habits or attributes of the morally good person. Excellences such as compassion, patience, and skill are habits of the character of the morally good nurse. For the nurse, virtues and excellences are those habits that affirm and promote the values of human dignity, well-being, respect, health, independence, and other values central to nursing. Both virtues and excellences, as aspects of moral character, can be either nurtured by the environment in which the nurse practices or they can be diminished or thwarted. All nurses have a responsibility to create, maintain, and contribute to environments that support the growth of virtues and excellences and enable nurses to fulfill their ethical obligations.

6.2 Influence of the environment on ethical obligations

All nurses, regardless of role, have a responsibility to create, maintain, and contribute to environments of practice that support nurses in fulfilling their ethical obligations. Environments of practice include observable features, such as working conditions, and written policies and procedures setting out expectations for nurses, as well as less tangible characteristics such as informal peer norms. Organizational structures, role descriptions, health and safety initiatives, grievance mechanisms, ethics committees, compensation systems, and disciplinary procedures all contribute to environments that can either present barriers or foster ethical practice and professional fulfillment. Environments in which employees are provided fair hearing of grievances, are supported in practicing according to standards of care, and are justly treated allow for the realization of the values of the profession and are consistent with sound nursing practice.

6.3 Responsibility for the healthcare environment

The nurse is responsible for contributing to a moral environment that encourages respectful interactions with colleagues, support of peers, and identification of issues that need to be addressed. Nurse administrators have a particular responsibility to assure that employees are treated fairly and that nurses are involved in decisions related to their practice and working conditions.

Acquiescing and accepting unsafe or inappropriate practices, even if the individual does not participate in the specific practice, is equivalent to condoning unsafe practice. Nurses should not remain employed in facilities that routinely violate patient rights or require nurses to severely and repeatedly compromise standards of practice or personal morality.

American Nurses' Association Code of Ethics for Nurses With Interpretive Statements—cont'd

6.3 Responsibility for the healthcare environment

As with concerns about patient care, nurses should address concerns about the health care environment through appropriate channels. Organizational changes are difficult to accomplish and may require persistent efforts over time. Toward this end, nurses may participate in collective action such as collective bargaining or workplace advocacy, preferably through a professional association such as the state nurses association, in order to address the terms and conditions of employment. Agreement reached through such action must be consistent with the profession's standards of practice, the state law regulating practice, and the Code of Ethics for Nursing. Conditions of employment must contribute to the moral environment, the provision of quality patient care, and the professional satisfaction for nurses.

The professional association also serves as an advocate for the nurse by seeking to secure just compensation and humane working conditions for nurses. To accomplish this, the professional association may engage in collective bargaining on behalf of nurses. While seeking to assure just economic and general welfare for nurses, collective bargaining, nonetheless, seeks to keep the interests of both nurses and patients in balance.

Provision 7: *The nurse participates in the advancement of the profession through contributions to practice, education, administration, and knowledge development.*

7.1 Advancing the profession through active involvement in nursing and in health care policy

Nurses should advance their profession by contributing in some way to the leadership, activities, and the viability of their professional organizations. Nurses can also advance the profession by serving in leadership or mentorship roles or on committees within their places of employment. Nurses who are self-employed can advance the profession by serving as role models for professional integrity. Nurses can also advance the profession through participation in civic activities related to health care or through local, state, national, or international initiatives. Nurse educators have a specific responsibility to enhance student's commitment to professional and civic values. Nurse administrators have a responsibility to foster an employment environment that facilitates nurses' ethical integrity and professionalism, and nurse researchers are responsible for active contribution to the body of knowledge supporting and advancing nursing practice.

7.2 Advancing the profession by developing, maintaining, and implementing professional standards in clinical, administrative, and educational practice

Standards and guidelines reflect the practice of nursing grounded in ethical commitments and a body of knowledge. Professional standards and guidelines for nurses must be developed by nurses and reflect nursing's responsibility to society. It is the responsibility of nurses to identify their own scope of practice as permitted by professional practice standards and guidelines, by state and federal laws, by relevant societal values, and by the Code of Ethics.

Continued

American Nurses' Association Code of Ethics for Nurses With Interpretive Statements—cont'd

7.2 Advancing the profession by developing, maintaining, and implementing professional standards in clinical, administrative, and educational practice—cont'd

The nurse as administrator or manager must establish, maintain, and promote conditions of employment that enable nurses within that organization or community setting to practice in accord with accepted standards of nursing practice and provide a nursing and health care work environment that meets the standards and guidelines of nursing practice. Professional autonomy and self-regulation in the control of conditions of practice are necessary for implementing nursing standards and guidelines and assuring quality care for those whom nursing serves.

The nurse educator is responsible for promoting and maintaining optimum standards of both nursing education and of nursing practice in any settings where planned learning activities occur. Nurse educators must also ensure that only those students who posses the knowledge, skills, and competencies that are essential to nursing graduate from their nursing programs.

7.3 Advancing the profession through knowledge development, dissemination, and application to practice

The nursing profession should engage in scholarly inquiry to identify, evaluate, refine, and expand the body of knowledge that forms the foundation of its discipline and practice. In addition, nursing knowledge is derived from the sciences and from the humanities. Ongoing scholarly activities are essential to fulfilling a profession's obligations to society. All nurses working alone or in collaboration with others can participate in the advancement of the profession through the development, evaluation, dissemination, and application of knowledge in practice. However, an organizational climate and infrastructure conducive to scholarly inquiry must be valued and implemented for this to occur.

Provision 8: *The nurse collaborates with other health professionals and the public in promoting community, national, and international efforts to meet health needs.*

8.1 Health needs and concerns

The nursing profession is committed to promoting the health, welfare, and safety of all people. The nurse has a responsibility to be aware not only of specific health needs of individual patients but also of broader health concerns such as world hunger, environmental pollution, lack of access to health care, violation of human rights, and inequitable distribution of nursing and health care resources. The availability and accessibility of high quality health services to all people require both interdisciplinary planning and collaborative partnerships among health professionals and others at the community, national, and international levels.

8.2 Responsibilities to the public

Nurses, individually and collectively, have a responsibility to be knowledgeable about the health status of the community and existing threats to health and safety. Through support of and participation in community organizations and groups, the nurse assists in efforts to educate the public, facilitates informed

American Nurses' Association Code of Ethics for Nurses With Interpretive Statements—cont'd

8.2 Responsibilities to the public—cont'd

choice, identifies conditions and circumstances that contribute to illness, injury and disease, fosters health life styles, and participates in institutional and legislative efforts to promote health and meet national health objectives. In addition, the nurse supports initiatives to address barriers to health, such as poverty, homelessness, unsafe living conditions, abuse and violence, and lack of access to health services.

The nurse also recognizes that health care is provided to culturally diverse populations in this country and in all parts of the world. In providing care, the nurse should avoid imposition of the nurse's own cultural values upon others. The nurse should affirm human dignity and show respect for the values and practices associated with different cultures and use approaches to care that reflect awareness and sensitivity.

Provision 9: *The profession of nursing, as represented by associations and their members, is responsible for articulating nursing values for maintaining the integrity of the profession and its practice, and for shaping social policy.*

9.1 Assertion of values

It is the responsibility of a professional association to communicate and affirm the values of the profession to its members. It is essential that the professional organization encourages discourse that supports critical self-reflection and evaluation within the profession. The organization also communicates to the public the values that nursing considers central to social change that will enhance health.

9.2 The profession carries out its collective responsibility through professional associations

The nursing profession continues to develop ways to clarify nursing's accountability to society. The contract between the profession and society is made explicit through such mechanisms as (a) the Code of Ethics for Nurses, (b) the standards of nursing practice, (c) the ongoing development of nursing knowledge derived from nursing theory, scholarship, and research in order to guide nursing actions, (d) educational requirements for practice, (e) certification, and (f) mechanisms for evaluating the effectiveness of professional nursing actions.

9.3 Intraprofessional integrity

A professional association is responsible for expressing the values and ethics of the profession and also for encouraging the professional organization and its members to function in accord with those values and ethics. Thus, one of its fundamental responsibilities is to promote awareness and adherence to the Code of Ethics and to critique the activities and ends of the professional association itself. Values and ethics influence the power structures of the association in guiding, correcting, and directing its activities. Legitimate concerns for the self-interest of the association and profession are balanced by a commitment to the social goods that are sought. Through critical self-reflection and self-evaluation, associations must foster change within themselves, seeking to move the professional community toward its stated ideals.

Continued

American Nurses' Association Code of Ethics for Nurses With Interpretive Statements—cont'd

9.4 Social reform

Nurses can work individually as citizens or collectively through political action to bring about social change. It is the responsibility of a professional nursing association to speak for nurses collectively in shaping and reshaping health care within our nation, specifically in areas of health care policy and legislation that affect accessibility, quality, and the cost of health care. Here, the professional association maintains vigilance and takes action to influence legislators, reimbursement agencies, nursing organizations, and other health professions. In these activities, health is understood as being broader than delivery and reimbursement systems, but extending to health-related sociocultural issues such as violation of human rights, homelessness, hunger, violence, and the stigma of illness.

The Caring Code

(Discussed in Chapter 13)

THEME	CARING BEHAVIOR
Caring assistance during admission	When I enter the ward, please ask me with genuine concern, "How are you feeling?" "How can I help you?"
	Be sensitive to my needs. For example, help me to lie down and then ask me about my problem.
	When you take me to my room, please introduce me to the environment and to my roommate(s).
	Introduce yourself and to the doctors and nurses responsible for me.
Professional caring behaviors	Help me take care of my hygiene. For example, change the sheets or give me a bath.
	Make me more comfortable. For example, help me turn over or find the proper position, or give me a massage.
	Pay attention to my safety. For example, help me get in and out of bed when necessary, or go to the bathroom.
	Inform me of daily diagnostic tests, therapy, and nursing plans to let me prepare myself for them.
	Before and after tests, therapy, and surgery, clearly explain what is happening, what I should do, and what to expect.
	When I am receiving fluids intravenously, please check the flow and the area around the insertion site and adjust it when needed without being asked.
	When I press the call button, please respond immediately.
	Perform nursing skills correctly. Do not hurt me or make me uncomfortable.
	Please make referrals to the personnel able to help me solve my problems.
	Teach me and demonstrate the skills I need to take care of myself. For example, how to apply pressure to my incision when I turn, how to cough, or how to apply hot compresses.
	Help me take my medicine and give my treatments when they are scheduled.
	Explain what my medicine is supposed to do and what side effects I might expect.
	Explain my condition to me and my family. For example, tell me and my family your reading of my vital signs.
	Teach me things to watch for after I am discharged. For example, how to take my medicine, signs that should be reported to the doctor, when I need to return for follow-up care, and how to take care of myself.

Continued

THEME	CARING BEHAVIOR
Caring in communication	Communicate with me in simple, clear language I can understand. For example, avoid using medical terms when discussing my condition with me or when I am present.
	Speak with me in a warm and caring tone of voice.
	Look at me when speaking to me.
	Wear a genuine smile.
	Give me time to ask questions.
	Encourage me to speak freely.
	Be patient with me. Avoid being impatient or irritated in tone or appearance.
	Listen patiently to my family and me.
Empathy	Let me know through your behavior and speech that you understand what I am going through during examinations and therapy. For example, "You look cold. Can I get you a blanket?"
	Believe me when I say I am in pain and when I express my personal feelings, such as feeling afraid or alone.
	When I am uncomfortable or sick, please try to help me feel more comfortable. For example, change my dressings when they are wet.
	Pay attention to my emotional state and find ways to help me feel better when needed.
	When I am upset, please be considerate and continue to take care of me.
	Provide a comfortable, quiet environment. For example, tell my roommates and visitors to keep their voices down.
	If I seem bored or restless, please make suggestions for some things I may do, such as reading, walking, or watching television. Please walk with me if I need help.
Sincerity	Please treat me like I am one of the family.
	Please act as though you really care about me. For example, do not make me feel like I am part of a routine or a cog in a machine.
	Keep promises to me or explain when they are broken.
	When you are busy or about to finish your shift, please continue to give me the care I need.
	In addition to necessary tests and therapy, please check in on me from time to time to let me know you did not forget me.
	Be concerned with my physical needs, such as appetite, digestion, special dietary needs, sleep habits, and bowel movements.
	Be gentle in your actions. For example, when you help me use the bedpan or turn over.
	Praise and encourage me. For example, say, "You are doing well."

THEME	CARING BEHAVIOR
	When I need it, use words and actions to support me through difficulties. For example, keep me company, hold my hand, and say, "You can do it" or "We're in this together."
Respect	Address me properly and make me feel respected.
	Respect my privacy at all times—during physical examinations, therapy, and nursing care. For example, draw the curtains or cover me in an appropriate manner.
	Respect my religious beliefs.
	Respect my customs and culture.
	Respect my individual privacy and keep my medical information privileged.
	Avoid criticizing my family or me behind my back.

From Lee-Hsieh, J., Kuo, C., & Tseng, H. (2005). Application and evaluation of a caring code in clinical nursing education. *Journal of Nursing Education, 44*(4), 177-184. Reprinted with permission from SLACK Incorporated.

Case Studies for Group Discussion

(Discussed in Chapter 14)

#1: Beginning Students Working With Elderly Clients in an Assisted Living Community

Case study: Momma Maria has lived independently in one of the apartments here for 5 years. Until recently, she came to the community dining room for her dinner, but prepared her own breakfast and lunch, managed her own medications, and light housework. Once a week, she rode the facility's bus to the grocery store to do her shopping, and often participated in community-planned activities such as trips to museums and malls. In the past several months, she has fallen three times: once in her apartment, once on a group excursion, and once getting off the bus.

Discussion questions

Today, let's talk about safety issues for the elderly.

1. What physiologic changes occur with aging that make this population vulnerable to falls?
2. Why are we concerned about falls in the elderly? What is the result of falls for them? *(Continue to refine and direct the discussion to identify the sequela of fall injury and hip fractures on overall quality of life and prognosis.)*
3. What additional information would we want about Momma Maria and her environment that would help guide our safety interventions? (i.e., physical assessment, medication evaluation, environmental assessment, diet; consider psychosocial issues and fiscal resources as well).

(At this point, discussion can be directed in any number of directions. Students can be given prompts in the form of "new data" from their assessment. For example, environmental hazards can be identified, or medications that might contribute to falls could be provided. The next questions follow one possible focus.)

4. So, one of the issues you've identified is problems with balance and flexibility that can contribute to Momma's falls. What are some exercises that might improve her balance and flexibility?
5. You also found that Momma's osteoarthritis is a factor in her mobility. What interventions might we explore to help with this problem?
6. You said that one of the reasons participation in these excursions is so important for Momma is the lack of social activities here. What might we do about that this term? What things might we initiate that would promote physical health and socialization and be sustainable after we leave?

Case Studies for Group Discussion—cont'd

#2: Exploring attitudes and beliefs about others

Case study: Imagine a day like this in the outpatient wound management clinic you have been working in. The morning schedule is full, as always, and a drug representative is slated to provide an in-service presentation on a new treatment approach during the lunch break from noon to 1:00 PM. Lunch is even being provided! The clinic is staffed today with one physician, one nurse practitioner who manages the clinic, one physician's assistant, two registered nurses, and of course, you, a student nurse. Efficiency is the order of the day; everyone wants to get to the meeting on time and enjoy a free lunch—someone says submarine sandwiches have been ordered! Patients are brought into the treatment rooms by the nurses and you for their initial assessments and dressing changes. The physician, physician's assistant, and nurse practitioner rotate through the rooms, treating and writing prescriptions as needed, and the nurses and you provide any needed discharge teaching. Many of the patients are being treated for diabetic ulcers. As you leave a room, you hear one nurse complain to the other "Some of these people are just filthy. They skip appointments and don't care for their wounds the way they are supposed to and then whine when their ulcers don't heal and their treatment takes longer! And now, we're going to be late for the meeting! It really pisses me off, but I guess it's to be expected."

Discussion questions

1. Based on these comments, what values, attitudes, and beliefs does this nurse hold?

    (Students will likely identify some of these: being compliant with care instructions; being responsible for one's own care; being clean; being efficient and on time; being with others like herself/himself. These provide the basis for the next question.)

2. How might these affect the care this nurse provides?

3. What kind of information about this nurse might help us understand where these values, attitudes, and beliefs came from?

    (This should open the door to matters of socioeconomic background and the influences of families, institutions, and cultural norms on values, beliefs, and attitudes.)

4. How might we enhance our own sensitivity to diversity when we are providing nursing care?

    (Activities such as this one provoke further individual reflection. Students might be directed next to their reflective journals to apply the results of the discussion from the last question to their own personal development.)

Case Study for Individual or Group Learning

(Discussed in Chapters 14 and 15)

Maternity nursing: gestational diabetes

Case studies relating to specialty areas can be used for individual written assignments or as group learning experiences. If they are to be completed individually and submitted as written assignments, they can be linked to articles, texts, or even web pages as part of the assignment. Under these circumstances, the directions must be very clear; if used with a group, it is possible further clarification will be needed.

Case study: Kathy Kopland is a 34-year-old primipara. She was overweight prior to her pregnancy and has a family history of type 2 diabetes mellitus. Her history is otherwise uneventful, and prior evaluations have been within normal limits. Today, at 22 weeks gestation, her postprandial blood sugar is abnormal, and her physician orders a glucose tolerance test. Kathy asks you, "So, if I do have diabetes, will I be taking pills like my Aunt Francis does?"

Discussion questions

1 How would you respond to Kathy's question?
2. What instructions will you give Kathy in preparation for her glucose tolerance test? What will you tell her to do prior to the test? Describe the procedure, using language Kathy will understand.

   If the results of the test confirm gestational diabetes, let's say her physician orders glargine insulin for basal use, with a sliding scale using Humulin N for mealtime coverage.
3. What types/groups of insulin are these? How do they differ in onset, peak, and duration? What is the rationale for ordering two different insulins?
4. Kathy asks you if this means she will be taking insulin forever now. How will you answer her?
5. During the course of her pregnancy, how will her risk for developing hyper- and hypoglycemia change?
6. What are the signs and symptoms of hyper- and hypoglycemia? What conditions can cause them?
7. What complications are Kathy and her baby at risk for because of her gestational diabetes?

   For an individual assignment, students could be instructed to go to the web page of the American Diabetes Association (http://www.diabetes.org) and find more information about gestational diabetes, including teaching materials for use with Kathy.

Faculty-Directed Independent Learning Experience:
Eye Surgery Center

(Discussed in Chapter 3)

Purpose: This one-day clinical experience is an opportunity to gain an understanding of surgical interventions for a variety of disorders of the eye. During this time, you will observe the nursing roles and collaboration among team members in a community-based surgical center and participate in selected aspects of the care provided. Following the experience, you will engage in guided reflection designed to facilitate additional learning and will share your insights with your colleagues in clinical conference.

Objectives
Upon completion of this assignment, the student will:
▣ Understand surgical interventions for a variety of disorders of the eye.
▣ Compare and contrast perioperative nursing roles and functions in the acute care setting to those in this community-based setting.
▣ Describe the collaboration of nurses with other team members.
▣ Perform preoperative assessments for two or more patients having different surgical interventions.
▣ Participate in discharge teaching and follow-through for two or more patients.

Preparation
▣ Review the anatomy of the eye.
▣ Read materials and review the links for this assignment posted on the course website.

Reflection activity
Following your experience, reflect on your learning in your journal. You may apply any of the techniques previously used, but address the following as well:
▣ What prior knowledge did you have to apply to this experience?
Reflecting now about the experience:
▣ What are your overall impressions?
▣ What preconceptions did you have? How were they supported or dispelled?
▣ What did you do well? *(Students will have previously learned that this includes all aspects of learning: what they know, what skills they did, and how they felt about the experience and their performance.)*
▣ What was this experience like from the patients' perspectives? *(Students will have previously learned that this is part of becoming more sensitive to patients by speculating what they thought and felt during a clinical encounter.)*
▣ What are your learning issues now? *(Learning issues are unanswered questions students have and topics they want and/or need to learn more about.)*
▣ Besides addressing the assignment objectives, what would you like to share with your student colleagues in conference about this entire experience?

Formal Graded Paper Addressing a Critical Incident

(Discussed in Chapter 15)

The purpose of this assignment is to provide the student with the opportunity to demonstrate his/her insight and awareness regarding a clinical situation (an incident) involving a patient that was critical to learning within the format of a formal, scholarly paper.

The paper will be graded according to the following guidelines:

I. **Description of the context of the incident (5 points):**
    Describe the background or the setting of the incident (clinical agency/unit, date, hour, location on the unit, others present/participating). Describe everything relevant to another person's understanding the incident.

II. **Clarity of the explanation of why you felt the incident was critical (10 points):**
    The incident chosen should represent a patient problem that is within the domain of the role of nursing. Explain why you considered the incident "critical" for your learning.

III. **Description of the responses to the incident (10 points):**
    Personal responses: Discuss what you were thinking/concerned about at the time; discuss your feelings/emotions at the time.
    Patient/family responses related/relevant to the critical incident): Include developmental responses, symptom responses, other responses of the patient to the critical incident, and any action that the patient took in response to the incident.

IV. **Description of actions and evaluation related to the critical incident (15 points):**
    Describe interventions taken; explain scientific rationale for interventions, if appropriate. Explain why interventions were or were not chosen; evaluate the effectiveness of interventions implemented. Describe the outcome (actual or anticipated) for the patient related to your analysis and interventions.

V. **Provision of theoretical rationale for decisions you made (20 points):**

VI. **Exploration of future actions (30 points):**
    Now, with the benefit of time, research, and reflection, what, if anything, would you do differently? How will your future practice be affected by this experience?

VII. **Format and style (10 points):**
    Papers must be written using APA format (*APA Manual*, 5th edition) and be clear, concise, and scholarly.

General Faculty Guidelines for Reflective Journaling

(Discussed in Chapter 11)

- Establish parameters for length of entries; emphasize that what is important is the quality of the content.
- Establish when entries are to be made (e.g., following the day of clinical), and when they must be submitted.
- Discourage detailed descriptions of clinical situations, what was observed or done; tell them to write only enough to provide a basis for the subsequent discourse.
- Encourage the identification and critique of assumptions.
- Encourage suitable application of theory, with an emphasis on thoughts, feelings, and pertinent actions.
- Maintain patient confidentiality by avoiding the use of individually identifiable health information (see Chapter 5).
- Assure student confidentiality; whether to share journal content should be the students' choice.
- Provide illustrative examples, using the selected format.

Getting to Know One Another: Ice Breakers

(Discussed in Chapter 10)

Introductions

Various name games encourage active, fun, and creative introductions. Always allow people to pass if they cannot think of something, and then return to them later. Start with yourself as a model.

- Introduce yourself with your favorite food (or pick something else, like favorite recreational activity). "Hello, I'm Alice, crab Louie salad." Have the group members do the same, working around the group.
- Introduce yourself with your name and an applicable rhyming descriptive adjective. "Hello, I'm Barbara and I'm bubbly." Have the group members do the same, working around the group.
- Introduce yourself as if you were a stew composed of your interests and activities. Use any unit of measurement; you can even use proportional units to convey the relative amounts of each. "Hi, I'm Marie—I'm one cup books, one cup woods and water, one cup music, and a pinch of handcrafts." Have the group members do the same, working around the group.
- Pair off, and have each person interview their partner, inquiring about their name, hobbies, family, favorite music, etc. Then go around the room, having the partners introduce one another using only three words to describe them. "This is Mark, smart, loving, and silly."
  - Have people describe their dream vacations and explain why they see them that way.
  - Have people choose an animal that best reflects their personality and explain why.
  - Have people tell the group something they would never guess about themselves. "Hi, I'm Bob, and I won a blue ribbon at the county fair for a quilt I made."

Activities

Lots of activities can be used to help create the set for the clinical course, while helping to diffuse some of the anxiety students may bring with them. Some of these are general, others more specific to nursing or clinical foci.

- For a course in pediatric nursing, have each student name their favorite toy as a child and explain their choice. This can be used as a springboard into a discussion about developmental stages.
- Identify the four corners of the room, labeling them as "Strongly agree," "Agree," "Disagree," and "Strongly disagree." Then give the group a statement, having each person move to the corner reflecting their answer. Have the group discuss their responses. Choose a statement appropriate to the situation, like "I'm afraid I might say the wrong thing to a patient" for a psych/mental health practicum, or "Young children intimidate me" for a pediatric nursing course.

Getting to Know One Another: Ice Breakers—cont'd

Activities—cont'd

■ Have the group stand very close together. Tell them to reach out their arms so everyone's hands are jumbled and intertwined. Tell them to grab one hand of a fellow student in each of their hands creating a human knot. Instruct them to use teamwork to untangle themselves to form a circle without letting go of any hands. Students may have to loosen a grip, but are not to release any hands. This "knotty" problem has several potential results: figure eight, two interlocking circles, or one big circle with the people facing in or out.

■ Have the students write down words or phrases that describe their feelings on this first day of the course. Gather the responses up, and then write them on a blackboard or overhead. Then ask the group what they think you, as the faculty, are feeling today (verbally or in writing). Put these up, ideally in a second column, noting the parallels between the two. Use this to open discussion of mutual expectations and responsibilities for learning in the course.

Guideline for Recording Critical Incidents

(Discussed in Chapter 15)

What constitutes a critical incident? Any one of the following:

- An incident in which you feel your intervention really made a difference in patient outcome, either directly or indirectly (by helping other staff members)
- An incident that went unusually well
- An incident in which there was a breakdown (i.e., things did not go as planned)
- An incident that was very ordinary or typical
- An incident that you think captures the quintessence of what nursing is all about
- An incident that was particularly demanding

What to include in your description of a critical incident:

- The context of the incident (e.g., location, time of day, significant people)
- A description of what happened
- Why the incident is "critical" to you
- What your concerns were at the time
- What you were thinking about as it was taking place
- What you were feeling during and after the incident
- What, if anything, you found most demanding about the situation

Benner, Patricia, *From novice to expert: Excellence and power in clinical nursing practice,* 1st ed. ©1984, pp. 300-302. Adapted by permission of Pearson Education, Inc., Upper Saddle River, NJ.

National Education Association Code of Ethics of the Education Profession

(Discussed in Chapter 7)

PREAMBLE

The educator, believing in the worth and dignity of each human being, recognizes the supreme importance of the pursuit of truth, devotion to excellence, and the nurture of the democratic principles. Essential to these goals is the protection of freedom to learn and to teach and the guarantee of equal educational opportunity for all. The educator accepts the responsibility to adhere to the highest ethical standards.

The educator recognizes the magnitude of the responsibility inherent in the teaching process. The desire for the respect and confidence of one's colleagues, of students, of parents, and of the members of the community provides the incentive to attain and maintain the highest possible degree of ethical conduct. The Code of Ethics of the Education Profession indicates the aspiration of all educators and provides standards by which to judge conduct.

The remedies specified by the NEA and/or its affiliates for the violation of any provision of this Code shall be exclusive and no such provision shall be enforceable in any form other than the one specifically designated by the NEA or its affiliates.

PRINCIPLE I

Commitment to the student

The educator strives to help each student realize his or her potential as a worthy and effective member of society. The educator therefore works to stimulate the spirit of inquiry, the acquisition of knowledge and understanding, and the thoughtful formulation of worthy goals.

In fulfillment of the obligation to the student, the educator—

Shall not unreasonably restrain the student from independent action in the pursuit of learning.

Shall not unreasonably deny the student's access to varying points of view.

Shall not deliberately suppress or distort subject matter relevant to the student's progress.

Shall make reasonable effort to protect the student from conditions harmful to learning or to health and safety.

Shall not intentionally expose the student to embarrassment or disparagement.

Shall not on the basis of race, color, creed, sex, national origin, marital status, political or religious beliefs, family, social or cultural background, or sexual orientation, unfairly—

a. Exclude any student from participation in any program

b. Deny benefits to any student

c. Grant any advantage to any student

Shall not use professional relationships with students for private advantage.

Shall not disclose information about students obtained in the course of professional service unless disclosure serves a compelling professional purpose or is required by law.

Adopted by the NEA 1975 Representative Assembly.
Retrieved from http://www.nea.org/aboutnea/code.html.

Continued

National Education Association Code of Ethics of the Education Profession—cont'd

PRINCIPLE II
Commitment to the profession
The education profession is vested by the public with a trust and responsibility requiring the highest ideals of professional service.

In the belief that the quality of the services of the education profession directly influences the nation and its citizens, the educator shall exert every effort to raise professional standards, to promote a climate that encourages the exercise of professional judgment, to achieve conditions that attract persons worthy of the trust to careers in education, and to assist in preventing the practice of the profession by unqualified persons.

In fulfillment of the obligation to the profession, the educator—

Shall not in an application for a professional position deliberately make a false statement or fail to disclose a material fact related to competency and qualifications.

Shall not misrepresent his/her professional qualifications.

Shall not assist any entry into the profession of a person known to be unqualified in respect to character, education, or other relevant attribute.

Shall not knowingly make a false statement concerning the qualifications of a candidate for a professional position.

Shall not assist a noneducator in the unauthorized practice of teaching.

Shall not disclose information about colleagues obtained in the course of professional service unless disclosure serves a compelling professional purpose or is required by law.

Shall not knowingly make false or malicious statements about a colleague.

Shall not accept any gratuity, gift, or favor that might impair or appear to influence professional decisions or action.

National Student Nurses' Association

Code of Academic and Clinical Conduct

(Discussed in Chapter 6)

Preamble

Students of nursing have a responsibility to society in learning the academic theory and clinical skills needed to provide nursing care. The clinical setting presents unique challenges and responsibilities while caring for human beings in a variety of health care environments.

The Code of Academic and Clinical Conduct is based upon an understanding that to practice nursing as a student is an agreement to uphold the trust with which society has placed in us. The statements of the Code provide guidance for the nursing student in the personal development of an ethical foundation and need not be limited strictly to the academic or clinical environment but can assist in the holistic development of the person.

A Code for nursing students

As students are involved in the clinical and academic environments, we believe that ethical principles are a necessary guide to professional development. Therefore, within these environments we:

- Advocate for the rights of all clients.
- Maintain client confidentiality.
- Take appropriate action to ensure the safety of clients, self, and others.
- Provide care for the client in a timely, compassionate and professional manner.
- Communicate client care in a truthful, timely and accurate manner.
- Actively promote the highest level of moral and ethical principles and accept responsibility for our actions.
- Promote excellence in nursing by encouraging lifelong learning and professional development.
- Treat others with respect and promote an environment that respects human rights, values and choice of cultural and spiritual beliefs.
- Collaborate in every reasonable manner with the academic faculty and clinical staff to ensure the highest quality of client care.
- Use every opportunity to improve faculty and clinical staff understanding of the learning needs of nursing students.
- Encourage faculty, clinical staff, and peers to mentor nursing students.
- Refrain from performing any technique of procedure for which the student has not been adequately trained.
- Refrain from any deliberate action or omission of care in the academic or clinical setting that creates unnecessary risk of injury to the client, self, or others.

Adopted by the 2001 House of Delegates; Nashville, TN.
From National Student Nurses' Association. Retrieved December 16, 2005, from http://www.nsna.org/press/pr_code.pdf.

Continued

National Student Nurses' Association—cont'd

Code of Academic and Clinical Conduct—cont'd

A Code for nursing students—cont'd

- Assist the staff nurse or preceptor in ensuring that there is full disclosure and that proper authorizations are obtained from clients regarding any form of treatment or research.
- Abstain from the use of alcoholic beverages or any substances in the academic and clinical setting that impair judgment.
- Strive to achieve and maintain an optimal level of personal health.
- Support access to treatment and rehabilitation for students who are experiencing impairments related to substance abuse and mental or physical health issues.
- Uphold school policies and regulations related to academic and clinical performance, reserving the right to challenge and critique rules and regulations as per school grievance policy.

Sample Anecdotal Notes Illustrating Key Components

(Discussed in Chapter 8)

Nursing 201 (Pediatric nursing clinical course)
Monday, September 13, 2004
Course orientation: All students present and have downloaded and printed course syllabus materials. Reviewed school policies related to conduct, due process, grievance procedure; course objectives, assignments, and evaluation tool with grading criteria and data sources. All policies and procedures documented in syllabus. Question and answer session. Two-hour block in the skills lab reviewing agency specific equipment with practice opportunities.

Tuesday, September 14, 2004
Orientation at St. Charles hospital: Included fire, disaster, kidnapping emergency protocols; problem-based charting review and agency chart forms; chemical/body fluid exposure management. Orientation to pediatric unit included introduction to nurse manager; student scavenger hunt (form in syllabus); review of unit-specific chart forms and policies/procedures.

Notes for Sylvia Dillon
9/14/04: Late to hospital orientation; stated car problems. Not wearing either uniform or lab coat per appearance standards of program documented in syllabus and unchanged from prior clinical courses. Located lab coat for her use today. Instructed to review clinical appearance policy and be in conformance for first patient care day 9/20.

    9/20/04: Appearance appropriate. Assignment: 2-year-old male first post-op day for inguinal hernia repair, developmentally delayed. Hesitant to touch child, initially ignored mother present in the room. Calculated IV drip correctly and able to explain rational for IV fluid constituents. Drsg change w/good technique; recognized when contaminated gauze pad. Performed developmental assessment with moderate assistance. Discussed comfort level with children, touching, communication skills. States today's problem d/t new clinical experience anxiety. Plan for next week: work with child therapist in playroom to increase comfort with children and assessment skills; teaching opportunity with child and parent(s) to work on communication skills.

Sample Approaches to Reflective Journaling

(Discussed in Chapter 11)

Some approaches to reflective journaling can be applied consistently throughout a given clinical course, while in other cases, specific directions may be used in association with aspects of the clinical experience.

Ah-hah journals

Have the students identify a critical clinical event, something they did not previously know, had not considered before, or something they found to be unexpected. Describe the ah-hah, the accompanying thoughts and feelings, and then endeavor to generalize the learned concepts for future application.

From Herrman, J.W. (2002). The 60-second nurse educator: Creative strategies to inspire learning. *Nursing Education Perspectives, 23*(5), 222-227.

Hide and seek critical thinking

To help students identify their critical thinking, provide the habits of the mind and skills with their definitions from the consensus definition of critical thinking by Scheffer and Rubenfeld. Have the students reflect upon their clinical experiences, seeking out examples of their use.

Adapted from Kennison, M.M., & Misselwitz, S. (2002). Evaluating reflective writing for appropriateness, fairness, and consistency. *Nursing Education Perspectives, 23*(5), 238-242.

Reflective questions

In their journals, have students briefly describe the most significant event that occurred during their day in the clinical setting, and then answer the following questions:

- What have I learned from this experience?
- How would I behave next time in a similar situation?
- In what ways do nursing and related theories explain the situation and provide guidance for action?

Adapted from Burrows, D.E. (1995). The nurse teacher's role in the promotion of reflective practice. *Nurse Education Today, 15,* 346-350.

A journaling framework

Identify learning goals in advance, and then evaluate them following the day's clinical experiences.

- Analyze the day's events.
- Critically connect theory to practice.
- Reflect upon cognitive learning experiences, and your attitudes and feelings associated with your clinical experience.
- Utilize collegiate and professional expectations for writing.

Adapted from Ruthman, J., Jackson, J., Cluskey, M., Flannigan, P., False, V.N., & Bunten, J. (2004). Using clinical journaling to capture critical thinking across the curriculum. *Nursing Education Perspectives, 25*(3), 120-123.

Sample Approaches to Reflective Journaling—cont'd

What? so what? what now?

Use these three questions as prompts for students' reflective journaling. "What?" directs them to describe what occurred in the experience. "So What"? guides them in their analysis of what occurred within the context of the situation and their knowledge. Assumptions are identified and evaluated. "What Now?" facilitates their examination of how to follow-up, either in terms of actions to take, questions they need to explore further, and/or self-knowledge they have attained.

From Eyler, J. (2002). Reflecting on service: Helping nursing students get the most from service-learning. *Journal of Nursing Education, 41*(10), 453-456. Reprinted with permission from SLACK Incorporated.

Focused fundamentals

For students beginning to learn reflection, in their first clinical course, students can be encouraged to set goals for the day, and then reflectively evaluate the outcomes. They should be guided to design their goals to address higher-level/more complex skills. Examples appropriate for this level student would be: communicate therapeutically with my patient while providing a bed bath and making an occupied bed; teach the patient alternative ways of managing pain; assess the patient's spiritual and cultural beliefs and practices to determine their influence on the care to be provided.

Setting-specific guidelines for pediatrics course

- How does this client's/patient's development correlate with the anticipated developmental stage?*
- How has the family adapted to this child's illness? What anticipatory guidance might you provide?*
- What self-care activities can the patient and/or family members assume during hospitalization? How do you think they would feel about such involvement?
- After spending a day with the hospital's child life therapist, what do you see as his/her role in holistic care of hospitalized children? In what ways can/do the nurses collaborate with this person?

Setting-specific guidelines for maternal-child course

- How do the results of your newborn assessment compare to those anticipated? What is the significance of any differences you found? What implications for your care can you derive from your results? What implications for teaching can you derive from your results?*
- In preparation for your assignment to labor and delivery, what psychosocial issues shape the care you will provide and how will you take them into consideration?*

*Adapted from Ruthman, J., Jackson, J., Cluskey, M., Flannigan, P., False, V.N., & Bunten, J. (2004). Using clinical journaling to capture critical thinking across the curriculum. *Nursing Education Perspectives, 25*(3), 120-123.

Continued

Sample Approaches to Reflective Journaling—cont'd

Setting-specific guidelines for maternal-child course—cont'd

■ What patient teaching did you see done by the nurses during your labor and delivery experience? What other teaching do you think could be done at this time? How do teaching/learning theories guide your selection of content and methods in this setting?

■ After interviewing a mother who chose to breast-feed and one who chose to bottle feed, summarize your findings. How did they make their decisions? How did culture affect their decisions?

Setting-specific guidelines for mental health course

■ Provide theoretical explanations and integrate the psychopathology of (depression, anxiety, childhood trauma) into the patient's current inability to meet self-care needs.*

■ How have family dynamics been affected by the client's illness?

Setting-specific guidelines for medical-surgical course

■ What is the patient's medical history? If it related to the current problem(s), explain how?*

■ For a patient with a chronic illness, describe how the family manages health care at home?*

■ How does the patient's current problem(s) relate to self-care practices? What are the implications for discharge teaching, and/or referrals?*

■ Using all your sources of data, explain how the patient's condition is improving/worsening.*

■ How has the patient's culture impacted (health maintenance, involvement in self-care in the hospital, discharge teaching)?

■ What examples of interdisciplinary collaboration have you observed? What collaborative opportunities did you observe that were missed?

■ Discuss how your physical assessment findings at the beginning of the shift impacted care decisions you made today.

---

*Adapted from Ruthman, J., Jackson, J., Cluskey, M., Flannigan, P., False, V.N., & Bunten, J. (2004). Using clinical journaling to capture critical thinking across the curriculum. *Nursing Education Perspectives, 25*(3), 120-123.

Setting-specific guidelines for community health course

■ How has homelessness affected your client's health (physical, emotional, spiritual...)?*

■ What referrals did you make today? How did you decide to make them? How did you choose where to direct them?*

■ You visited a new agency today. How do the services provided impact clients in this community?*

■ What are the differences in health teaching for a group of senior citizens at the community center different from teaching an individual patient an acute care setting? Use teaching/learning theories to guide your discussion.

■ Is there a culture of homelessness? Use relevant theory to support your conclusions.

Sample Approaches to Reflective Journaling—cont'd

Setting-specific guidelines for leadership/management course

- How would you evaluate your time management skills? What changes will you make and why?*
- What sources of power did you see demonstrated? What were the results? What implications can you draw to guide your own practice?*
- Describe a decision you made today. What prompted the decision? What was the result (positive or negative)? How will this experience influence your decision-making in the future?*
- During your experience as team leader, what delegation decisions did you make? What were the bases for them? What did you learn from them to provide guidance for future delegation decisions?*
- Describe a conflict you observed. Use conflict management theories to analyze the situation. What have you learned from this experience to guide your future practice?
- What type of leader is the nurse manager on your unit? The charge nurse? Using the applicable leadership theories, examine your observations of the effectiveness of these individuals. Using leadership theory to support your conclusions, discuss the leadership skills a nurse needs to be an effective team leader. In order for you to fulfill this role, what skills do you think you need to develop? How might you do this?

*Adapted from Ruthman, J., Jackson, J., Cluskey, M., Flannigan, P., False, V.N., & Bunten, J. (2004). Using clinical journaling to capture critical thinking across the curriculum. *Nursing Education Perspectives, 25*(3), 120-123.

Setting-specific guidelines for a critical care experience

- What collaborative behaviors did you observe between nurses and physicians, pharmacists, therapists, or other health care practitioners?
- What feelings do you think the patient's family was experiencing?
- What was the nature of interactions between nurses and the patient's family members?
- How did the nurses demonstrate caring to the patient?
- What characteristics do you think a nurse should possess to work in this type of setting?

Setting-specific guidelines for an operating room experience

- Prior to the administration of general anesthesia, what was done to make an adult patient physically and emotionally more comfortable? A child?
- What behaviors did the team demonstrate that were directed toward maintaining patient safety?
- How did you feel about the interactions between the members of the team during the procedure?

Sample Checklist of Psychomotor Skills and Site of Evaluation for a Medical-Surgical Nursing Course

(Discussed in Chapter 12)

SKILL	REQUIRED IN CLINICAL	COMPETENCY MAY BE EVALUATED IN LRC	MAY BE TESTED ALTERNATELY
Basic ECG interpretation	■	■	
Blood administration	■	■	
Urinary catheterization	■		■
Care of central venous access devices		■	■
Closed chest drainage	■		■
Enterostomal care	■	■	
Insulin therapy		■	■
IV medications		■	■
IV therapy	■		■
Nasogastric intubation	■		■
Respiratory suctioning	■		■
Total parenteral nutrition	■		■
Arterial blood gases	■		■
Care of dialysis accesses	■		■
Hemodynamic monitoring	■	■	
Care of a patient on a ventilator	■	■	
Care of a patient in traction	■	■	
Spinal analgesia	■	■	

Sample Clinical Course Syllabus

(Discussed in Chapter 10)

ADULT MEDICAL-SURGICAL NURSING PRACTICE

This clinical practicum course, taken following the Foundations in Nursing Practice practicum, provides students with opportunities to apply medical-surgical nursing concepts to adult patients. Experiences will be provided in both hospital and out-patient settings, as well as in the learning resources center. Seminars for group learning experiences and written assignments also will facilitate student learning.

Course objectives
- Demonstrate an understanding of theoretical concepts and their appropriate application to patient care situations.
- Apply critical thinking skills in clinical problem solving situations.
- Discuss the application of current and relevant research to the practice of nursing.
- Provide safe nursing care.
- Demonstrate the behaviors of a professional nurse in all interactions.

Required reference materials
The textbook used in the accompanying theory course will be used in this course. In addition the drug handbook and laboratory diagnostics text available in the Student Bookstore must be brought to the clinical setting. Students are required to also have the clinical supplies required in the previous clinical practicum (i.e., stethoscopes, bandage scissors, hemostat, tape measure, and calculator).

Course evaluation
Formal course evaluations that include student input will be conducted at midterm and at the conclusion of the course, and will use the course evaluation tool. *(NOTE: The applicable evaluation instrument(s) should always be included with the syllabus.)* Grades will be provided at the conclusion of the course based on the system provided in the evaluation tool. Students will be given regular feedback on their performance and will make their own contributions to the process.

*(**NOTE:** There are additional materials that should be a routine part of the course syllabus and others that are optional. These have been discussed throughout this text and include topics such as descriptions of safe/unsafe practice, process for seeking disability accommodations, students' legal and ethical responsibilities in patient care, student behavioral guidelines, individual faculty member's teaching philosophy, and directions for written and individual assignments.)*

Sample Concept Maps

(Discussed in Chapter 15)

Season (winter, summer)
Forecast (rain, temperature)

Clean clothes
Matching/coordinated

What's the weather?

What's available?

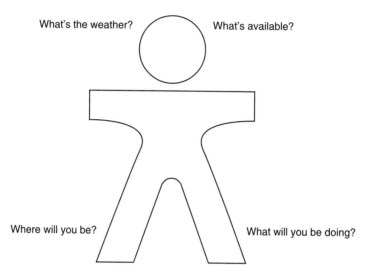

Where will you be?

What will you be doing?

Transportation
• walking
• bus
• car—distance from parking lot
Air-conditioned room
Walking between campus building

Just attending class
Practicing in the LRC
Volleyball at lunch
Dinner and a movie after school

Learning mind map: What will I wear to school today?

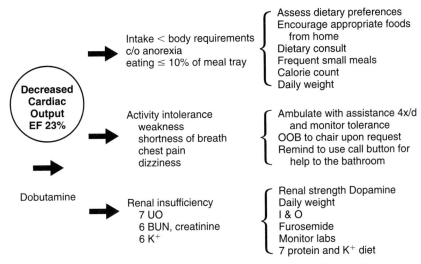

An 18-year-old with viral cardiomyopathy producing systolic heart failure.

Sample Notice of Unsatisfactory Performance

(Discussed in Chapter 8)

NOTICE OF UNSATISFACTORY PERFORMANCE

Student: Suzanne Smith   **Course:** Nursing 112   **Date:** 9/24/04

Area of Deficiency:

Objective 1: Communicate the integration of interrelationships between theoretical concepts and patient data.

In her written clinical preparation and in discussion with faculty, Suzanne has been unable to identify the etiology of her patient's diagnosis and unable to correctly and/or adequately relate the pathophysiologic basis of the disease process to her patient's status. She has been given verbal and written feedback for 2 weeks, without sufficient improvement.

Plan: Suzanne must meet course expectations for this objective at a minimal level at her next clinical experience day. She is to reread the articles regarding concept mapping and the samples provided. She is to meet with her study partner after gathering information regarding her patient assignment for assistance in completing the written clinical preparation and verbal quizzing of the relationship of the disease process to the manifestations and laboratory data. If she is unable to meet minimal expectations at this time, she will remain on this unit, forfeiting her scheduled operating room rotation. If she is still unable to meet minimal expectations after an additional 2 weeks of the course, she will fail this course objective, resulting in course failure.

Faculty signature: _____

Student signature: _____

Sample Objective Exemplars for a Graded Clinical Course

(Discussed in Chapter 8)

Objective III: Communicate the application of relevant literature and research to the practice of nursing (10% of total grade).

For the grade of C/C+ (73%-79%)

This grade represents an adequate ability to communicate the application of literature and research to nursing practice. Current literature is most often used to prepare for clinical or address the learning needs of the student. Outdated sources are sometimes used although current items are available. Gaining a breadth of knowledge and viewpoint is not commonly the purpose for literature review; "because it is required" is usually the impetus. When the literature is consulted, usually only the minimum number of articles, or one viewpoint, is studied. Reviewing literature for the purpose of meeting self-identified knowledge gaps is rarely initiated. There is little evidence of intellectual perseverance in pursuit of knowledge (i.e., if issues, topics, or answers to questions are not quickly found, the student gives up). The student prefers and most commonly uses nonresearch articles and has difficulty understanding and interpreting research studies and prefers not to make the effort. The student is often unable to describe how to incorporate research findings into practice. Sharing and dialoguing about research findings with clinical staff is not initiated.

For the grade of B-/B/B+ (80%-89%)

This grade represents an above average ability to communicate the application of literature and research related to nursing practice. Current literature is often used to prepare for clinical or address learning needs of the student. The student occasionally reviews the literature on relevant topics to gain a breadth of knowledge and viewpoint. When the literature is consulted, many articles and viewpoints are studied. Patient care problems are often the impetus for literature review. The student consistently identifies own gaps in knowledge and sometimes uses the literature to formulate answers to questions. There is some evidence of intellectual perseverance; some effort is made to answer the hard questions. The student occasionally reviews articles describing research studies and at times can describe how to incorporate findings into practice.

For the grade of A-/A (90%-100%)

This grade represents an outstanding ability to communicate the application of literature and research related to nursing practice. Current literature is consistently used to prepare for clinical or address learning needs of the student. The student often reviews the literature on relevant topics to gain a breadth of knowledge and viewpoint. When the literature is consulted, many articles and viewpoints are studied. Patient care problems and a desire to understand more completely is often the impetus for literature reviews. The student consistently identifies own gaps in knowledge, and frequently uses the literature to formulate answers to questions. There is substantial evidence of intellectual perseverance; significant effort is made to answer the hard questions. The student often reviews articles describing research studies and can describe how to incorporate findings into practice. The student also begins to identify areas of practice that could benefit from nursing research.

Sample Objective Exemplars for a Pass-Fail Clinical Course

(Discussed in Chapter 8)

Objective 2: Demonstrate critical thinking in the management of holistic nursing care of adults experiencing acute and chronic illnesses.

- Present a strong beginning level understanding of nursing skills and abilities necessary when caring for adults with acute and chronic illnesses.
- Build upon prior knowledge and, with the use of the skills checklist as a guide, seek opportunities to perform the necessary skills.
- Consistently articulate the significance of patient data.
- Make appropriate health care decisions based on legal, ethical, and professional standards, using agency policies and procedures.
- Implement individualized plans of care, including needed revisions, specific to patient needs and incorporating information from the history and physical, physician's progress notes, and current physical assessment and laboratory findings.
- Prioritize decisions based on pertinent patient findings, theoretical knowledge base, and collaboration with other health care members on an ongoing basis.
- Use a daily organization tool to ensure all nursing responsibilities are completed within an acceptable time frame.
- Communicate with instructor and primary care nurse any changes in patient status, plan of care, or personal concerns.

Some Approaches for Obtaining Formative Clinical Teaching Evaluation

(Discussed in Chapter 19)

1. Quantitative scaling:

I would appreciate your input concerning my teaching at this point in the term to guide me during the remainder of the term. For each of the following statements, please mark your response as:

      1 = Strongly Disagree; 2 = Disagree; 3 = Agree; 4 = Strongly Agree.

I feel I can approach (name) with any learning concern.	1	2	3	4
I feel I am encouraged to actively participate in group discussions.	1	2	3	4
I find the feedback given provides clear direction for my learning.	1	2	3	4
I understand the learning goal of course assignments.	1	2	3	4
I am treated fairly and with respect	1	2	3	4
My learning goals are being met	1	2	3	4

Comments:

2. Qualitative approach:

Your specific responses to the following questions will help me grow as a teacher.

- What have I done that has most helped you meet your own personal learning goals related to this course?

- As I have given you feedback in your learning, what have I done well? What could I do better?

- How have the assignments helped you learn in this course?

- How have I demonstrated caring and trust in our relationship?

Student Clinical Preparatory Sheet for a Medical-Surgical Nursing Course*

(Discussed in Chapter 15)

Patient room #:

Acute diagnosis:

Chronic health problems:

Surgery done or planned:

Procedures done or planned:

Significant psychosocial, cultural, or spiritual issues:

Medications: *(Meds you will be administering, including any PRN meds you may need to administer)*

Attach an additional page if needed.

NAME OF MEDICATION	ROUTE	TIME	NURSING ACTION OR MONITORING THAT NEEDS TO OCCUR

*Concept map is also required.

Patient care goals for the day (2-3):

1.

2.

3.

Interventions: *(Include all patient care activities [treatments, teaching, etc] that you will do or collaborate on to facilitate the meeting of your goals)*

*Concept map is also required.

A Summative Clinical Teaching Evaluation

(Discussed in Chapter 19)

Instructor name:

Course number and name:

Term:

Please respond to items 1-15 using the following scale:
    1 = Strongly Disagree, 2 = Disagree, 3 = Agree, 4 = Strongly Agree.
    It would be most helpful if you could provide an example to substantiate your selection.

1. Facilitated instructor-student interaction   1   2   3   4

2. Provided feedback in a timely manner to keep   1   2   3   4
me aware of my performance and progress in
the course

3. Clearly presented appropriate guidelines for   1   2   3   4
progression in the course

4. Was knowledgeable and skilled in the clinical   1   2   3   4
area

5. Helped me relate theoretical knowledge to the   1   2   3   4
clinical experience

6. Conducted meaningful clinical conferences   1   2   3   4
that supported the course objectives

7. Demonstrated an attitude of mutual respect   1   2   3   4

Designed by Emerson, R.J., Gass, G., & Severtsen, B., Washington State University College of Nursing/Intercollegiate College of Nursing.

Continued

A Summative Clinical Teaching Evaluation—cont'd

8. Served as a role model of professional nursing	1	2	3	4
9. Demonstrated enthusiasm in clinical instruction	1	2	3	4
10. Was available to assist me in the clinical area	1	2	3	4
11. Encouraged the development of my critical thinking skills	1	2	3	4
12. Made assignments that were appropriate in promoting my application of theory into clinical practice	1	2	3	4
13. Was aware of my strengths and limitations and assisted me appropriately	1	2	3	4
14. Encouraged research-based practice	1	2	3	4
15. Supervised students at the appropriate level to support autonomy but assure the safety of patients/clients	1	2	3	4

Please write your responses to questions 16-18.

16. What behaviors of the instructor contributed the most to your learning in this course?

A Summative Clinical Teaching Evaluation—cont'd

17. What behaviors of the instructor detracted the most from your learning in this course?

18. What suggestions do you have to enhance the overall quality of instruction of this course?

Any additional comments?

Epilogue

In 1562, at the age of 87, having accomplished the carving of *David* and the *Pietà* from marble, painted the ceiling of the Sistine Chapel, participated in the erection of St. Peter's basilica in Rome, and much more, Michelangelo Buonarroti was quoted as saying Ancoro imparo, or "I am still learning." The commitment to lifetime learning by clinical nurse educators is an acknowledgment of both the temporal nature of knowledge and the potential for improvement in all of us. Admitting fallibility while caring deeply about what and who we teach, being open to change and willing to risk, and sharing successes with our peers, clinical nurse educators leave their mark on their students, their profession, and the future of health care and society.

Index

3